D0282706

FUNDAMENTAL ASPECTS AND RECENT DEVELOPMENTS IN OPTICAL ROTATORY DISPERSION AND CIRCULAR DICHROISM

FUNDAMENTAL ASPECTS AND RECENT DEVELOPMENTS IN OPTICAL ROTATORY DISPERSION AND CIRCULAR DICHROISM

Proceedings of NATO Advanced Study Institute held at Tirrenia (Pisa), 5–18 September 1971

Editors: F. Ciardelli and P. Salvadori

University of Pisa

Contributors:

J. Badoz	D. N. Kirk	P. Salvadori
E. R. Blout	W. Klyne	P. M. Scopes
B. Bosnich	M. Legrand	G. Snatzke
J. Brahms	S. F. Mason	I. Tinoco, Jr.
B. Briat	A. Moscowitz	O. E. Weigang, Jr.
F. Ciardelli	P. Pino	F. Snatzke (formerly
M. Kajtár	J. S. Rosenfield	Werner-Zamojska)

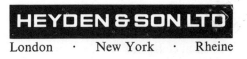

HEYDEN & SON LTD

London   ·   New York   ·   Rheine

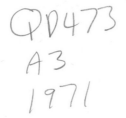

Heyden & Son Ltd., Spectrum House, Alderton Crescent, London NW4 3XX.
Heyden & Son Inc., 225 Park Avenue, New York, N.Y. 10017, U.S.A.
Heyden & Son GmbH, 4440 Rheine/Westf., Münsterstrasse 22, Germany.

Library of Congress Catalog Card No. 72–97936

ISBN 0 85501 060 6

Printed in Great Britain by William Clowes & Sons, Limited,
London, Colchester and Beccles.

CONTENTS

Chapter 2.3—Approaches to the Prediction of Cotton Effects: Organic Compounds O. E. Weigang, Jr

Chapter 2.4—Calculation of Circular Dichroism and Optical Rotatory Dispersion of Polymers I. Tinoco, Jr

SECTION 3—Relationship of Chiroptical Properties (ORD and CD) with Structure

Chapter 3.1—The Carbonyl Chromophore: Saturated Ketones W. Klyne and D. N. Kirk

Chapter 3.2—The Carbonyl Chromophore: Unsaturated Ketones and Lactones G. Snatzke and F. Snatzke (formerly Werner-Zamojska)

Chapter 3.3—The Carboxyl and Related Chromophores W. Klyne and P. M. Scopes

Chapter 3.4—Aromatic Chromophores   G. Snatzke, M. Kajtár, and F. Snatzke (formerly Werner-Zamojska)

Chapter 3.5—Other Chromophores   G. Snatzke and F. Snatzke (formerly Werner-Zamojska)

Chapter 3.6—Optical Activity and Molecular Dissymmetry in Coordination Compounds   S. F. Mason

Chapter 3.7—Exciton Circular Dichroism in Metal Complexes
B. Bosnich

Chapter 3.8—Induced Optical Activity
B. Bosnich

SECTION 4—Use of ORD and CD in Conformational Analysis

Chapter 4.1—Generalities   on   Low-molecular-weight   Organic Compounds
M. Legrand

Chapter 4.2—Use of Solvent and Temperature Effects
M. Legrand

Chapter 4.3—Recent Advances in Optical Activity Investigation of Nucleic Acids and Polynucleotides
J. Brahms

Chapter 4.4—ORD and CD in Conformational Analysis of Synthetic High Polymers   P. Pino

Chapter 4.5—Polypeptides and Proteins   E. R. Blout

SECTION 5—Special Topics

Chapter 5.1—Faraday-effect Spectroscopy   B. Briat

Chapter 5.2—Current Problems and Future Developments in ORD and CD Instrumentation   J. Badoz

FOREWORD

A NATO Summer School on ORD and CD organized by Dr. G. Snatzke was held at Bonn (BRD) in September 1965 and the proceedings were published in 1967. The success of the School and the value of the published proceedings made it inevitable that another similar meeting would be held in due course.

The next meeting, now called an Advanced Study Institute, was organized by Dr. F. Ciardelli and Dr. P. Salvadori of Pisa (Italy); it was held at Tirrenia near Pisa in September 1971, and the pattern was essentially the same as that of the Bonn Meeting. There were twenty-two main papers by invited specialists from all over the world, and about forty contributed papers; several 'round table' discussions were held, some of them far into the night; problem sessions were held on two afternoons, and there were demonstrations of equipment by four manufacturers.

This Volume presents to a wider public the text of the main papers, which provide a balanced survey of the present state of affairs in the ORD/CD field, with some suggestions regarding future development. Those who attended the Meeting certainly learnt much from the papers, and even more from personal discussion with colleagues on the spot. We hope that readers of this book will find the survey equally valuable.

Regarding the place of ORD and CD, now called the 'chiroptical techniques', in chemistry I cannot do better than reproduce *verbatim* a paragraph from the Foreword to the Bonn volume by a colleague and friend, Professor Guy Ourisson of Strasbourg.

'For the study of chiral substances, and maybe soon for that of non-chiral substances with magnetic circular dichroism, the two methods of study of the Cotton Effect have become *routine*. It is hardly easier to dispense with them than with IR or UV. True, the information they provide is limited and does not compare in wealth with that given by NMR or MS. But, usually, this information *cannot be obtained simply by any other method.*'

This is all still true; perhaps magnetic CD has not progressed as quickly as we had hoped. Today there is a growing realization of the fact that the chiroptical techniques provide a *sensitive* probe, as well as a *chiral* probe, of molecular structure.

The key to further progress in this field lies in closer contact between theoretical workers, empirical workers and the manufacturers of instruments; for the widespread use of any physical technique in organic chemistry we are dependent on reliable, commercially available, equipment, which is fairly simple to handle.

Again I express to the authorities of NATO and to our colleagues in Pisa the thanks of chemists for these discussions which we enjoyed at Tirrenia and which are in large measure reproduced here.

W. KLYNE

INTRODUCTION

This book takes its origin from the Advanced Study Institute (ASI) on ORD and CD held in Tirrenia on 6–18 September 1971; the main reasons for the publication are to allow the non-participants to benefit from the work described and the lectures given.

The aim of this book is, as was that of the ASI, to provide a general picture of the present state of the progress of ORD and CD from both the theoretical and the experimental viewpoints and to focus the future trends of these techniques and their possible development.

The tremendous growth of the research in the chiroptical field precludes exhaustive reviews and all contributions have been devoted mainly to the more important topics and significant examples. As a consequence many basic principles are employed without an introduction.

Considering these points, we have written an introductory Section mainly for the benefit of students approaching the subject without a basic knowledge of ORD and CD. We hope that the more advanced reader will appreciate our aim and will excuse us if this section is not as original as the others.

In addition, the division of the book is non-classical and notable differences, even more formal than substantial, from the general plan of the Proceedings of the analogous ASI held at Bonn are apparent.

The divisions between organic and inorganic chemistry as well as those between polymers and low molecular weight compounds are becoming more and more artificial in many fields of chemical research, especially in the area of optical activity. The overlapping of different fields has been found to be extremely fruitful in a number of cases. Similarly, not only is the study of low molecular weight models of great importance for a better understanding of macromolecular properties, but also the investigation of the latter has been found to be of notable assistance in obtaining information on the conformational isomerism of low molecular weight flexible molecules.

In regard to chiroptical properties, the former division between configurational and conformational optical activity as well as conformational and solvation optical activity are also no longer as relevant as they were formerly since they often overlap and attempts to separate them have often a heuristic significance only, even if some classes of compounds are known where one of these aspects is dominant.

At present, the classical division is still in part valid and cannot be completely disregarded. Therefore in planning this book we have attempted initially to combine classical and newer concepts; it is, however, certain that the situation has not crystallized and better division can be expected in the future.

Accordingly, all chapters dealing with theoretical aspects of optical activity have been collected in Section 2, independent of the type of molecules considered.

A general discussion on the development of classical physical theories and quantum theories is reported in the first chapter (Chapter 2.1) by Mason, which is followed by the chapter (Chapter 2.2) by Rosenfield and Moscowitz dealing with the application of CD data to the assignment of electronic transitions. In the next Chapters, 2.3 and 2.4, by Weigang and Tinoco respectively, generalized models are proposed for the prediction of chiroptical properties of low and high molecular weight organic compounds. Similar approaches for coordination compounds are discussed by Mason and by Bosnich in Chapters 3.6 and 3.7 of Section 3.

The latter includes contributions devoted mainly to the effect of structure and configuration, not neglecting conformation, on chiroptical properties of organic and inorganic compounds.

Section 3 covers the organic chromophores which are at present more extensively investigated from the experimental and theoretical viewpoint, such as the carbonyl chromophore, the carboxyl chromophore, the aromatic chromophore, the olefin chromophore, the nitrogen- and sulphur-containing chromophores (Chapters 3.1 and 3.3 by Klyne *et al.* and Chapters 3.2, 3.4 and 3.5 by Snatzke and coworkers). Essentially, these chapters indicate the progress made in the assignment of configuration and some rules are reported relating ORD and CD data to the spatial arrangement of atoms and bonds in chiral molecules.

Similar problems in coordination chemistry are discussed by Mason (Chapter 3.6) and by Bosnich (Chapter 3.7). This Section includes also a chapter (3.8) on induced optical activity in inorganic and organic compounds.

The investigation of the chiroptical properties is one of the most useful tools for obtaining information about conformational equilibria. Accordingly Section 4 includes two chapters (4.1 and 4.2) by Legrand on the general aspects of the problem in organic compounds and several significant examples and possible applications are discussed; similar aspects for coordination compounds are treated in Chapter 3.6 of Section 3. The final three chapters by Brahms, Pino and Blout of Section 4 deal with polymers. These ORD and CD studies are of considerable assistance in solving the problem of the conformation of macromolecules in solution of biologically important polymers and in some cases of synthetic stereoregular polymers.

Frequently it is observed that the CD (or ORD) spectrum shows more structure than the respective absorption spectrum and accordingly the former has been a useful means of aiding the assignment of electronic transitions. In this respect the MCD (or MORD) spectrum is frequently able to reveal further structural details of chiral molecules by inducing optical activity in nonchiral molecules and hence providing even more information about the origin of electronic transitions. Thus, in Chapter 5.1 by Briat, a comprehensive picture is presented of application of MORD and MCD to organic and inorganic molecules.

Finally Section 5 includes a chapter by Badoz (Chapter 5.2) on instrumentation which reports the present status and the expected developments of ORD and CD equipment.

Before concluding, we wish to express our warm thanks to Professors E. R. Blout, W. Klyne, S. F. Mason, P. Pino and G. Snatzke who shared with us the hard job of the scientific organization of the ASI by agreeing to be members of the Scientific Advisory Committee. Particular thanks are due to Professor P. Pino for his continuous encouragement and for his helpful assistance. We are also very grateful to the speakers and contributors for their cooperation and especially indebted to Professor S. F. Mason for the suggestions given during the preparation of the general plan of the book. Moreover we would like to express our appreciation to Professor F. Woldbye for introducing the final general discussion of the A.S.I. and to our colleagues of the Institute of Organic Chemistry and of Industrial Organic Chemistry of the University of Pisa for their friendly assistance. Finally we wish to acknowledge the generous financial support by the NATO Scientific Affairs Division and by the Consiglio Nazionale delle Ricerche (C.N.R.).

F. CIARDELLI AND P. SALVADORI*

* Present addresses:
   Istituto di Chimica Organica Industriale (F. CIARDELLI)
   Istituto di Chimica Organica–Nucleo di Ricerca del C.N.R. (P. SALVADORI)
   Università di Pisa
   Via Risorgimento, 35,
   56100 Pisa, Italy

General Aspects of Chiroptical Techniques

An Introduction to Chiroptical Techniques: Basic Principles, Definitions and Applications

P. SALVADORI and F. CIARDELLI

University of Pisa, Italy

1.1.1 Introduction

Many of the basic principles we discuss have already been covered by several recent books[1-6] and reviews[7-12] to which the reader is referred for more details. Nevertheless, it appeared useful to collect the main definitions, with related references, in the same chapter and to introduce some basic principles which are in our view necessary for a better understanding of the following chapters. For the reader without previous experience, this chapter should provide a basic background for deriving stereochemical information from ORD and CD. Therefore, in this section the units and conventions used are described and the relationship between chemical structure and chiroptical properties is discussed from a phenomenological point of view. Finally, some applications of these techniques are summarized.

For completeness it would be necessary to discuss also the physical origin of optical activity and the relative theoretical approaches, but this will not be attempted here as these aspects are treated by Mason in Chapter 2.1. It would be impossible at present, as well as beyond the scope of this book, to collect all papers devoted to chiroptical properties. However, in order to give the reader the opportunity to study further the very advanced and recent examples of each topic treated, an Appendix is included which gives titles, authors and, where possible, the relevant literature reference of the short communications which were presented at the Tirrenia ASI.

1.1.2 Optical Rotatory Power and Ellipticity

Taking into account the phenomenological aspects, the influence of an optically active absorbing medium on a linearly polarized radiation wave of electromagnetic radiation[13] can be described in the following way. A linearly polarized light beam results from two circular components with opposite rotation senses but with the same amplitude and with the same wavelength (in phase).[14,15]

The left and right circularly polarized components pass through the optically active medium with different speeds and are also differently absorbed to an extent depending on the *circular birefringence* $(n_L - n_R)$ and *circular dichroism* $(k_L - k_R)$ exhibited by the medium, respectively.[7,9,16,17] As a consequence the components,

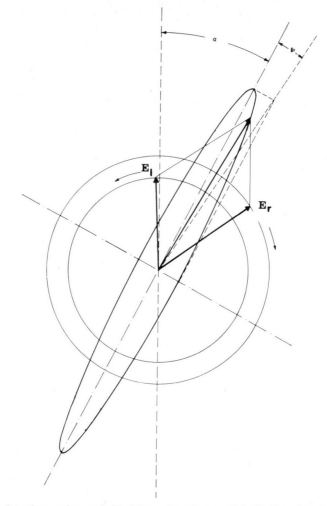

Fig. 1. Rotation angle α and ellipticity angle ψ for an originally linearly polarized light beam (direction of polarization vertical) emerging from an optically active absorbing medium.

having different amplitudes and a change of phase, combine to produce a wave which is elliptically polarized (Fig. 1).

The major axis of elliptical vibrations is rotated with respect to the polarization plane of incident light by an angle α, the *optical rotation*, and the arc-tangent of the ratio of minor to major axis of elliptical vibration is called the *angle of ellipticity* ψ.

The angles of rotation and ellipticity measured are related to the refractive indices and absorption coefficients for left and right circularly polarized light by the following equations:[7,9,14,15]

$$\alpha = \frac{\pi}{\lambda}(n_L - n_R) \qquad [1]$$

$$\psi = \frac{\pi}{\lambda}(k_L - k_R) \qquad\qquad [2]$$

where λ is the wavelength of incident light *in vacuo*, $n_L(k_L)$ and $n_R(k_R)$ are the refractive (absorption) indices for left and right circularly polarized light, respectively, and α and ψ are given in radians per unit length, measured in the same units as wavelength. If for a given optically active compound $k_L > k_R$, circular dichroism is positive and the rotation angle is positive at longer wavelengths where $n_L > n_R$ and negative at shorter λ where $n_L < n_R$.[15, 18] The opposite is obviously true for the enantiomeric molecule.

Optical rotation and ellipticity are measured generally on pure liquids or solutions, even if measurements in the vapour and in the solid state are possible and have been performed in several cases. They depend on wavelength, temperature, cell-path length and enantiomeric purity of the sample examined. For solutions, further effects may arise from the solvent nature and from concentration.

Standards, which eliminate dependence on path length and on density for a pure liquid or concentration for a solution, are obtained by the use of specific quantities. The *specific optical rotation* and the *specific ellipticity* for a given temperature and wavelength, indicated as superscript and subscript respectively, are expressed in the case of a pure compound as:

$$[\alpha]_\lambda^T = \alpha/ld \qquad\qquad [3]$$

and

$$[\psi]_\lambda^T = \psi/ld \qquad\qquad [4]$$

where l is the length of the cell in dm and d the density of the compound in grams per millilitre. For solutions, the analogous quantities are given by equations [5] and [6]

$$[\alpha]_\lambda^T = 100\alpha/lc \qquad\qquad [5]$$

$$[\psi]_\lambda^T = 100\psi/lc \qquad\qquad [6]$$

where c is the concentration in grams of solute per dl of solution. The solvent used, the concentration and the enantiomeric purity of the sample should be stated.

These specific quantities are given not in radians per unit length but in radians $\times$ length^2 $\times$ gram^{-1}. In order to correct for the effect on rotatory power of the different refractive index of solvent and solute, equation [7] has been proposed[19]

$$([\alpha]_\lambda^T)_0 = [\alpha]_\lambda^T \frac{3}{n^2 + 2} \qquad\qquad [7]$$

where n is the refractive index of the solvent at the temperature T and wavelength λ.

The effect of the solvent is, however, much more complex, as the molecules of solute are more or less solvated and solutions of the same compound in different solvents can be regarded in principle as containing different solute molecules.[20]

The dependence on temperature derives from the following factors: change of density or concentration, variation of position of the equilibria between different conformers and different association species, as well as various other electronic or vibrational changes in the chromophore. If the 'L' enantiomer predominates, the percent enantiomeric purity, EP, is given by

$$EP = \frac{N_L - N_D}{N_L + N_D} \times 100 \qquad [8]$$

where N_L and N_D are the numbers of molecules having opposite absolute configuration,[21] respectively. In general EP is numerically equal to the optical purity OP given by equation [9]:

$$OP = \frac{[\alpha]}{[\alpha]_{max}} \times 100 \qquad [9]$$

$[\alpha]_{max}$ being the specific rotatory power of an optically pure enantiomer measured in the same conditions as $[\alpha]$. However, it must be pointed out that if the specific optical activity of a single enantiomer of a given molecule does not linearly depend on concentration, OP is different from EP.[22]

For the purpose of comparison between compounds of different molecular weights molar optical rotation $[\Phi]_\lambda^T$ and molar ellipticity $[\theta]_\lambda^T$ are advantageous, since the comparison is made on a mole basis. The molar quantities are related to the corresponding specific quantities through equations [10a] and [10b]:

$$[\Phi]_\lambda^T = \frac{[\alpha]_\lambda^T \times M}{100} \qquad [10a]$$

and

$$[\theta]_\lambda^T = \frac{[\psi]_\lambda^T \times M}{100} \qquad [10b]$$

where M is the molecular weight of the optically active compound examined. As the specific quantities are ten times larger than the c.g.s. unit, the molar quantities are ten times smaller.

In the case of polymers, M is the molecular weight of the repeating unit, provided that the average molecular weight of the polymer is high enough to ensure the independence of the rotatory power from the chain length.[23,24]

According to equation [5], the observed specific rotatory power is an average value for all the individual rotatory powers of the N species present in the system:

$$[\alpha]_\lambda^T = \sum_1^N \frac{W_i}{W_t} [\alpha]_i \qquad [11]$$

where W_t is the total weight of the solute and W_i the weight of the ith species having $[\alpha]_i$. Equation [11] is valid if no interactions occur between the different chiral species present in the system. Correspondingly, the molar rotatory power is given by

$$[\Phi]_\lambda^T = \frac{[\alpha]_\lambda^T \times \bar{M}}{100} = \sum_1^N \frac{W_i}{W_t} \times \frac{[\alpha]_i \times \bar{M}}{100} \qquad [12]$$

$\bar{M} = \sum_i N_i M_i / N$ being the number average molecular weight. As $W_i = N_i M_i$ and $W_t = \sum_i N_i M_i$, we get

$$[\Phi]_\lambda^T = \sum_{i}^{N} \frac{N_i}{N} \times \frac{M_i}{100} \times [\alpha]_i = \sum_i^N X_i[\Phi]_i \qquad [13]$$

X_i being the molar fraction of the ith species.

Equation [13] is particularly important to establish a relationship between rotatory properties and conformational equilibrium in the case of flexible compounds existing in N different conformations which have in general different rotatory power (see Chapters 4.1 and 4.2).

In equation [2] the absorption indices k_L and k_R can be replaced by the molecular extinction coefficients ε_L and ε_R by the relation

$$k = \frac{2 \cdot 303}{4\pi} \times \lambda c \varepsilon$$

where c is the concentration of the absorbing solute in moles per litre and λ is in centimetres. The molar ellipticity can then be expressed as a function of the *molar coefficient of dichroic absorption* $\Delta\varepsilon$:

$$[\theta] = 2\cdot303 \left(\frac{4500}{\pi}\right)(\varepsilon_L - \varepsilon_R) = 3300\,(\varepsilon_L - \varepsilon_R) = 3300\Delta\varepsilon \qquad [14]$$

$[\theta]$ and $\Delta\varepsilon$ are used equally in practice, but the former has the advantage of being of the same order of magnitude as $[\Phi]$ (see below).

1.1.3 Optical Rotatory Dispersion (ORD) and Circular Dichroism (CD)

Variations, as a function of wavelength, of optical rotation angle and ellipticity angle as well as of the related quantities are called *Optical Rotatory Dispersion* (ORD) and *Circular Dichroism* (CD), respectively.

ORD and CD curves are reported by plotting, respectively, specific or molar optical rotation and molar ellipticity, or $\Delta\varepsilon$, versus wavelength or frequency. An optically active compound gives a curve which shows a characteristic feature in the region of the isotropic absorption band known as the *Cotton effect*[25, 26] (see Fig. 2). In the ideal case of an electronic transition well separated from all others of the same molecule, a positive Cotton effect has the form shown in Fig. 2.

A positive Cotton effect measured in the ORD has a positive optical rotation at longer wavelength values and negative at shorter wavelengths. $[\Phi]_\lambda$ decreases in absolute value with increase of the distance from the peak and from the trough. However the effect of an optically active band is marked outside the region of the Cotton effect, thus producing overlapping contributions from different transitions in real cases.[27] Well outside the absorption region, the ORD curve can be mathematically described by the Drude equation.[15, 28] In the case of an isolated transition, as in the ideal situation depicted above, this equation is the well-known, one-term, Drude equation

$$[\Phi]_\lambda = \frac{K}{\lambda^2 - \lambda_0^2} \qquad [15]$$

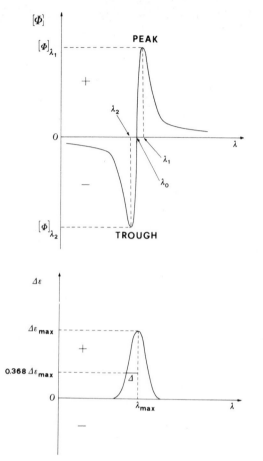

Fig. 2. Positive Cotton effect for an isolated electronic transition in ORD and CD spectra.

λ_0, the *dispersion constant* being very close to the wavelength of the considered optically active transition and K the so-called *rotation constant*. If several optically active transitions contribute to the optical rotation in a given spectral region, equation [15] assumes the more complex form

$$[\Phi]_\lambda = \sum_i K_i/(\lambda^2 - \lambda_i^2) \qquad [16]$$

The Drude equation does not hold in the absorption region, since $[\Phi]_\lambda$, as observed, does not go to ∞ for $\lambda = \lambda_i$. In this region the modified equation [17] is used where the damping factor G has been introduced

$$[\Phi]_\lambda = \frac{K(\lambda^2 - \lambda_0^2)}{(\lambda^2 - \lambda_0^2)^2 + G\lambda^2} \qquad [17]$$

Equations [15]–[17] have been used largely where the poor penetration of the available instruments does not allow measurements in the Cotton effect region. They are however becoming more and more obsolete, due to the considerable improvement in instrumentation.

In ORD curves the Cotton effect can be well characterized by the following parameters. In order to avoid possible confusion with absorption spectra, the term *peak* is used for a maximum and *trough* for a minimum.[29] If the peak is located at longer wavelength than the corresponding trough, the Cotton effect is designated as positive (Fig. 2), in the opposite case negative. The difference between the molecular rotation at the extremum (peak or trough) of the longer wavelength, $[\Phi]_{\lambda_1}$, and the molecular rotation at the extremum of the shorter wavelength, $[\Phi]_{\lambda_2}$, divided by 100 gives the *amplitude, a*

$$a = \frac{[\Phi]_{\lambda_1} - [\Phi]_{\lambda_2}}{100} \qquad [18]$$

The difference in nanometres between the wavelength of the extremum of the Cotton effect at the longer wavelength (λ_1) and that at the shorter wavelength (λ_2) is called *breadth, b*

$$b = \lambda_1 - \lambda_2 \qquad [19]$$

The shape of a positive Cotton effect in the CD spectrum is reported in Fig. 2.

A circular dichroism band is commonly described in terms of four parameters:[27] the wavelength of the maximum circular dichroism (λ_{max}), the maximum value of dichroic absorption or of molar ellipticity ($\Delta\varepsilon_{max}$ or $[\theta]_{max}$, respectively), the half-width of the band Δ, and the rotational strength R, which derives from the area under the CD band, defined[30] as

$$R_K = \frac{3hC}{8\pi^3 N} \int_0^\infty \frac{\psi_K(\lambda)}{\lambda} \, d\lambda \qquad [20]$$

where h is the Planck constant, c is the speed of the light, N is the number of absorbing molecules per cubic centimetre of solution and ψ_K is the partial ellipticity for the Kth transition. In terms of the partial molecular quantities, R_K is given by

$$R_K \approx 0\cdot696 \times 10^{-42} \int_0^\infty [\theta_K(\lambda)] \frac{d\lambda}{\lambda} = 0\cdot229 \times 10^{-38} \int_0^\infty \Delta\varepsilon_K(\lambda) \frac{d\lambda}{\lambda} \qquad [21]$$

If we assume that this transition takes place between the electronic states a and b, the rotatory strength can be written[31] as

$$R_K = I_m(a|\mu_e|b)(b|\mu_m|a) \qquad [22]$$

that is, the imaginary part of the scalar product of the electric μ_e and magnetic μ_m dipole transition moments. For practical purposes equation [21] can be written[9]

$$R_K = \rho . \mu . \cos\gamma \qquad [23]$$

where ρ and μ are, respectively, the absolute magnitudes of the electric and magnetic transition moments, and γ is the angle between the directions of the two moments. In general, an optically active molecule shows several optically active bands to each of which a different rotational strength is related. The sum of all these rotational strengths vanishes identically.[31,32]

ORD and CD are connected through Kronig–Kramers integral transforms;[7] thus for the *K*th transition we have

$$[\Phi_K(\lambda)] = \frac{2}{\pi} \int_0^\infty [\Theta_K(\lambda_1)] \frac{\lambda_1}{\lambda^2 - \lambda_1^2} d\lambda_1 \qquad [24]$$

$$[\Theta_K(\lambda)] = -\frac{2}{\pi\lambda} \int_0^\infty [\Phi_K(\lambda_1)] \frac{\lambda_1^2}{\lambda^2 - \lambda_1^2} d\lambda_1 \qquad [25]$$

Useful semiquantitative expressions, [26] and [27], have been derived from Kronig–Kramers transforms which relate the amplitude *a* of the Cotton effect to the maximum dichroic absorption or ellipticity[4,33]

$$a \approx 40{\cdot}28 \, \Delta\varepsilon_{max} \qquad [26]$$

$$a \approx 0{\cdot}0122 \, [\Theta]_{max} \qquad [27]$$

1.1.4 ORD and CD Curves and their Nomenclature

In practice, ORD curves of the type reported in Fig. 3 are more familiar for people dealing with optical activity problems.

Lowry[16,34] defined *normal rotatory dispersion curves* as those which show no change of sign, no maxima or minima and no points of inflexion; *anomalous curves* are those which show one or more of these features. The terms simplex and complex have been used to distinguish between normal curves which do or do not follow a one-term Drude equation.

Because of the difficulties encountered in fitting mathematical equations, Djerassi and Klyne[29] suggested the name plain curves for all normal curves whether or not they can be described by a one-term Drude equation.

In our view, ORD curves can be divided in the following groups:

(a) *Plain* (or normal) *curves* when the absolute value of the rotatory power increases regularly with decreasing wavelength (Fig. 3A).
(b) *Complex* (or anomalous) *curves* if they show changes in sign, maxima or minima (pseudoextrema), or inflexion points due to superimposition of plain curves of different sign (Fig. 3B).
(c) *Cotton effect curves* when there are anomalies associated with the presence of optically active absorption bands. Curves of the type C, D, E, and F in Fig. 3 are called *single Cotton effect curves* and their combinations, for instance G, are called *multiple Cotton effect curves*.

Because of the improvement of ORD instrumentation, enabling measurements to be made at shorter and shorter wavelengths, the last type is coming to be the commonest type of ORD curve encountered in practice. The nomenclature of absorption spectroscopy is used to indicate the characteristic points of circular dichroism curves.[35] But circular dichroism data in contrast to absorption spectroscopy are

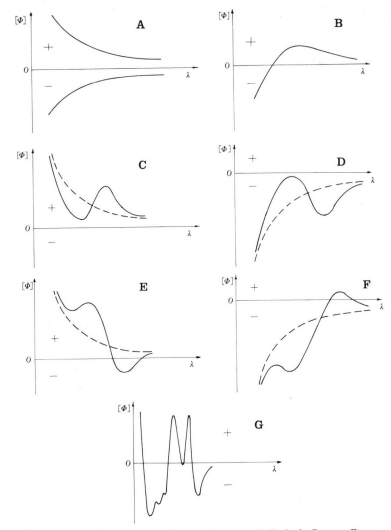

Fig. 3. ORD curves: A, plain curve; B, complex curve; C–F, single Cotton effect curve; G, multiple Cotton effect curve.

quantities requiring sign. Accordingly we speak of positive maxima, positive inflexion points and positive minima for a curve of the type shown in Fig. 4A, and of negative maxima, negative inflexion points and negative minima in the case of Fig. 4B. The point of inflexion derives from the overlapping of two optically active bands having different intensities and occurring at similar frequencies as shown in Fig. 4C for two overlapping bands of the same sign; the values of λ_{max} and $\Delta\varepsilon_{max}$ of each band cannot be directly deduced from the characteristic points of the curve but the resolution into the component bands is necessary to evaluate these data.[27] The same procedure must clearly be adopted to calculate the rotatory strengths.

A similar situation arises when a negative and a positive CD band overlap as shown in Fig. 4D. In fact, it has been established[36] that two overlapping gaussian curves of opposite sign give a resultant curve with peaks appreciably shifted from the true position of either component band and with reduced intensity. The term *bisignate CD curve* has been introduced by Klyne (see Chapters 3.1 and 3.3) for

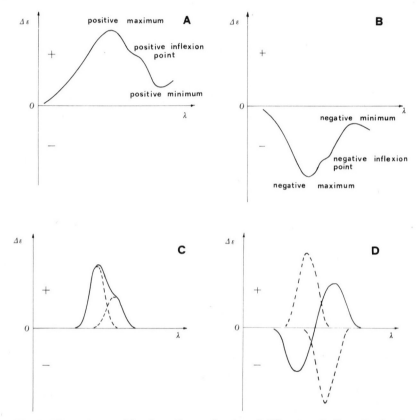

Fig. 4. CD spectra resulting from the overlapping of different optically active bands: (———) experimental curve; (– – – –) resolved curve.

CD curves consisting of two bands having opposite sign, whatever their origin. Moreover, the term *couplet* has been used to indicate bisignate CD curves of equal rotational strength within both branches, being due to exciton splitting.[37]

An additional characteristic of CD curves is given in some cases by the presence of a vibrational fine structure. Moscowitz[27] has noted that this fine structure can often be ignored and replaced by a suitably smoothed out curve. In fact, especially in solution, few vibrational profiles appear. This smoothing out process must be disregarded when looking for information concerned primarily with the force constants of the vibrational sublevels.[38]

1.1.5 Critical Comparison Between ORD and CD

Although ORD and CD give equivalent information, there are many points which differentiate the two techniques and offer particular advantages in certain cases.

The most remarkable specific characteristic of ORD is the *background* or *skeleton effect*. This effect arises from the shape of dispersion curves. The observed optical rotation at a given wavelength results from several contributions due to near and far Cotton effects, the entity of each contribution depending on position, sign and amplitude of the corresponding Cotton effect. If from one side this produces some complications giving rise to complex curves as shown in Fig. 3, from the other side it can be of considerable help in some cases. These cases usually have the common characteristic that their optical rotation cannot be investigated in the absorption region because of the too low dissymmetry factor[9] $\Delta\varepsilon/\varepsilon$ ($\approx 4R/D$) or because of instrumental limitations. The background rotation in spectral regions separated from those of the Cotton effect will give information on its position, sign and shape, taking into account equations of the Drude or Moffitt type.[39,40] Another case to mention is that of an optically active compound exhibiting a weak Cotton effect superimposed on a strong skeleton optical rotation (Fig. 3). Here also, ORD can provide useful structural information.[41]

As CD is an absorption phenomenon, the shape of the curve is such that its contribution is detectable only in the close vicinity of the isotropic absorption maximum. Therefore, there are in practice no background effects and, provided the frequency separation is large enough, it is possible to evaluate more accurately the rotational strength of individual electronic transitions. As previously shown, overlapping among different bands can also occur, but in these cases the resolution into single bands is much easier than with ORD. CD measurements are also to be preferred for the interpretation of vibrational fine structure and for low temperature and vapour phase measurements.

Having pointed out the main similarities and relative advantages of these two chiroptical techniques, we can conclude that the relative merits are often dependent on the type of instrument used, on the nature of compound examined and on the type of information required. The recent progress in instrumentation (see Chapter 5.2) has led to instruments with greater penetration making CD more and more preferred.

Looking back at the Bonn Meeting and making a comparison with the present one we can conclude, as Woldbye did during his introduction to the final discussion at the Tirrenia A.S.I., that it seems that CD has overcome ORD.

1.1.6 Optical Activity and Structure: the Optically Active Chromophores

Optical activity is associated with electronic transitions occurring in a chiral environment such that the scalar product of the electric and magnetic transition dipole moment is non-zero.

In many cases the electrons involved in a given transition belong to a particular grouping of atoms designated the chromophore. The separation into chromophoric and non-chromophoric moieties is only a matter of convenience.

As the pertinent electrons are mainly localized in the region of the chromophore, symmetry considerations are applied in first approximation to the chromophore itself, neglecting the rest of the molecule. However, in order to predict the possibility that a given compound exhibits optical activity, symmetry considerations must be extended to the whole molecule. On the basis of symmetry considerations, optically active chromophores have been classified by Moscowitz[42] into two main groups:

(i) inherently symmetric but dissymmetrically perturbed chromophores;
(ii) inherently dissymmetric chromophores.

If the point group of the chromophore possesses at least one secondary symmetry element, case (i) holds, showing that in this instance symmetric means achiral. On the other hand, if this point group lacks a secondary element of symmetry, the chromophore is inherently dissymmetric or, better, inherently chiral. It seems therefore more convenient (see Chapters 3.2 and 3.4) to call 'inherently achiral but chirally perturbed chromophores' those of group (i) and 'inherently chiral chromophores' those of the group (ii).

Any optical rotation associated with electronic transitions of chromophores belonging to group (i) arises from a chiral perturbation due to the environment. A classical example of this type is given by the carbonyl chromophore in saturated ketones which possesses two orthogonal reflection planes and hence it is, *per se*, inherently achiral. (For a more detailed discussion on this chromophore the reader is referred to Chapter 3.1.) The 290-nm transition is optically inactive in the acetone molecule and in all other ketones where the two alkyl or aryl groups are achiral, but optically active in ketones in which at least one of the two groups bound to the carbonyl is chiral. For instance, in optically active *sec.*-butylethylketone the asymmetric carbon atom is able to perturb chirally the 290-nm transition of the symmetric carbonyl chromophore which is now optically active.[43, 44] Chromophores of this group, some of which are reported in Table 1, exhibit a rotatory strength which in general does not exceed $\sim 10^{-40}$ c.g.s. units.

To the second group belong chromophores lacking a secondary element of symmetry,[45] so that even in isolation their transition would manifest optical activity. In other words, there is no secondary element of symmetry to preclude optical activity and there is no need to invoke the perturbation of the chromophore by a chiral environment. However, a chiral disposition of the substituents, for instance an asymmetric carbon atom, is necessary in some cases to stabilize one chiral form over the enantiomeric form.

The inherently chiral chromophores (Table 2) exhibit rotational strength of the order of 10^{-38} c.g.s., that is one hundred times larger than inherently achiral chromophores. It is worth mentioning that the contribution to the magnitude of the rotational strength arising from the chromophore usually, but not necessarily, outweighs possible contributions due to the chiral perturbation by molecular surroundings. A third class of optically active chromophores is formed by homoconjugated systems[46] such as β,γ-unsaturated ketones, non-conjugated dienes and so on, where the molecule contains at least two inherently achiral chromophores separated by more than one single but interacting bond and chirally disposed to each other. The properties of these systems resemble those of inherently chiral chromophores including the order of magnitude of the rotational strength.

It must be emphasized that the value of the rotational strength allows the correct

Table 1

Some Examples of Inherently Achiral Chromophores

Chromophoric system	Related compounds	Ref.
$\diagdown$C$=$C$\diagdown$	Unstrained olefins	*a*
(benzene ring)	Benzene derivatives	*b*
$\diagdown$C$=$O	Saturated ketones, aldehydes	*c*
$\diagdown$O	Ethers, alcohols	*d*
—C$\diagdown$$\overset{O}{\diagup}$$_{O-}$	Carboxylic acids, esters	*e*
$\diagdown$S—C$\equiv$N	Thiocyanates	*f*
$\diagdown$C$\diagdown$$\vert$$\diagup$C$\diagdown$ S	Episulphides	*g*

a A. I. Scott and A. D. Wrixon, *Tetrahedron* **26**, 3695 (1970); C. C. Levin and R. Hoffmann, *J. Amer. Chem. Soc.* **94**, 3446 (1972). *b* P. Crabbé and W. Klyne, *Tetrahedron* **23**, 3449 (1967); G. Snatzke, M. Kajtár and F. Werner-Zamojska, This book, Chapter 3.4. *c* P. Crabbé, *Optical Rotatory Dispersion and Circular Dichroism in Organic Chemistry*. Holden-Day, San Francisco, 1965; W. Klyne and D. N. Kirk, This book, Chapter 3.1; L. Lardicci, P. Salvadori, C. Botteghi and Pino, *Chem. Commun.* 381 (1968); D. N. Kirk, W. Klyne, W. P. Mose and E. Otto, *Chem. Commun.* 35 (1972). *d* P. Salvadori, L. Lardicci, G. Consiglio and P. Pino, *Tetrahedron Lett.* 5343 (1966); D. N. Kirk, W. P. Mose and P. M. Scopes, *Chem. Commun.* 81 (1972). *e* W. Klyne and P. M. Scopes, This book, Chapter 3.3; J. P. Jennings, W. Klyne and P. M. Scopes, *J. Chem. Soc.* 294, 7211, 7229 (1965). *f* C. Djerassi, D. A. Lightner, D. A. Schooley, K. Takeda, T. Komeno and K. Kuriyama, *Tetrahedron* **24**, 6913 (1968). *g* K. Kuriyama, T. Komeno and K. Takeda, *Tetrahedron* **22**, 1039 (1966).

classification of a chromophoric system only if a particular well-known transition is considered.

As pointed out by Moscowitz *et al.*,[12] the critical point of this classification lies in the separation of two chromophoric systems combined in one molecule, that is to consider them as isolated or interacting. The criterion of conjugation can fail as in homoconjugated systems where distant groups interact.

Table 2

Some Examples of Inherently Chiral Chromophores

Compounds	Chromophoric systems	Ref.

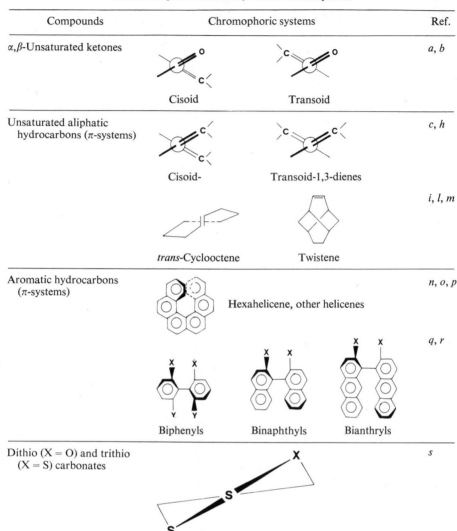

α,β-Unsaturated ketones	Cisoid Transoid *a, b*
Unsaturated aliphatic hydrocarbons (π-systems)	Cisoid- Transoid-1,3-dienes *c, h*
	trans-Cyclooctene Twistene *i, l, m*
Aromatic hydrocarbons (π-systems)	Hexahelicene, other helicenes *n, o, p*
	Biphenyls Binaphthyls Bianthryls *q, r*
Dithio (X = O) and trithio (X = S) carbonates	*s*

[a] C. Djerassi, R. Records, E. Bunnenberg, K. Mislow and A. Moscowitz, *J. Amer. Chem. Soc.* **84**, 870 (1962). [b] See Chapter 3.2, and references therein. [c] A. Moscowitz, E. Charney, U. Weiss and H. Ziffer, *J. Amer. Chem. Soc.* **83**, 4661 (1961). [d] U. Weiss, H. Ziffer and E. Charney, *Tetrahedron* **21**, 3105 and 3121 (1965). [e] E. Charney, *Tetrahedron* **21**, 3127 (1965). [f] G. Snatzke, E. Kovats and G. Ohloff, *Tetrahedron Lett.* 4551 (1966). [g] A. W. Burgstahler and R. C. Barkhurst, *J. Amer. Chem. Soc.* **92**, 7601 (1970). [h] P. Crabbé and A. Guzman, *Chem. Ind.* 851 (1971). [i] A. Moscowitz and K. Mislow, *J. Amer. Chem. Soc.* **84**, 4605 (1962). [l] A. C. Cope and S. Mehta, *J. Amer. Chem. Soc.* **86**, 5626 (1964). [m] A. F. Drake, Dissertation, King's College, London, 1972. [n] O. E. Weigang, Jr, J. A. Turner, and P. A. Tronard, *J. Chem. Phys.* **45**, 1126 (1966). [o] M. S. Newman, R. S. Darlak and L. Tsai, *J. Amer. Chem. Soc.* **89**, 6191 (1967). [p] S. F. Mason, *Proc. Roy. Soc.* **A297**, 3 (1967); W. S. Brickell, A. Brown, C. M. Kemp and S. F. Mason, *J. Chem. Soc.* A756 (1971). [q] K. Mislow, in G. Snatzke, Ed., *ORD and CD in Organic Chemistry*. Heyden, London, 1967, p. 153. [r] S. F. Mason, in G. Snatzke, Ed., *ORD and CD in Organic Chemistry*. Heyden, London, 1967, p. 71. [s] D. A. Lightner, C. Djerassi, K. Takeda, K. Kuriyama and T. Komeno, *Tetrahedron* **21**, 1581 (1965).

The general practicability of such separation has been recently questioned[47] and it is accepted that the above classification is artificial from the theoretical point of view, but very useful for interpretation of ORD and CD data and for obtaining stereochemical information.

Another classification has been made by Snatzke,[48] who has suggested that the molecule may be divided into 'spheres', starting with the chromophore and then going to the more remote atoms (see also Chapters 3.2 and 3.4). The first sphere is the chromophore itself, and the 'chiral first sphere' coincides with Moscowitz's inherently dissymmetric chromophore. The second sphere is the ring, in which the chromophore is included or attached in the case of cyclic compounds, and the third sphere comprises rings or groups attached to the second sphere and so on. It is clear that the sphere with pronounced dissymmetry nearest to the chromophore mainly determines the Cotton effects and that the more remote ones have only minor influence.

The aforementioned classifications of optically active chromophoric systems are usually limited to low-molecular-weight organic molecules; as far as chiral metal complexes and polymers are concerned, less clear situations can arise owing to the complexity of these molecules. In the former case the problem is particularly difficult because of the proximity of electronic transitions from the organic ligands and from the metal and because of the metal-ligand charge transfer excitations. Indeed, it is not easy to recognize the ORD and CD contributions deriving from a single chromophoric system in this type of molecule.

As pointed out by Mason in Chapter 3.6 of this book, the three types of electronic excitation have mainly been considered individually. This approach is in several cases facilitated by the small mixing energies and the large frequency separations, which allow the identification of the Cotton effects associated with each type of excitation. It is worth mentioning at this point that the d → d electronic transitions of lowest energy have been used to relate the stereochemistry to the chiroptical properties of metal complexes.[49] Moreover, as far as the Cotton effects arising from the organic ligands are concerned these are not simply those expected for an isolated ligand molecule. In fact, in several cases there is coupling of individual excitations in the different ligand molecules present in the coordination complex with a definite relative stereochemical position (see Chapter 3.6).

In polymers the problem of the identification of chromophoric systems can usually be approached successfully by comparison with suitable low-molecular-weight models.[50] The importance of this type of information is exhaustively discussed in Chapters 2.4, 4.3, 4.4 and 4.5.

If the low-molecular-weight model is a structural model (that is, closely resembling the chemical structure of the monomeric residue), two limiting cases can occur:

(i) the monomeric residues can be considered as electronically isolated, and model and polymer exhibit chiroptical properties associated with the same chromphores;[50]

(ii) the monomeric residues in the macromolecules interact through bonds or space, giving chromophoric systems markedly different from those of the model (see Chapters 4.3, 4.4 and 4.5).

The second group is more interesting, because chiroptical properties can give more information on the macromolecule conformation. In addition one can properly speak in this case of an inherently chiral chromophoric system associated with the macro-molecular structure, that is with repetition of a simple chromophoric system along the helical chain having a predominant screw sense.

1.1.7   Main Applications of Chiroptical Techniques

ORD and CD have become as routine as other spectroscopic techniques, such as infrared, nuclear magnetic resonance and mass spectrometry. The two methods for studying Cotton effects are more limited with respect to the other techniques, but the information they give cannot be simply obtained in any other way. They are largely used to obtain stereochemical and spectroscopical information on chiral molecules, and even achiral by the use of MORD and MCD.

The most popular application of optical activity measurements is the determina-tion of absolute, or relative, configuration. In this field, ORD and CD have completely replaced methods based on the sign of the rotatory power at a given wavelength, for instance the sodium D-line, the indications being more reliable. In fact, as pointed out in the preceding section, the rotatory power at a wavelength far from the absorp-tion region results from many contributions of different Cotton effects and the sign can change from one term to another of a homologous series even without changing absolute configuration.

Despite the efforts of many scientists the *a priori* calculation of optical activity of a given molecule is still far from being possible and any prevision must be based on experimental data.

The non-empirical determination of absolute configuration is, however, possible in some particular cases. Examples are reported for organic molecules containing two non-coplanar chromophores and then an inherently chiral chromophore.[52] Similar approaches have also been reported for some coordination complexes (see Chapters 3.6 and 3.7) and for biological polymers (see Chapters 2.4 and 4.3).

In the other cases attempts have been made to develop semiempirical as well as empirical *sector rules*[47,53,54] based on wide sets of experimental data. In order to minimize complications arising from the presence of different conformers, these data have been selected mainly by considering those from cyclic compounds having possibly a rigidly fixed conformation.

The proliferation of these rules was very great indeed after the proposal of the *octant rule* for saturated ketones.[54] In recent years especially, attempts to rationalize the increasing number of available data on previously not accessible chromophores have led to the proposal of other, in general empirical, sector rules, some of which have subsequently been shown to be invalid or else have been successively modified to accommodate new results. In any case one must be careful in drawing conclusions from these rules even if supported by a large number of data. An exhaustive review of all sector rules is beyond the scope of this chapter and for several would have only historical value. Some recent examples are summarized in Table 3. For a more de-tailed discussion and examples, the reader is referred to Section 3 of this book.

Before passing to other applications it seems useful to summarize briefly the method used to develop a sector rule. First of all, the type of electronic promotion occurring in the transition examined must be known. Next the molecule is divided into spatial regions and sectors by the nodal planes of the orbitals involved—ground- and ex-cited-state orbitals. The distribution of the substituents in these regions can be

Table 3

Examples of Recently Proposed Sector Rules

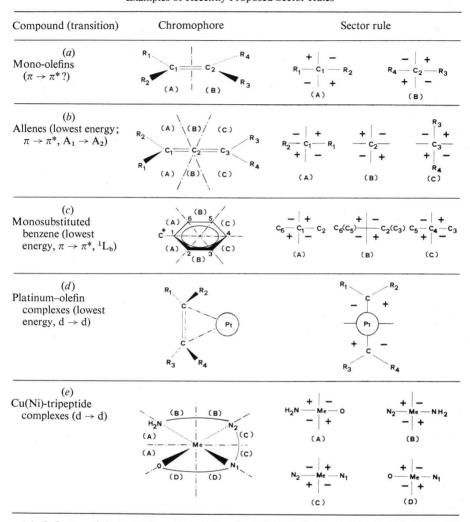

Compound (transition)	Chromophore	Sector rule
(a) Mono-olefins ($\pi \to \pi^*$?)		
(b) Allenes (lowest energy; $\pi \to \pi^*$, $A_1 \to A_2$)		
(c) Monosubstituted benzene (lowest energy, $\pi \to \pi^*$, ^1L_b)		
(d) Platinum–olefin complexes (lowest energy, d → d)		
(e) Cu(Ni)-tripeptide complexes (d → d)		

[a] A. I. Scott and A. D. Wrixon, *Tetrahedron* **26**, 3695 (1970). [b] P. Crabbé, E. Velarde, H. W. Anderson, S. D. Clark, W. R. Moore, A. F. Drake and S. F. Mason, *Chem. Commun.* 1261 (1971). [c] G. Snatzke and P. C. Ho, *Tetrahedron* **27**, 3645 (1971). [d] A. I. Scott and A. D. Wrixon, *Tetrahedron* **27**, 2339 (1971). [e] R. B. Martin, J. M. Tsangaris and J. Wen Chang, *J. Amer. Chem. Soc.* **90**, 821 (1968).

deduced if the configuration and conformation of the molecule are known. By collecting CD (or ORD) data on a large number of compounds, and considering the capability of the substituents as electron donors and the probable mechanism of the electron promotion, the type and position of the substituents can be related to the sign of the rotational strength induced by each in the transition examined. The observed rotational strength is an average value of these contributions which can have different magnitude and opposite sign, therefore an order of priority of the substituents is also needed.

Other correlations have been used for configurational assignments,[55] but that based on sector rules seems to be at present the most useful, particularly in the cases in which it is based on a firm theoretical basis.

As pointed out in the preceding discussion, the conformation should be known, and possibly unique, to allow prediction of optical rotatory properties. Conversely, the conformational equilibria can be investigated by the sector rules when the absolute configuration is known. This leads to a second important application of ORD and CD. In fact, chiroptical properties are extremely sensitive to conformational changes and if there is no variation of optical activity with changing temperature[56] or solvent[20] this is a firm indication of high conformational rigidity. On the other hand, a solvent effect in rigid molecules is taken as an indication of solvation.[57] A discussion of this application, and many pertinent examples, can be found in Chapter 3.6 for metal complexes, Chapters 4.1 and 4.2 for low-molecular-weight organic compounds and Chapters 4.3, 4.4 and 4.5 for polymers.

CD has been also widely used for investigating spectroscopic problems, and particularly for assignment of electronic transitions.

CD, in fact, exhibits better resolution in general than UV-absorption, mainly owing to the fact that CD bands can have a negative or a positive sign. A recent example is given in Chapter 2.2, dealing with the assignment of electronic transitions in dialkyl sulphides.

Information on solute/solvent interactions can be obtained by measuring the CD and ORD of a solution of an achiral compound containing a suitable chromophore in an optically active solvent which does not absorb in the same region. The presence of optically active bands associated with the solute (induced optical activity) will unequivocally demonstrate solvation by the dissymmetric solvent molecules. Examples of induced optical activity are known both in organic[58] and in inorganic chemistry (Chapter 3.8).

A different type of induced optical activity is used for investigating macromolecular conformation. This is simply obtained by including in the same macromolecule an optically active monomer with an achiral one.

The presence of chiral stereo-ordered macromolecular conformations can be proved by the presence of optical activity induced in the latter monomer units by the chiral monomer units[59, 60] (see Chapters 4.4 and 4.5).

No less important is the use of chiroptical techniques for investigating the occurrence of asymmetric induction when a new chiral centre is formed under the control of a chiral environment. A recent example is given by the complex formation of chiral olefins with platinum. In fact it has been demonstrated[61] that the predominant absolute configuration of the C_2 carbon atom of chiral α-olefins in *cis*-dichloro-(olefin)(amine)Pt^{II} complexes is determined by the asymmetric carbon atom of the non-complexed olefin.

The examples reported do not cover all possible applications of ORD and CD, but give an indication of the importance of these techniques. For other examples the reader is referred to the following chapters, as well as to the literature cited therein.

1.1.8 Appendix

As already stated in the introductory remarks, it has not been possible to report an exhaustive survey of all literature concerning CD and ORD published since the 1965 Bonn A.S.I.

As far as the topics treated in the present book are concerned, an up to date picture is given covering literature till the end of 1971 and, in several cases, early 1972.

More recent examples in particular fields are given by the short communications presented at the Tirrenia 1971 A.S.I. Therefore, a list of these is given below, including publication details where known.

C1. Theory of Chirality Functions[62]
C2. Mo–Ci-calculations on the Optical Activity of α,β-Unsaturated Ketones and of α- and β-Diketones[63]
C3. New Considerations on Induced Dipole Moments as observed in CD Studies[64]
C4. An Approach to General Principles that govern the Interaction between Two Functional Groups: Spectroscopic Applications[65]
C5. Theoretical Interpretation of the CD of Adenine Nucleosides[66]
C6. Optical Activity of Flow-oriented Deoxyribonucleic Acid[67]
C7. Exciton Selection Rules and the Optical Activity Tensor for the Two Transitions of Poly-L-glutamic Acid[68]
C8. CD in Co(III) Amine Outersphere Complexes: Perturbed CD/Induced CD[69]
C9. The CD of some Trichelate Complexes of Ni(III) with 1,2-Diamines[70]
C10. Investigation of Simple and Mixed Chelation of Copper with Amino Acids by Spectrophotometry, Polarimetry and CD[71]
C11. CD of Co(III) Complexes of Linear Tetramines[72]
C12. Stereochemical Aspects of the Complexation of Chiral Olefins to Pt(II)[73]
C13. Optical Activity of Heteroannular Cisoid Dienes[74]
C14. Chiroptical Properties of Non-planar Polyenes[51]
C15. Mathematical and Dimensional Relationships in CD[75]
C16. Chiroptical Properties of Sulfur Chromophore[76]
C17. CD in the Vacuum UV Region[77]
C18. Interpretation of the Solvent Dependent CD associated with the Thiobenzamide Chromophore[78]
C19. CD of Oriented Systems[79]
C20. Optical Activity of Symmetric Compounds in Chiral Media: Induced CD Studies[80]
C21. ORD in the Infrared Region[81]
C22. CD of 3,3'-Bithienyls[82]
C23. Optically Active Aromatic Chromophores: Chiroptical Studies of some 1-Substituted 2-Phenyl-cyclohexanes[83]
C24. Chiroptical Properties of Nitroaryl Chromophore[84]
C25. The CD of an Optically Active Benzene Chromophore[85]
C26. On the Optically Active ^{1}B Transition in High Molecular Weight Aromatic Hydrocarbons[86]
C27. The CD of some Pyridine Alcohols[87]
C28. CD of some α-Substituted Steroid Lactones[88]
C29. CD Spectra of Tea Flavins[89]

References

1. G. Snatzke, Ed., *ORD and CD in Organic Chemistry*. Heyden, London, 1967.
2. C. Djerassi, *Optical Rotatory Dispersion*. McGraw-Hill, New York, 1960.
3. L. Velluz, M. Legrand and M. Grosjean, *Optical Circular Dichroism*, Verlag Chemie GMB, Academic Press, 1965.
4. P. Crabbé, *Optical Rotatory Dispersion and Circular Dichroism in Organic Chemistry*. Holden-Day, San Francisco, 1965.
5. D. J. Caldwell and H. Eyring, *The Theory of Optical Activity*. Wiley-Interscience, New York, 1971.
6. P. Crabbé, *An Introduction to the Chiroptical Methods in Chemistry*. Mexico, 1971.
7. A. Moscowitz, *Advan. Chem. Phys.* **4**, 67 (1962).
8. I. Tinoco, Jr, *Advan. Chem. Phys.* **4**, 113 (1962).
9. S. F. Mason, *Quart. Rev. Chem. Soc.* **17**, 20 (1963).
10. J. H. Brewster, *Topics Stereochem.* **2**, 1 (1967).
11. H. Eyring, H. C. Liu and D. Caldwell, *Chem. Rev.* **68**, 525 (1968).
12. C. W. Deutsche, D. A. Lightner, R. W. Woody and A. Moscowitz, *Ann. Rev. Phys. Chem.* **20**, 407 (1969).
13. J. R. Partington, *Advanced Treatise on Physical Chemistry*, Vol. IV. Longmans Green, London, 1953, p. 290.
14. A. Fresnel, *Ann. Chim. Phys.* **28**, 147 (1825).
15. P. Drude, *Lehrbuch der Optik*. Hirzel, Leipzig, 1900, p. 379. English translation: Dover, New York, 1959.
16. T. M. Lowry, *Optical Rotatory Power*. Dover, New York, 1964.
17. W. Heller, 'Polarimetry', in A. Weisberger, Ed., *Physical Methods of Organic Chemistry*, Vol. 1, Part II. Interscience, New York, 1949, p. 1491.
18. S. F. Mason, *Chem. Brit.* 245 (1965).
19. W. Kauzman, F. B. Clough and I. Tobias, *Tetrahedron* **13**, 57 (1961).
20. A. Moscowitz, in G. Snatzke, Ed., *ORD and CD in Organic Chemistry*. Heyden, London, 1967, p. 329.
21. E. L. Eliel, *Stereochemistry of Carbon Compounds*. McGraw-Hill, New York, 1962, p. 87.
22. A. Horeau, *Tetrahedron Lett.* 3121 (1969).
23. M. Goodman, A. S. Verdini, C. Toniolo, W. D. Phillips and F. Bovey, *Proc. Natl. Acad. Sci. U.S.A.*, **64**, 444 (1969).
24. P. L. Luisi and F. Pezzana, *Eur. Polym. J.* **6**, 259 (1970).
25. A. Cotton, *C.R.H. Acad. Sci.* **120**, 989 and 1044 (1895).
26. S. Mitchell, *The Cotton Effect*. Bell, London, 1933.
27. A. Moscowitz, in C. Djerassi, Ed., *Optical Rotatory Dispersion*. McGraw-Hill, New York, 1960, p. 150.

28. W. Heller, *J. Phys. Chem.* **62**, 1569 (1958).
29. C. Djerassi and W. Klyne, *Proc. Chem. Soc.* 55 (1957).
30. W. Moffitt and A. Moscowitz, *J. Chem. Phys.* **30**, 648 (1959).
31. E. U. Condon, *Rev. Mod. Phys.* **9**, 432 (1937).
32. W. Kuhn, *Z. Phys. Chem.* **4**, B, 14 (1929).
33. K. Mislow and E. M. Richards, *Ann. N. Y. Acad. Sci.* **93**, 457 (1962), and references cited therein.
34. T. M. Lowry, *J. Chem. Soc.* **125**, 2511 (1924).
35. C. Djerassi and E. Bunnenberg, *Proc. Chem. Soc.* 299 (1963).
36(a) K. M. Wellman, P. H. A. Laur, W. S. Briggs, A. Moscowitz and C. Djerassi, *J. Amer. Chem. Soc.* **87**, 66 (1965).
36(b) Th. Bürer, *Helv. Chim. Acta* **46**, 2388 (1963).
37. G. Haas, P. B. Hulbert, W. Klyne, V. Prelog and G. Snatzke, *Helv. Chim. Acta* **54**, 491 (1971).
38(a) R. D. Gillard and P. R. Mitchell, *Trans. Faraday Soc.* **65**, 2611 (1969).
38(b) R. T. Klingbiel and H. Eyring, *J. Phys. Chem.* **74**, 4543 (1970).
39. W. Moffitt and Jen Tsi Yang, *Proc. N.Y. Acad. Sci.* **42**, 597 (1956).
40. J. Y. Cassin and Jen Tsi Yang, *Biopolymers* **9**, 1475 (1970).
41. C. Djerassi, *Proc. Chem. Soc.* 314 (1964).
42. A. Moscowitz, *Tetrahedron* **13**, 48 (1961).
43. C. Djerassi and L. E. Geller, *J. Amer. Chem. Soc.* **81**, 2789 (1959).
44. L. Lardicci, P. Salvadori, C. Botteghi and P. Pino, *Chem. Commun.* 381 (1968).
45. H. H. Jaffé and M. Orchin, *Symmetry in Chemistry*. Wiley, New York, 1965.
46. K. Mislow, in G. Snatzke, Ed., *ORD and CD in Organic Chemistry*, Heyden, London, 1967, p. 153.
47. E. G. Höhn and O. E. Weigang, Jr, *J. Chem. Phys.* **48**, 1127 (1968).
48. G. Snatzke and P. C. Ho, *Tetrahedron*, **27**, 3645 (1971), and references cited therein.
49(a) S. F. Mason, *J. Chem. Soc. A*, 667 (1971).
49(b) C. J. Hawkins, *Absolute Configuration of Metal Complexes*. Wiley, New York, 1971.
50. P. Pino, F. Ciardelli and M. Zandomeneghi, *Ann. Rev. Phys. Chem.* **21**, 561 (1970).
51. O. Pieroni, F. Matera and F. Ciardelli, *Tetrahedron Lett.* 597 (1972).
52. S. F. Mason, *Chem. Ind.* 1286 (1964).
53. J. A. Schellman, *J. Chem. Phys.* **44**, 55 (1966).
54. W. Moffitt, R. B. Woodward, A. Moscowitz, W. Klyne and C. Djerassi, *J. Amer. Chem. Soc.* **83**, 4013 (1961).
55. J. A. Mills and W. Klyne, 'The Correlations of Configurations', in W. Klyne, Ed., *Progress in Stereochemistry*, Vol. 1. Butterworths, London, 1954, 177.
56. G. Snatzke, Ed. *ORD and CD in Organic Chemistry*. Heyden, London, 1967, p. 335.
57. A. Rassat, in G. Snatzke, Ed., *ORD and CD in Organic Chemistry*. Heyden, London, 1967, p. 314.
58. L. D. Hayward and R. N. Totty, *Chem. Commun.* 676 (1969).
59. C. Carlini, F. Ciardelli and P. Pino, *Makromol. Chem.* **119**, 244 (1968).
60. P. Pino, C. Carlini, E. Chiellini, F. Ciardelli and P. Salvadori, *J. Amer. Chem. Soc.* **90**, 5025 (1968).
61. R. Lazzaroni, P. Salvadori and P. Pino, *Chem. Commun.* 1164 (1970).
62(a) E. Ruch and A. Schonhofer, *Theor. Chim. Acta* **19**, 225 (1970). (b) E. Ruch, *Accounts Chem. Res.* **5**, 49 (1972).
63. W. Hug and G. Wagnière, *Helv. Chim. Acta* **54**, 633 (1971).
64. D. E. Francis, to be published in *J. Amer. Chem. Soc.* and *J. Coordination Chem.*
65. J. Hudec, to be published.
66. C. A. Bush, *J. Amer. Chem. Soc.* **95** (1973).
67. S. Y. Wooley and G. Holzwarth, *J. Amer. Chem. Soc.* **93**, 4066 (1971).
68. J. Hofrichter and J. A. Schellman, to be published.
69. B. Nordén, *Acta Chem. Scand.* **23**, 2925 (1969); **24**, 1703 (1970); **25**, 2516 (1971); **26**, 111 (1972).
70. M. J. Harding, S. F. Mason and B. J. Peart, to be published in *J. Chem. Soc.*
71. M. M. Petit-Ramel and M. R. Paris, *Colloque International CNRS*, N. 191, Paris, 27–31 octobre 1969.
72. B. Bosnich and J. MacB. Harrowfield, *J. Amer. Chem. Soc.* **94**, 989 (1972).
73. P. Salvadori, R. Lazzaroni and C. Bertucci, to be published.
74. E. Charney, J. M. Edwards, U. Weiss and H. Ziffer, *Tetrahedron* **28**, 973 (1972).
75. L. Verbit, to be published.

76. P. Laur, 'Steric Aspects of Sulfur Chemistry', in A. Senning, Ed., *Sulfur in Organic and Inorganic Chemistry*, Vol. III. M. Dekker, New York, in press.
77(a) W. C. Johnson, Jr, *Rev. Sci. Instrum.* **42**, (1972); (b) R. G. Nelson and W. C. Johnson, Jr, *J. Amer. Chem. Soc.* **94**, 3343 (1972).
78(a) G. C. Barrett, *J. Chem. Soc. C*, 1123 (1969); (b) G. C. Barrett and P. R. Cousins, *J. Chem. Soc.* Perkin I, (1972).
79. B. Nordén, *Acta Chem. Scand.* **25**, 357 (1971); **26**, 842 (1972).
80. L. D. Hayward, to be published.
81. E. H. Korte and B. Schrader, *Angew. Chem.* **84**, 218 (1972).
82. R. Hakansson and E. Wiklund, *Acta Chem. Scand.* **25**, 2109 (1971).
83. L. Verbit and H. C. Price, *J. Amer. Chem. Soc.* **94**, 5143 (1972).
84. P. Laur, to be published.
85. S. D. Allen and O. Schnepp, to be published in *J. Chem. Phys.*
86. F. Ciardelli, P. Salvadori, C. Carlini and E. Chiellini, *J. Amer. Chem. Soc.*, **94**, 6536 (1972).
87. G. Gottarelli and B. Samori, *Tetrahedron Lett.* 2055 (1970).
88. K. Noack, *Helv. Chim. Acta*, in the press.
89. P. D. Collier, T. Bryce, R. Mallows, P. E. Thomas, D. J. Frost, O. Korver and C. K. Wilkins, *Tetrahedron*, in the press.
90. H. Wolf and H. Scheer, *Proc. N.Y. Acad. Sci.*, in the press.
91. N. D. Jones, E. E. Helmy, R. J. K. Taylor and A. C. F. Edmonds, *Chem. Commun.* 1401 (1971); *J. Chem. Soc.* (Perkin Transactions).
92. G. Snatzke and S. H. Doss, *Tetrahedron* **28**, 2539 (1972).
93. J. T. Roberts and R. J. Kitz, to be published.
94. C. Toniolo, D. Nisato, L. Biondi and A. Signor, *J. Chem. Soc.* (Perkin I) 1179 and 1182 (1972).
95. C. Toniolo, F. Filira and C. Di Bello, *Biopolymers*, in the press.
96. A. Wollmer and G. Buse, *F.E.B.S. Letters* **16**, 307 (1971).
97. R. Koberstein and H. Sund, *F.E.B.S. Letters* **19**, 149 (1971).
98(a) W. Voelter, G. Kuhfittig, O. Oster and E. Bayer, *Chem. Ber.* **104**, 1234 (1971); (b) W. Voelter, *V. Int. Conf. Organomet. Chem.* Moscow, 1971, Vol. II, p. 248.
99. B. Jirgensons and S. Capetillo, to be published.
100. K. Jacobsohn, *Enzymologia*, in the press.

Theoretical and Semiempirical Calculation of Optical Activity

The Development of Theories of Optical Activity and of their Applications

S. F. MASON

King's College, London WC2R 2LS, U.K.

2.1.1 Classical Stereochemistry

The colours observed by Arago (1811) on propagating white light parallel to the optic axis of a quartz crystal placed between crossed polarizers[1] were found by his colleague Biot (1812) to arise from two distinct effects, firstly, the rotation of the plane of polarization of monochromatic light and, secondly, the dispersion of that rotation with respect to wavelength.[2] The latter effect was shown[3] to follow an approximate inverse square relationship between the rotation, α, and the wavelength, λ, $\alpha = k/\lambda^2$ (Biot's law). Of more chemical significance was Biot's discovery (1815) of optical rotation by natural products in solution or in the fluid phase,[4] indicating that the rotation was a molecular effect.

The significance was long term, for half a century elapsed before the advent of classical stereochemistry. Avogadro's hypothesis[5] (1811), which might have provided immediately, through definitive valencies, a theory of molecular structure, foundered on Newton's interpretation of Boyle's law. To account for the law, Newton had supposed that like atoms repel one another according to a linear inverse-distance law which, as Dalton pointed out, precluded the existence of diatomic or polyatomic elementary molecules. Dalton's law of partial pressures[6] indicated that repulsive forces did not obtain between unlike atoms, every gas being a vacuum to every other gas, so that di- and poly-heteroatomic molecules were allowed species.

Such views were current until the 1860s when the sheer pressure of organic chemistry,[7] with its plethora of isomerisms, radicals and types, demanded a structural systematization. For this purpose Kekulé called the Karlsruhe conference of 1860, where Cannizzaro[8] expounded, and ultimately obtained agreement to, his method of determining valencies, atomic and molecular weights based on Avogadro's hypothesis.

Meanwhile, Pasteur (1848) had long since arrived at the general stereochemical criterion for a chiral molecular structure. Biot, and Haüy before him, had noted the hemihedral facets of quartz crystals, but it was Herschel[9] who made the significant observation that all laevorotatory quartz crystals are morphologically identical and are enantiomorphous in the disposition of the hemihedral facets to dextrorotatory quartz crystals which, in turn, form an isomorphous class. One of the many isomerisms identified by the 1840s was that between (+)-tartaric acid and the corresponding racemate. Mitscherlich found that crystals of corresponding salts of the two acids are, in general, morphologically distinct, but the sodium ammonium salts were exceptional, the crystals being identical, apparently in all respects. Biot confirmed this apparent result[10] but Pasteur[11] by hand-picking isolated from the racemate two distinct sets of crystals, one laevorotatory with facets 'hemihedral to the left', and the other dextrorotatory with facets 'hemihedral to the right', the latter being identical to the crystals of sodium ammonium (+)-tartrate. The specific rotations of the two sets of crystals in solution were equal in magnitude and opposite in sign, from which Pasteur inferred that the macroscopic enantiomorphism of the dextro- and laevorotatory crystals is reproduced in the microscopic stereochemistry of the (+)- and (−)-tartaric acid molecules. Pasteur coined the term 'dissymmetric' to describe all such cases, microscopic or macroscopic, where a structure is not superposable by translations or rotations upon its mirror image.

Early stereochemical conceptions in the 1860s tended to be two-dimensional, which was adequate and productive in aromatic chemistry, notably that of benzene and its derivatives, but structural applications to aliphatic chemistry during this period were less remarkable. With the principle of dissymmetry, Le Bel and van't Hoff (1874) completed the conceptual framework of classical organic stereochemistry. Le Bel[12] largely confined his attention to the rationalization of known chemical properties, whereas van't Hoff[13] employed the three-dimensional atomic model to predict isomerisms, both optical and geometrical, then unknown, notably in the cumulene and spiran series.

The progress of classical inorganic stereochemistry appears to have been retarded in some respects by the organic success. It was a temptation, which Blomstrand and Jörgensen did not successfully resist, to regard the ammonia groups of a metal amine complex as the analogues of the methylene groups of a paraffin chain. Werner[14] took over from the organic stereochemists, not the detailed structural conclusions as analogies, but the general concepts and procedures. For a given coordination number only a limited set of regular geometrical structures are feasible, e.g. hexagonal, octahedral or trigonal prism for six-coordination, and, for each structure, reduction in symmetry through mono-, di-, or poly-substitution generates a defined number and type, geometrical or optical, of permitted isomers. Exploration and characterization of the prevalence of isomers then establishes the particular geometry of the coordination sphere. In a *tour de force* Werner resolved[15] the tetranuclear hexol $[Co\{(OH_2)Co(NH_3)_4\}_3]Br_6$, asserting an inorganic autonomy and freeing the subject of optical activity from the mystique of the asymmetric carbon atom, with vitalist overtones, which had accrued since the 1870s.

2.1.2 Classical Physical Theories

The principal features of optical rotation were discovered not only before the emergence of classical stereochemistry but also before the general acceptance of the transverse wave theory of light. In a crucial experiment Arago and Fresnel (1816) found that parallel-polarized light rays gave an interference pattern, whereas two rays with a mutual perpendicular polarization did not. Young (1817) suggested to

Arago the transverse-wave explanation for the result, and with Young's suggestion Fresnel was able to account for all optical effects then known, including optical rotation.[16]

Fresnel ascribed optical rotation to the circular birefringence of optically active media. Plane-polarized radiation, regarded as the resultant of a left- and a right-circularly polarized component with equal amplitudes, undergoes a rotation if one component is retarded relative to the other on propagation through a transparent medium. The angle of rotation, α, at the wavelength, λ, for unit pathlength in the unit-system measuring λ, is

$$\alpha = (n_L - n_R)\,\pi/\lambda \qquad [1]$$

where n_L and n_R are the refractive indices for left- and right-circularly polarized light, respectively. Fresnel's equation [1] was confirmed by Babinet[17] for quartz, $(n_L - n_R) = 7 \cdot 11 \times 10^{-5}$ at the sodium D-line, and for a variety of optically active media by subsequent workers.

Fresnel himself obtained evidence for his interpretation by demonstrating that the two circular components were separated by a combination of (+)- and (−)-quartz prisms from a ray of plane-polarized or unpolarized light, and by investigating the properties of circularly-polarized light obtained with a quarter-wave plate or a Fresnel rhomb.[18] As a physical model Fresnel suggested that the molecules of an optically active medium have a helical structure, but he was not able to show that such a structure would produce a differential retardation of the left and right circular components of polarized light.

The first attempt to formulate a theory of optical rotation in terms of the general equations of wave motion was made by MacCullagh[19] (1837). His model is not explicit but the forms of his equations imply that a ponderable particle in an optically active molecule is constrained to vibrate through a helical path so that the particle responds differentially to the forces impressed upon it by the medium of the luminiferous ether transmitting left and right circular light vibrations. MacCullagh deduced Biot's inverse square law of rotatory dispersion from his treatment. However, Biot's dispersion law is implicit in Fresnel's equation [1].

MacCullagh's theory and, more particularly, Fresnel's helix model, were extensively developed both prior and subsequent to Maxwell's electromagnetic theory of radiation (Partington[20] listed some forty papers on the subject over the period between MacCullagh and the first quantum treatment). Goldhammer[21] (1892), starting from a more developed elastic-solid ether theory, due to Boussinesq[22] (1865), showed in effect that MacCullagh's molecular parameter singular to optically active media was equivalent in the electromagnetic theory to the molecular polarizability, β, which connects the electric moment of the molecule, μ, with the time-derivative of the magnetic radiation field, H, and the magnetic moment, m, with the time-derivative of the electric radiation field, E

$$\mu = \alpha E - \frac{\beta}{c}\frac{\partial H}{\partial t} \qquad [2]$$

and

$$m = \frac{\beta}{c}\frac{\partial E}{\partial t} \qquad [3]$$

The helix model came to a fruition, which was regarded by subsequent classical theorists as imperfect, with Drude[23] (1892) who related optical activity to the helical motion of a charged particle in a dissymmetric molecule under the electromagnetic radiation field and derived the successful dispersion relation

$$[M]_\lambda = \sum_i A_i/(\lambda^2 - \lambda_i^2) \tag{4}$$

where the λ_i are resonance wavelengths and the A_i are constants. The relation of a right-handed helical charge displacement with positive optical activity, and a left-handed path with a negative rotation, appeared to offer some prospect of determining absolute stereochemical configuration, a problem then coming to the fore with Fischer's configurational convention[24] (1891).

However, Drude's theory was regarded as unsound by Born[25] and by Kuhn,[26] amongst others,[18,20] on the principal ground that a single particle has no appreciable extension whereas optical rotation depends upon a non-zero phase difference between the different parts of the radiation field incident upon spatially distinct regions of the dissymmetric molecule. From the classical standpoint a rigorous one-particle theory of optical activity was not possible. Born showed[25] that a minimum of four non-coplanar coupled isotropic oscillators is required classically to produce optical activity. Kuhn found[26] that two coupled anisotropic oscillators sufficed to produce rotation if the principal directions of the anisotropies were neither coplanar nor mutually orthogonal and perpendicular to the vector along the line of centres. In both models the overall charge displacement produced by the radiation field has a helical form, but the optical rotation depends upon a spatial separation between the coupled oscillators which cannot be neglected in comparison with the wavelength of the radiation, in contrast to the treatment of many other molecule–radiation interactions where the molecular size is taken as negligible.

2.1.3 Circular Dichroism

In the classical as in the quantum theory, the circular birefringence of a medium in the transparent wavelength regions implies circular dichroism at absorption frequencies. However, the study of circular dichroism up to the time of Cotton[27] (1895) appears fragmentary. Biot had observed linear dichroism in tourmaline crystals,[28] and Billet[29] (1859) predicted an analogous differential absorption of left and right circular light in an optically active medium, apparently unaware that circular dichroism in amethyst quartz had been previously reported by Haidinger[30] (1847). The result was confirmed by Dove (1860) and subsequent workers.[18,20]

Cotton's optical studies of solutions containing copper(II) and chromium(III) (+)-tartrate demonstrated the anomalous form of the dispersion of the optical rotation at absorption frequencies and a concomitant ellipticity in the transmitted radiation, due to the circular dichroism. The two main aspects of the Cotton effect stimulated studies of the rotatory dispersion–absorption relations, notably, by Natanson,[31] Bruhat,[32] and, particularly, Kuhn.[33]

During the 1930s Kuhn[33] established detailed analytical relations between circular dichroism and rotatory dispersion, on the assumption of a Gaussian band-shape with tabulated functions for numerical analysis, and approximations expressing the CD band maximum in terms of the rotations at the anomalous ORD extrema,

$$4028(\varepsilon_L - \varepsilon_R)_{max} = [M]_{(v_1)} - [M]_{(v_2)} \tag{5}$$

and the CD band-width Δv in terms of the frequencies of the ORD extrema, v_1 and v_2,

$$\Delta v = 0.925(v_2 - v_1) \qquad [6]$$

with $v_2 > v_1$.

Kuhn defined a rotatory strength for an absorption band as the difference between the oscillator strength for left and right circular radiation $(f_L - f_R)$, and the dissymmetry factor as the ratio of the rotatory strength to the average oscillator strength, f

$$g = (f_L - f_R)/f = (\varepsilon_L - \varepsilon_R)/\varepsilon \qquad [7]$$

He established the classical sum rules that

$$\sum_i f_i = n \qquad [8]$$

where n is the number of oscillators (electrons), and

$$\sum_i g_i f_i / v_i = 0 \qquad [9]$$

As the sum [9] of the rotatory oscillator strengths vanishes, the rotation tends to zero at high and at low frequencies since, outside the absorption region

$$\alpha = \frac{Ne^2 v^2}{2mc} \sum_i \frac{g_i f_i}{v_i(v_i^2 - v^2)} \qquad [10]$$

Kuhn indicated that, since the rotation at a given frequency represents a sum of contributions from all of the optically active absorption bands in the spectrum of a dissymmetric molecule [10], a knowledge of the absolute stereochemical configuration of the molecule is to be sought from the Cotton effect of a particular absorption band, or set of bands, rather than from the sign and the magnitude of the D-line rotation. To this end Kuhn applied his anisotropic coupled oscillator model to a number of particular cases and measured the corresponding ORD and CD and absorption spectra. While correct in principle, these applications remained inconclusive. There were two prime limitations. Firstly, the principal directions of the anisotropies of chromophores, i.e. the polarization directions of the electronic transitions, were not well established in his period. Secondly, for reasons of experimental accessibility, chromophores with large g-factors in the region of the lowest-energy absorption were especially studied, e.g. the carbonyl, azide, and nitrite chromophores. These transitions involve one-centre rotatory charge displacements which were not considered in Kuhn's model. Such displacements were associated with the classical one-particle models which entailed the spatial-extension problem.

2.1.4 Quantum Theories

The quantum-mechanical treatment of optical activity was initiated by Rosenfeld[34] (1928) who showed that the rotatory polarizability β of [2] and [3] is represented by a sum over all electronic transitions of the rotational strengths, R_{oa}, at the frequency, v_a

$$\beta = \frac{c}{3\pi h} \sum_a \frac{R_{oa}}{(v_a^2 - v^2)} \qquad [11]$$

The rotational strength is defined by the scalar product of the electric and magnetic dipole moment of the transition

$$R_{oa} = \text{Im}\{\langle o| \hat{\mu} |a\rangle . \langle a| \hat{m} |o\rangle\} \tag{12}$$

and the sum of the rotational strengths over the spectrum vanishes, as in the classical case [9].

Since the wave function corresponding to a classical particle is spatially extended, the primary classical objection to a one-particle theory of optical activity is circumvented in the quantum theory. The one-electron charge density in a given molecular orbital, or the transition charge density connecting two such orbitals, is extended over the several atoms and bonds of the dissymmetric molecule and encounters a radiation field with a phase difference between spatially distinct regions which is equal in magnitude, but opposite in sign for left and right circular radiation. The enantiomeric molecule has an inequality of phase difference for left and right circular radiation between the corresponding spatial regions of reversed sign for the same frequency.

Thus one of the earliest applications was the one-electron theory of optical rotatory power due to the Princeton group[35] (1937). Another was the reformulation of the coupled oscillator model by Kirkwood[36] (1937) who gave an expression for the monochromatic rotation of a dissymmetric molecule in terms of its geometrical configuration and the polarizability tensors of its constituent groups. These are the immediate ancestors of virtually all current treatments of optical activity. At the time, attention concentrated upon the calculation of D-line rotations, which in part was predicated by taking the asymmetric carbon atom, in the particular manifestation of 2-butanol,[35,36] as the paradigm of optical activity, but the tradition extended to the nitrite[35] and carbonyl[37] chromophore for which Cotton-effect data were available.[18,33,38]

The reorientation towards the analysis of specific Cotton effects came with a second wave of the quantum theory of optical activity, centring on Moffitt[39] (1956), stimulated by the revival of organic ORD studies,[40] soon to be followed by both organic and inorganic CD investigations.[41-48] Moffitt initiated the analysis of the d-electron Cotton effects of metal complexes, using the one-electron theory and a static-field mechanism,[39] the polypeptide α-helix rotatory dispersion employing the coupled-excitation model,[39] and with co-workers examined the vibronic problem[49] and introduced the use of sector rules for the correlation of structure with optical activity.[50]

Moffitt and Moscowitz[41,49] drew a useful distinction between optically active molecules containing an inherently dissymmetric chromophore and those with a symmetric chromophore in a chiral molecular environment. The distinction cuts across and, to a degree, supersedes the old division into one-particle and coupled oscillator models. In the case of the inherently dissymmetric chromophore, of which the helicenes[51-57] are paradigmatic, the rotational strengths considered have a one-electron provenance, but the analysis proceeds through a coupling scheme involving the individual bond transition moments. The model and the procedure employed in the calculation of the CD spectrum of a helicene[56] (Fig. 1) and of a typical two-chromophore coupled-oscillator system[58] (Fig. 2) are in no fundamental way distinct.

In the case of the symmetric chromophore in a dissymmetric molecular environment the one-electron and the coupled-excitation treatments lead to different models.

Taking the carbonyl n → π* transition as paradigmatic, it is possible to regard the excitation as basically one-electron in character, taking place between states so perturbed by the static Coulombic field of the substituents that the zero-order magnetic moment is augmented by a first-order electric moment with a collinear

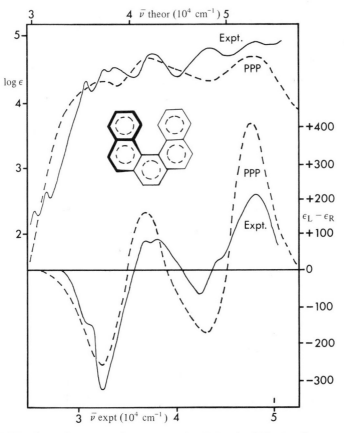

Fig. 1. The absorption spectra (upper curves) and circular dichroism (lower curves) of [5]-helicene. The full curves refer to the experimental spectra for the (−)-isomer and the broken curves to the theoretical spectra for the *M*-configuration illustrated, calculated by the Pariser–Parr–Pople method using the dipole velocity procedure.

component.[37] Alternatively the charge distribution of the magnetic-dipole transition correlates Coulombically an electric dipole induced in the substituent, and the collinear component of the induced dipole provides, with the zero-order magnetic moment, a non-vanishing rotational strength.[59,60]

Both the static field and the dynamic-coupling mechanisms for the optical activity of a symmetric chromophore in a chiral molecular environment afford sector rules and these, in principle, provide a distinction between the two models. In the static-field case the effective component of the Coulombic potential due to the substituent has a pseudoscalar form in the point group of the symmetric chromophore, and the particular pseudoscalar function providing a sector rule is determined by the form of the chromophoric states mixed under the perturbation.[61]

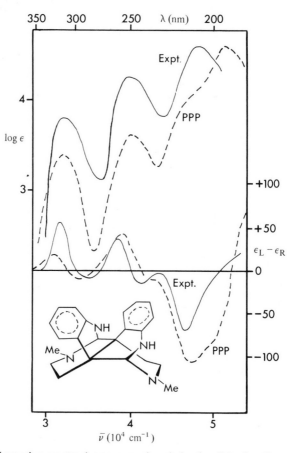

Fig. 2. The absorption spectra (upper curves) and circular dichroism (lower curves) of calycanthine. The full curves refer to the experimental spectra of the natural product and the broken curves to the theoretical curves for the configuration illustrated, calculated by the Pariser–Parr–Pople method using the dipole velocity procedure.

In the dynamic coupling case the sector rule follows from the geometric factor describing the angular dependence of the Coulombic potential between the leading electric multipole of the chromophoric transition and the induced dipole of the substituent.[60] The lowest-order charge distribution on the substituent is a dipole in the dynamic-coupling case but it may be a monopole in the static-field case. Thus the simplest sector rule is of lower order in the power of the substituent coordinates for static field than the dynamic-coupling mechanism, e.g. an XY quadrant rule for the $n \rightarrow \pi^*$ carbonyl transition is permitted in the static-field case whereas an XYZ

octant rule, or other third-power rules for anisotropic perturbers,[60] is the lowest-order rule allowed in the dynamic-coupling case.

The one-electron theory of optical activity and subsequent treatments of a symmetric chromophore in a chiral molecular environment focused attention upon magnetic-dipole transitions, marking them off from the general amorphous class of forbidden excitations. A large g-factor came to be recognized as indicative of a

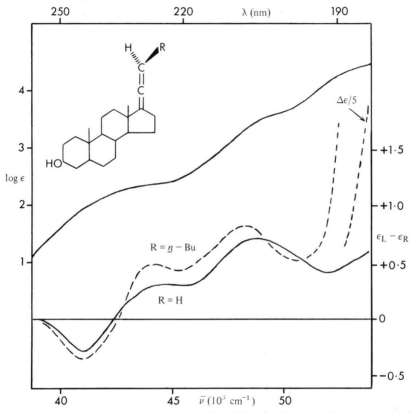

Fig. 3. The absorption spectra (upper curve) and circular dichroism (lower curves) of 17-allenic steroids in iso-octane solution.

magnetic-dipole transition, and a comparison of the rotational strength with the increment in the dipole strength due to dissymmetric substitution gave values for the magnetic transition moments of the right order.[43]

Although there are evident gaps and imperfections in our detailed knowledge of magnetic and electric dipole optical activity, the general principles underlying the analysis of zero- and first-order rotational strengths connected with magnetic and electric dipole transitions are fairly well understood. This is not yet the case for transitions which have appreciable rotational strengths but no zero-order magnetic or electric dipole moment.

The problem is illustrated by the CD spectra of chiral allenes (Figs. 3 and 4). The allene chromophore has four one-electron excited $\pi \to \pi^*$ configurations, giving excited states which π-SCF and all-valence electron calculations place in the general energy-order, $B_2 > B_1 > A_2$, with the fourth state, A_1, at a position varying from one calculation to another. The leading moments of transitions from the A_1 ground

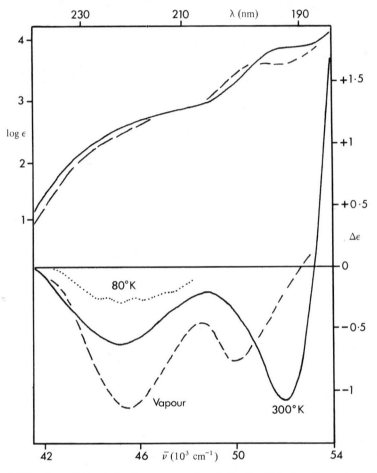

Fig. 4. The absorption spectra (upper curves) and circular dichroism (lower curves) of (*S*)-(+)-1,3-dimethylallene in the vapour phase (— — — — —), in iso-octane at 300°K (————) and in EPA at 80°K (· · · · · · · ·).

state are the z^2 component of an electric quadrupole for the excited A_1 state, the z-component of a magnetic dipole and the xyz-component of an electric octopole for the A_2 state, the xy-component of an electric quadrupole for the B_1 state, and, finally, the z-component of an electric dipole for the B_2 state. The coordinate frame is that depicted (Fig. 5). Dissymmetric allenes give three or, in favourable cases, four CD bands in the quartz ultraviolet region (Figs. 3 and 4). These CD bands have rotational strengths of the same order, approximately 10^{-40} c.g.s., but one or two of these arise from transitions with neither an electric nor a magnetic dipole moment.

One approach to an analysis of the rotational strengths of the 'forbidden' transitions is vibronic coupling with the magnetic- and electric-dipole allowed excitations.[49,62-64] Another is suggested by a consideration of the optical activity exhibited by chiral 1,3-dialkylallenes (Fig. 4) where the substituents are cylindrically symmetrical and lie in a nodal plane of the π_x or the π_y system. Here the rotational strength of the magnetic- and the electric-dipole allowed transitions cannot arise by a first order process and the CD spectrum suggests that the mechanism involved is common to at least one of the quadrupole transitions.

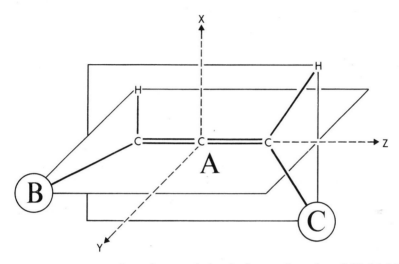

Fig. 5. The allenic coordinate frame and the absolute configuration of (S)-$(+)$-1,3-dimethylallene for B = C = Me.

In the first order the static-field and the dynamic-coupling mechanisms are distinct, but, on proceeding to second order, cross-terms appear.[48] However, by setting appropriate terms to zero, a pure static-field or dynamic-coupling analysis becomes feasible. The static-field rotational strengths of 1,3-dimethylallene are zero in the second as in the first order since cylindrically symmetrical substituents in the π-nodal planes of the allene chromophore generate a potential devoid of a pseudoscalar component or of components with symmetries which contain B_1 of D_{2d} in their direct product.

Dynamic-coupling is a possible mechanism for the origin of the observed circular dichroism (Fig. 4). For a chiral allene consisting of the allene chromophore (A) and cylindrically symmetrical substituents (B) and (C) in the 1- and 3-position (Fig. 5) the pure dynamic-coupling rotational strength (R_{oa}) of the allenic transition $(o \rightarrow a)$ is, in the second order,

$$R_{oa} = \pi \bar{v}_a [(\beta\bar{\alpha})_B (\beta\bar{\alpha})_C \, M_{oa} \, G_{BC}]^2 \, G_{AB} \, G_{AC} \, R_{BC} (\vec{e}_{BC} \, \vec{e}_C \times \vec{e}_B) \qquad [13]$$

where β is the anisotropy and $\bar{\alpha}$ the mean polarizability of the substituent at the frequency $\bar{v}_a$ of the chromophore transition o $\rightarrow$ a with the leading electric multipole M_{oa}. The geometric factor governing the radial and angular dependence of the Coulombic potential between the multipole M_{oa} of the chromophore (A) and the electric dipole induced in the substituent (B) or (C) is G_{AB} and G_{AC}, respectively, G_{BC} being the corresponding factor for the potential between the latter dipoles, which are separated by the distance R_{BC}. Of the unit vectors, $\vec{e}_{BC}$ is directed from (B) to (C) and $\vec{e}_B$ and $\vec{e}_C$ are orientated along the principal polarizability direction of the substituent (B) and (C), respectively. An energy ratio with a minimum value of unity and a maximum value of 2 is omitted from [13].

In the model which equation [13] expresses, the electronic states of the allene chromophore are hard and remain unmixed under the perturbation due to the substituents. The leading electric multipole of a chromophoric transition correlates Coulombically the electric dipoles induced in the two substituents, and the rotational strength arises entirely from the coupling of the two induced dipoles. The moments of the allenic transitions do not contribute to the rotational strengths even in the dipole-allowed cases. The relevant components of the induced substituent dipoles are orthogonal to the magnetic moment of the $A_1 \rightarrow A_2$ allenic transition, and each is coplanar with the electric dipole of the $A_1 \rightarrow B_2$ transition. In this model it is immaterial whether the chromophoric transition is dipole-allowed or 'forbidden', as a rotational strength of much the same magnitude arises from the induced substituent dipoles in either case. However, the values estimated for (S)-$(+)$-1,3-dimethylallene are almost an order lower in magnitude than those observed (Fig. 4), the expected signs for this isomer being positive for $R(B_2)$ and $R(A_2)$ and negative for $R(B_1)$ and $R(A_1)$. An alternative model, perhaps more realistic, in which the chromophoric states are softer and mix under the second-order perturbation of the induced substituent dipoles, singles out the magnetic and electric dipole allenic transitions, giving $R(B_2)$ and $R(A_2)$ values of an order of magnitude larger than those observed (Fig. 4) and signs which are positive and negative, respectively, for (S)-$(+)$-1,3-dimethylallene.

In addition to the problem of the rotational strengths of electronic transitions forbidden in dipole radiation fields, there remains the almost perennial question of the origin of the optical activity of the asymmetric carbon atom. It should be possible to tackle the latter problem spectroscopically in the near future. With the new vacuum ultraviolet instruments the measurement of the CD spectrum of a simple chiral carbon derivative with four cylindrically symmetrical substituents is now feasible. The tetrahedral carbon atom has its centenary in 1974. By that time we should have the measurements and, hopefully, a more fundamental understanding of the traditional paradigm for optical activity.

References

1. D. F. J. Arago, *Mémoires de l'Institut* **12**, part 1, 93 (1811).
2. J. B. Biot, *Mémoires de l'Institut* **13**, part 1, 218 (1812).
3. J. B. Biot, *Ann. Chim. (Paris)* **9**, 382 (1818); **10**, 63 (1818).
4. J. B. Biot, *Bull. Soc. Philomath. Paris* 190 (1815).
5. A. Avogadro, *J. Phys. (Paris)* **73**, 58 (1811).
6. J. Dalton, *Mem. Manchester Lit. Phil. Soc.* **5**, part 2, 538 (1802).

7. Wöhler wrote to Liebig about 1840: 'Organic chemistry nowadays almost drives me out of my mind. To me it appears as a primeval tropical forest full of the most remarkable things, a dreadful endless jungle into which one does not dare to enter, for there seems no way out'.
8. S. Cannizzaro, *Nuovo Cimento* **7**, 321 (1858).
9. J. Herschel, *Trans. Cambridge Phil. Soc.* **1**, 43 (1820).
10. J. B. Biot, *C.R.H. Acad. Sci.* **19**, 719 (1844).
11. L. Pasteur, *C.R.H. Acad. Sci.* **28**, 477 (1849).
12. J. A. Le Bel, *Bull. Soc. Chim. Fr.* **22**, 337 (1874).
13. J. H. van't Hoff, *Chemische Constitutie van Organische Verbindingen*. Utrecht, 1874; *Chemistry in Space*. Oxford, 1891.
14. A. Werner, *Neuere Anschauungen auf dem Gebiete der anorganischem Chemie*, Brunswick, 1905; *Chem. Ber.* **45**, 121 (1912).
15. A. Werner, *C.R.H. Acad. Sci.* **159**, 426 (1914); *Chem. Ber.* **47**, 3087 (1914).
16. A. Fresnel, *Ann. Chim.* **28**, 147 (1825).
17. J. Babinet, *C.R.H. Acad. Sci.* **4**, 900 (1837).
18. T. M. Lowry, *Optical Rotatory Power*. Longmans Green, London, 1935.
19. J. MacCullagh, *Trans. Roy. Irish Acad.* **17**, 461 (1837).
20. J. R. Partington, *An Advanced Treatise on Physical Chemistry*, Vol. 4. Longmans Green, London, 1953, p. 336.
21. D. A. Goldhammer, *J. Phys.* (*Paris*) **1**, 205, 345 (1892).
22. J. Boussinesq, *C.R.H. Acad. Sci.* **61**, 19 (1865); *J. Math.* (*Paris*) **13**, 313, 425 (1868).
23. P. Drude, *The Theory of Optics* (translated by C. R. Mann and R. A. Millikan, 1902). Dover Reprint, New York, 1959, p. 400.
24. E. Fischer, *Chem. Ber.* **24**, 2683 (1891).
25. M. Born, *Ann. Phys. Leipzig.* **55**, 177 (1918).
26. W. Kuhn, *Z. Phys. Chem.* **B20**, 325 (1933).
27. A. Cotton, *C.R.H. Acad. Sci.* **120**, 989, 1044 (1895); *Ann. Chim.* **8**, 347 (1896); *Z. physikal. Chem.* **21**, 158 (1896).
28. J. B. Biot, *Bull. Soc. Philomath Paris* 26 (1815).
29. A. Billet, *Traité d'Optique Physique* **2**, 7 (1859).
30. W. Haidinger, *Ann. Phys. Leipzig* **70**, 531 (1847).
31. L. Natanson, *Bull. Acad. Pol.* 764 (1908); *J. Phys. Radium* [4] **8**, 321 (1909).
32. G. Bruhat, *Ann. Phys. Paris* **3**, 232, 417, 469 (1915).
33. Bibliography and summary in W. Kuhn, *Ann. Rev. Phys. Chem.* **9**, 417 (1958).
34. L. Rosenfeld, *Z. Phys.* **52**, 161 (1928).
35. E. U. Condon, W. Altar and H. Eyring, *J. Chem. Phys.* **5**, 753 (1937); E. Gorin, J. Walter and H. Eyring, *J. Chem. Phys.* **6**, 824 (1938).
36. J. G. Kirkwood, *J. Chem. Phys.* **5**, 479 (1937).
37. W. J. Kauzmann, J. E. Walter and H. Eyring, *Chem. Rev.* **26**, 339 (1940).
38. S. Mitchell, *The Cotton Effect*. Bell, London, 1933.
39. W. Moffitt, *J. Chem. Phys.* **25**, 467, 1189 (1956).
40. C. Djerassi, *Optical Rotatory Dispersion*. McGraw-Hill, New York, 1960.
41. A. Moscowitz, *Advan. Chem. Phys.* **4**, 67 (1962).
42. I. Tinoco, Jr, *Advan. Chem. Phys.* **4**, 113 (1962).
43. S. F. Mason, *Quart. Rev. Chem. Soc.* **17**, 20 (1963).
44. L. Velluz, M. Legrand and M. Grosjean, *Optical Circular Dichroism*. Academic Press, New York, 1965.
45. P. Crabbé, *Optical Rotatory Dispersion and Circular Dichroism in Organic Chemistry*. Holden-Day, London, 1965.
46. G. Snatzke, Ed., *Optical Rotatory Dispersion and Circular Dichroism in Organic Chemistry*. Heyden, London, 1967.
47. C. J. Hawkins, *Absolute Configuration of Metal Complexes*. Wiley-Interscience, New York, 1971.
48. D. J. Caldwell and H. Eyring, *The Theory of Optical Activity*. Wiley-Interscience, New York, 1971.
49. W. Moffitt and A. Moscowitz, *J. Chem. Phys.* **30**, 648 (1959).
50. W. Moffitt, R. B. Woodward, A. Moscowitz, W. Klyne and C. Djerassi, *J. Amer. Chem. Soc.* **83**, 4013 (1961).
51. A. Moscowitz, Thesis, Harvard, 1957; *Tetrahedron* **13**, 48 (1961).

52. D. D. Fitts and J. G. Kirkwood, *J. Amer. Chem. Soc.* **77**, 490 (1955).
53. J. H. Brewster, *Topics Stereochem.* **2**, 40 (1967).
54. O. E. Weigang, Jr, J. A. Turner and P. A. Trouard Dodson, *J. Chem. Phys.* **45**, 1126 (1966); **49**, 4248 (1968).
55. M. S. Newman, R. S. Darlak and L. Tsai, *J. Amer. Chem. Soc.* **89**, 6191 (1967).
56. W. S. Brickell, A. Brown, C. M. Kemp and S. F. Mason, *Tetrahedron* **22**, 629 (1966); *Mol. Phys.* **20**, 787 (1971); *J. Chem. Soc. A*, 751, 756 (1971).
57. G. Wagnière, *Aromaticity, Pseudo-Aromaticity and Anti-Aromaticity.* Jerusalem Symposia III, Israel Acad. Sci., Jerusalem, 1971, p. 127.
58. W. S. Brickell, S. F. Mason and D. R. Roberts, *J. Chem. Soc. B*, 691 (1971).
59. M. P. Kruchek, *Opt. Spectrosc.* **17**, 294 (1964); **30**, 481 (1971).
60. E. G. Höhn and O. E. Weigang, Jr, *J. Chem. Phys.* **48**, 1127 (1968).
61. J. A. Schellman, *J. Chem. Phys.* **44**, 55 (1966); *Accounts Chem. Res.* **1**, 144 (1968).
62. O. E. Weigang, Jr, *J. Chem. Phys.* **43**, 71, 3609 (1965).
63. D. J. Caldwell, *J. Chem. Phys.* **51**, 984 (1969).
64. S. E. Harnung, E. C. Ong and O. E. Weigang, Jr, *J. Chem. Phys.* **55**, 5711 (1971); M. D. Frank-Kamenetskii and A. V. Lukashin, *Opt. Spectrosc.* **30**, 585 (1971).

Optical Activity Data as an Aid in the Assignment of Electronic Transitions: Application to Dialkyl Sulphides

J. S. ROSENFIELD and A. MOSCOWITZ

Department of Chemistry
University of Minnesota
Minneapolis, Minnesota 55455, U.S.A.

2.2.1 Introduction

To date, the interpretation of natural optical activity data has been directed primarily toward the acquisition of stereochemical information. For the case of molecules containing inherently symmetric but dissymmetrically perturbed chromophores,[1] this information can sometimes, within certain limitations, be succinctly summarized in terms of sign-determining regions of space, e.g. the Octant rule for the lowest lying singlet transition in saturated ketones,[2] and the Quadrant rule for the lowest singlet in amides.[3] In such instances, symmetry or group theoretical considerations[4] can provide the minimum number of such spatial regions. Indeed, they are just those regions delineated by the intersecting symmetry planes of the pertinent chromophore. However, these domains may be further subdivided because of nodal surfaces associated with the orbitals involved in the electronic transition of interest. When such is the case, specification of the sign-determining regions requires some detailed knowledge of the relevant orbitals, i.e. it is necessary to be able in some degree to assign the electronic transition giving rise to the absorption band and the circular dichroism band under consideration.

Unfortunately, for polyatomic systems, the number of transitions that have been unequivocally assigned is really quite small. The nature of the difficulties involved is exemplified nicely by the case of the 290-nm transition in saturated ketones. The papers of McMurry and Mulliken[5] stand as testimony to the thorough examination and interpretation of data required in order to achieve the assignment that is today so casually referred to as 'n → π*'.

It is the purpose of the present contribution to emphasize that optical activity data can be useful for assigning electronic transitions. Actually, the situation may be viewed as the converse of the problem of delineating the sign-determining spatial regions when given a specification of the pertinent electronic transition. Namely, the circular dichroism data, for a given electronic transition in a series of compounds containing a common chromophore, place constraints on the possible nature of the orbitals involved, in addition to those constraints provided by considerations of energy and absorption intensity. Hence, given these additional constraints, one can apply them in the task of assigning the nature of a particular electronic promotion.

The present work illustrates one possible approach, in the specific case of cyclic dialkyl sulphides, which we discuss from the point of view of the inherently symmetric but dissymmetrically perturbed chromophore. First, an analysis of the experimental data and symmetry considerations lead to tentative assignments of the three lowest lying singlets in dialkyl sulphides. Then, order of magnitude calculations of the absorption intensity and the optical activity of some conformationally rigid sulphides of known absolute configuration test the assignments and permit a fuller understanding of the optical properties of these transitions.

2.2.2 Absorption and Circular Dichroism Data

Dialkyl sulphides exhibit three absorption bands in the region from 200 to 240 nm.[6, 7] There is a band at approximately 200 nm with an oscillator strength of about 0·06, which is relatively. structureless in the vapour phase. Methyl sulphoxide[7] and hydrogen sulphide[6] show bands at 200 nm of approximately the same intensity as that in methyl sulphide. In addition, compounds in which the carbons bonded to sulphur are replaced by silicon and germanium, for example in $(R_3Si)_2S$, where R is a methyl group, exhibit a band with roughly the same wavelength and intensity.[8]

Sulphides show another band at about 220 nm, with an oscillator strength of about 0·016. The vibrational structure of this band, exhibited in the vapour-phase spectrum, has been assigned[6] to progressions and combinations of the symmetrical C–S–C stretch and the parallel methyl rock (symmetry a_1) built on the 0—0 transition. In solution, this band appears as a shoulder to the 200 nm transition. In addition, there is a third, very weak band at about 240 nm, with $\varepsilon_{max} \approx 20$. In cyclic sulphides, this band red shifts as the ring size decreases; it appears at about 265 nm in the three-membered ring episulphides.[7]

Optical rotatory dispersion and circular dichroism properties are known in the range 200 to 240 nm for some dissymmetric sulphides.[9–11] In *cyclic* sulphides, three Cotton effects are observed in this spectral region, at about 200, 220 and 240 nm. As is the case in the absorption spectrum, the long wavelength circular dichroism band red shifts from about 235 nm in the six-membered ring sulphides to about 265 nm in episulphides.[12, 13] The rotational strengths observed are of the order of 10^{-40} c.g.s.

In summary, there are at least three optically active low-energy transitions in dialkyl sulphides. These are: a very weak band, $\varepsilon_{max} \approx 20$, at 240 nm; a band, $f \approx 0·016$, at 220 nm; and a moderately strong band, $f \approx 0·06$, at 200 nm.

2.2.3 Assignments Based on Symmetry Considerations

We describe our model sulphide chromophore, the sulphur atom plus its neighbouring carbons, with a basis set consisting of the 3s, 3p, 3d, and 4s Slater type AOs on sulphur, plus one $2sp^3$ hybrid orbital centred on each carbon atom, directed toward the sulphur atom. This primitive C–S–C sulphide chromophore has local symmetry C_{2v} (Table 1). The hybrids are denoted by c_1 (centred on C_1) and c_2 (centred on C_2). The coordinate system and the labelling of atoms are shown in Fig. 1. In order to

Table 1

C_{2v} Character Table (The Coordinate System is that of Fig. 1)

C_{2v}	E	$C_2(y)$	$\sigma_v(yz)$	$\sigma_v'(xy)$
A_1	1	1	1	1
A_2	1	1	−1	−1
B_1	1	−1	1	−1
B_2	1	−1	−1	1

discuss the constraints that the absorption and optical activity data place on the nature of the orbitals involved in these transitions, we form crude MOs by taking linear combinations of the AOs. These MOs are listed in Table 2 in approximate order of the orbital energies, which are determined by the number of nodes. The ordering of the 3d and 4s levels is arbitrary. The symmetry designations refer to the

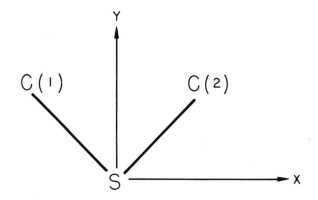

Fig. 1. Coordinate system of sulphide chromophore (z axis is toward reader).

irreducible representations of C_{2v} given in Table 1. In Table 3, we give the possible transitions corresponding to promotions from the three highest filled orbitals, together with the directions of the electric and magnetic dipole transition moments, μ and m, respectively.

The sign and magnitude of the circular dichroism band associated with the transition o → i is determined by the rotational strength R_{oi}:

$$R_{oi} = \text{Im}[\langle o| \boldsymbol{\mu}|i\rangle . \langle i| \boldsymbol{m}|o\rangle]$$

From the point of view of the dissymmetrically perturbed symmetric chromophore, we can say that the dissymmetrically disposed substituents perturb the wave functions of the erstwhile isolated chromophore in such a way that there is some electric and magnetic dipole transition moment in a common direction. Looking at Table 3, we see that for our case of a C_{2v} isolated chromophore, some perturbation V must cause the mixing of an A_1 excited state with an A_2 state, or of a B_1 with a B_2 state, in order to produce a non-zero rotational strength. It is assumed the perturbation V arises from the neutral carbon and hydrogen atoms making up the extrachromophoric framework of the molecule.[14-17] A feature of V which plays an important role in our considerations is that, since it is a one-electron operator, it cannot mix, in first order, configurations which differ in more than one orbital.

In looking for the assignments, it is reasonable to confine our attentions to promotions from the highest filled orbital, the lone pair $b_1(3p_z)$. In defence of this we note that sulphones, which have no non-bonding electrons on sulphur, are transparent in the region of the spectrum we are considering. Actually, we did test sets of assignments, other than those we shall discuss, but could find none which were consonant with both the absorption and optical activity data.

Table 2

Crude MOs Constructed as Linear Combinations of the AO Basis Set[a, b]

Orbital designation	Linear combination	Symmetry
——— 4s		a_1
——— $3d_{xy}$		b_2
——— $3d_{x^2-y^2}$		a_1
——— $3d_{yz}$		b_1
——— $3d_{xz}$		a_2
——— $3d_{z^2}$		a_1
——— a_1^*	$3s + 3p_y - (c_2 + c_1)$	a_1
——— b_2^*	$3p_x - (c_2 - c_1)$	b_2
XX ——— b_1	$3p_z$	b_1
XX ——— $2a_1$	$3s - 3p_y - (c_2 + c_1)$	a_1
XX ——— b_2	$3p_x + (c_2 - c_1)$	b_2
XX ——— $1a_1$	$3s + 3p_y + (c_2 + c_1)$	a_1

[a] The energy increases from bottom to top. [b] X denotes that the orbital is occupied in the ground state.

Let us first consider the 240-nm transition. Since it is so very weak in absorption, but exhibits rotational strengths of the order of 10^{-40} c.g.s. in dissymmetric sulphides, we want a transition which is electric dipole forbidden, magnetic dipole allowed. There is only one lone pair promotion which qualifies, $b_1 \rightarrow b_2^*$. This transition has a magnetic dipole moment in the y direction, and could become optically active by a first-order mixing with $b_1 \rightarrow 3d_{yz}$ and $b_2 \rightarrow b_2^*$. These are, in fact, the only states in our manifold that can mix with the $b_1 \rightarrow b_2^*$ state (symmetry A_2) to give optical activity in first order, for they are the only A_1 states that differ by no more than a single orbital from the $b_1 \rightarrow b_2^*$ state.

Looking next at the 220-nm band, we note that the oscillator strength indicates an electric dipole allowed transition. The experimentally observed vibrational structure of the absorption band shows a progression in the C–S–C symmetric stretching frequency. This suggests that the equilibrium carbon–sulphur bond length changes on going from the ground to the excited state. So a plausible assignment of this band would be a promotion to the antibonding orbital, a_1^*, rather than to the atomic-like 3d or 4s. The transition $b_1 \rightarrow a_1^*$ has an electric dipole moment in the z direction, and a magnetic dipole moment in the x direction. Examining Table 3, we see that it could become optically active by a first order mixing only with $b_1 \rightarrow 3d_{xz}$ and $b_2 \rightarrow a_1^*$.

Table 3

Electric and Magnetic Dipole Moments of Transitions

Transition	State Symmetry	μ	m
$b_1 \rightarrow b_2^*$	A_2	0	y
$b_1 \rightarrow a_1^*$	B_1	z	x
$b_1 \rightarrow 3d_{z^2}$	B_1	z	0
$b_1 \rightarrow 3d_{xz}$	B_2	x	0
$b_1 \rightarrow 3d_{yz}$	A_1	y	0
$b_1 \rightarrow 3d_{x^2-y^2}$	B_1	0	0
$b_1 \rightarrow 3d_{xy}$	A_2	0	0
$b_1 \rightarrow 4s$	B_1	z	0
$2a_1 \rightarrow b_2^*$	B_2	x	z
$2a_1 \rightarrow a_1^*$	A_1	y	0
$2a_1 \rightarrow 3d_{z^2}$	A_1	y	0
$2a_1 \rightarrow 3d_{xz}$	A_2	0	y
$2a_1 \rightarrow 3d_{yz}$	B_1	z	x
$2a_1 \rightarrow 3d_{x^2-y^2}$	A_1	y	0
$2a_1 \rightarrow 3d_{xy}$	B_2	x	z
$2a_1 \rightarrow 4s$	A_1	y	0
$b_2 \rightarrow b_2^*$	A_1	y	0
$b_2 \rightarrow a_1^*$	B_2	x	z
$b_2 \rightarrow 3d_{z^2}$	B_2	x	0
$b_2 \rightarrow 3d_{xz}$	B_1	z	x
$b_2 \rightarrow 3d_{yz}$	A_2	0	y
$b_2 \rightarrow 3d_{x^2-y^2}$	B_2	x	z
$b_2 \rightarrow 3d_{xy}$	A_1	y	0
$b_2 \rightarrow 4s$	B_2	x	0

Finally, we focus on the 200-nm band. The oscillator strength f of this band indicates that it is electric dipole allowed. The relative insensitivity of the position and intensity of the band to the nature of the atoms bonded to sulphur suggests an atomic-like 3p $\rightarrow$ 3d or 3p $\rightarrow$ 4s on sulphur. The electric-dipole-allowed lone pair promotions of this sort are $b_1 \rightarrow 3d_{z^2}$, $b_1 \rightarrow 3d_{xz}$, $b_1 \rightarrow 3d_{yz}$, and $b_1 \rightarrow 4s$. We calculated the oscillator strengths of the promotions 3p $\rightarrow$ 3d and 3p $\rightarrow$ 4s, and found that, although the oscillator strengths were very sensitive to the effective nuclear charge Z of the 3d and 4s orbitals, one could find a reasonable value of Z_{3d} (in the neighbourhood of 1·5) for which the f value of 3p $\rightarrow$ 3d agreed with experiment for the 200-nm transition. However, f values for the 3p $\rightarrow$ 4s transition were at least an order of magnitude smaller than the experimental ones for either of the electric dipole allowed transitions, when Z_{4s} was varied between 0 and 2.

To examine the information that the optical activity data yield in this case, we note that the transition $3p_z \rightarrow 4s$ has μ in the z direction and is magnetic dipole forbidden. We note from Table 3 that there is no state with which $b_1 \to 4s$ can mix, in first order, to give some magnetic moment in the z direction. However, one can see that some of the $b_1 \to 3d$ transitions can become optically active by first-order mixings. From these considerations, which take into account both the absorption and the optical activity data, we prefer the assignment $b_1 \to 3d$ for the 200 nm band.

As a result of these qualitative arguments, we come to the following tentative conclusions. The very weak 240-nm transition is assigned to the electric dipole forbidden, magnetic dipole allowed $b_1 \to b_2^*$. The 220-nm transition is assigned to the electric dipole allowed $b_1 \to a_1^*$. The band at 200 nm is assigned to an atomic-like $b_1 \to 3d$ promotion (which one we cannot say). The orbital b_1 is a non-bonding $3p_z$ sulphur orbital, b_2^* and a_1^* are orbitals antinodal in the plane of the C–S–C chromophore and antibonding between the sulphur and carbon atoms.

2.2.4 Oscillator and Rotational Strength Calculations

A. Outline of Calculations

In order to test the assignments, and to inquire further into the nature of these transitions, order of magnitude calculations of oscillator and rotational strengths were performed. First, molecular orbitals for the isolated sulphide chromophore were obtained by a Wolfsberg–Helmholz type calculation.[18] Then the effect on the isolated sulphide chromophore wrought by the dissymmetric molecular environment provided in a series of relatively rigid optically active compounds was treated by perturbation methods. The perturbation operator V was the potential energy of an electron in the field of the incompletely shielded carbon and hydrogen atoms of the molecules.[14-17] Finally, oscillator and rotational strengths were calculated and compared with experiment. Details of the calculations may be found in reference 19.

The compounds considered were the five-membered ring sulphides, (8R,9R)-*trans*-2-thiahydrindan (I) and A-nor-2-thiacholestane (II), and six-membered ring sulphides 1,8,8-trimethyl-3-thiabicyclo-[3,2,1]-octane (III) and 3-thia-5α-cholestane (IV).

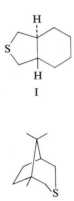

I

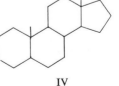

II

III

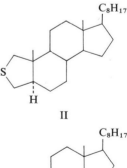

IV

B. The $b_1 \rightarrow b_2^*$ Transition

This is the electric dipole forbidden, magnetic dipole allowed promotion which we have tentatively assigned to the very weak band at 240 nm. The two promotions it can mix with in first order to become optically active are $b_1 \rightarrow 3d_{yz}$ and $b_2 \rightarrow b_2^*$. The calculations showed that the contribution of the $b_2 \rightarrow b_2^*$ state to the rotational strengths of the $b_1 \rightarrow b_2^*$ transition was three orders of magnitude low, as well as being of the wrong sign in some of the compounds. The mixing, however, with the $b_1 \rightarrow 3d_{yz}$ transition yielded the correct sign and order of magnitude for the rotational strengths of all four compounds. The resulting rotational strengths, calculated with the first order perturbed wavefunctions of the $b_1 \rightarrow b_2^*$ transition, are given in Table 4. The calculations support the assignment of the 240-nm band to the promotion $b_1 \rightarrow b_2^*$, and indicate that the optical activity of this band arises from a borrowing of electric dipole moment from a higher lying $b_1 \rightarrow 3d_{yz}$ transition.

Table 4

Calculated Rotational Strengths of the $b_1 \rightarrow b_2^*$ Transition[a]

Compound	R_{calc}	R_{exp}
I	−0·64	−4·0[b]
II	1·75	4·0[b]
III	−0·91	−0·7[c]
IV	1·23	1·8[d]

[a] Rotational strengths (R) in units of 10^{-40} c.g.s. [b] Reference 9. [c] Determined from CD spectra taken by R. Nagarajan, assuming Gaussian shape. [d] Determined from CD spectra taken by L. Verbit, assuming Gaussian shape.

C. The $b_1 \rightarrow a_1^*$ Transition and the $b_1 \rightarrow 3d$ Transition

The transition $b_1 \rightarrow a_1^*$ is our candidate for the band at 220 nm, which has an oscillator strength of 0·016. The oscillator strength of this transition was calculated with the molecular orbitals for the isolated chromophore, and the resulting value of 0·012 compares well with experiment. The two first-order mixings which could lead to optical activity are $b_1 \rightarrow 3d_{xz}$ and $b_2 \rightarrow a_1^*$. The calculation showed that the mixing of the $b_1 \rightarrow a_1^*$ and $b_2 \rightarrow a_1^*$ promotions were orders of magnitude too small to account for the observed rotational strengths. The $b_1 \rightarrow a_1^*$ and $b_1 \rightarrow 3d_{xz}$ mixing, although large enough in magnitude, did not lead to correctly signed rotational strengths in some of the compounds. Hence a more elaborate calculation was performed, in which the eight lone-pair promotions were mixed in a degenerate perturbation type of calculation. The resulting oscillator and rotational strengths for the perturbed $b_1 \rightarrow a_1^*$ promotion are shown in Table 5. The signs of R are correct, but the magnitudes are not especially good, particularly in the case of the five-membered ring compounds, I and II.

Table 5

Calculated Oscillator Strengths (f) and Rotational Strengths (R) of the $b_1 \rightarrow a_1^*$ and $b_1 \rightarrow 3d$ Transition[a]

Compound	$b_1 \rightarrow a_1^*$			$b_1 \rightarrow 3d$		
	f	R_{calc}	R_{exp}	f	R_{calc}	R_{exp}
I	0·012	0·02	4·0[b]	0·035	−0·14	−4·0[b]
II	0·017	−0·42	—[b, c]	0·033	0·46	4·0[b]
III	0·034	−0·82	−2·4[d]	0·074	1·51	1·9[d]
IV	0·008	0·39	1·3[e]	0·067	−1·20	−1·4[e]

[a] Rotational strengths in units of 10^{-40} c.g.s. [b] Reference 9. [c] The CD spectrum shows no band at 220 nm in this compound. [d] Determined from CD spectra taken by R. Nagarajan, assuming Gaussian shape. [e] Determined from CD spectra taken by L. Verbit, assuming Gaussian shape.

The promotion $b_1 \rightarrow 3d$ is the assignment we prefer for the 200 nm band with experimental oscillator strength 0·06. Our starting Wolfsberg–Helmholz 3d orbitals were nearly degenerate, and the degenerate perturbation type of calculation mentioned above served to order these levels, as well as to provide the mixings required for optical activity. Oscillator and rotational strengths are given in Table 5 for the lone pair promotion to the lowest 3d level. The particular linear combination of 3d AOs is dependent on the compound: for the five-membered ring sulphides I and II, the lowest 3d level is predominantly $3d_{x^2-y^2}$ and $3d_{z^2}$, while for the six-membered ring sulphides III and IV it is mainly $3d_{yz}$ and $3d_{x^2-y^2}$. The effective nuclear charge of the sulphur 3d orbital, Z_{3d}, was chosen to produce the agreement in oscillator strengths (the value chosen was $Z_{3d} = 1·5$). The rotational strengths have the correct sign in all compounds, and the magnitudes in the six-membered ring sulphides III and IV are good. However, as was the case for the $b_1 \rightarrow a_1^*$ transition, the magnitudes are low for the five-membered ring sulphides I and II.

It should be noted that we found that the precise magnitudes, and even some of the signs, of the rotational strengths of the three transitions were critically dependent on the exact values of the molecular orbital coefficients. In particular, the coefficients of the 3d AOs in the antibonding orbitals, b_2^* and a_1^*, were important. (A fuller discussion may be found in reference 19.) Thus, a strict quantitative accounting of the optical activity must await much more precise wave functions than those we have employed. Nevertheless, it does appear that one can account at least for the signs of the rotational strengths by considering only the mixing of states that arise from the non-bonding b_1 orbital.

2.2.5 Conclusion

The three lowest energy transitions in saturated dialkyl sulphides have been assigned on the basis of symmetry considerations, combined with an examination of the constraints provided by the optical absorption and optical activity data. The assignments arrived at are:

    (1) the very weak band at about 240 nm: the electric dipole forbidden, magnetic dipole allowed transition, $b_1(3p_z) \rightarrow b_2^*$;

(2) the band at about 220 nm: the electric dipole allowed $b_1(3p_z) \rightarrow a_1^*$ promotion;

(3) the band at 200 nm: the transition $b_1(3p_z) \rightarrow 3d$, where 3d is a linear combination of sulphur 3d orbitals. The particular linear combination may vary from compound to compound.

The proposed assignments are at variance in some instances with others previously offered. In particular, Thompson and coworkers[6] assigned the 240-nm band to the electric dipole forbidden transition $3p_z \rightarrow 3d_{xy}$ on sulphur, the 220-nm band to the transition $3p_z \rightarrow 3d$ (unspecified), and the 200-nm band to the $3p_z \rightarrow 4s$ promotion. We agree with the assignment of Clark and Simpson[7] as regards the 240-nm band. However, they assigned the 220-nm band to an intensity cancelling combination of the $b_1 \rightarrow b_2^*$ and $a_1 \rightarrow a_1^*$ promotions, and the 200-nm band to an intensity enhancing combination of the $b_2 \rightarrow a_1^*$ and $a_1 \rightarrow b_2^*$ promotion. However, our own assignments appear more compatible with the optical activity data than these alternative ones.

References

1. A. Moscowitz, *Proc. Roy. Soc. A* **297**, 16 (1967).
2. W. Moffitt, R. B. Woodward, A. Moscowitz, W. Klyne and C. Djerassi, *J. Amer. Chem. Soc.* **83**, 4013 (1961).
3. J. A. Schellman, *Accounts Chem. Res.* **1**, 144 (1968).
4. J. A. Schellman, *J. Chem. Phys.* **44**, 55 (1966).
5. H. L. McMurry and R. S. Mulliken, *Proc. Natl. Acad. Sci. U.S.A.* **26**, 312 (1940); H. L. McMurry *J. Chem. Phys.* **9**, 231 (1941).
6. S. D. Thompson, D. G. Carroll, F. Watson, M. O'Donnell, S. P. McGlynn, *J. Chem. Phys.* **45**, 1367 (1966).
7. L. B. Clark and W. T. Simpson, *J. Chem. Phys.* **43**, 3666 (1965).
8. C. W. N. Cumper, A. Melnikoff and A. I. Vogel, *J. Chem. Soc. A* 242 (1966).
9. P. Laur, H. Haüser, J. E. Gurst and K. Mislow, *J. Org. Chem.* **32(2)**, 498 (1967).
10. R. M. Dodson. Private communication.
11. P. Salvadori, *Chem. Commun.* 1203 (1968).
12. C. Djerassi, H. Wolf, D. A. Lightner, E. Bunnenberg, K. Takeda, T. Kumeno and K. Kuriyama, *Tetrahedron* **19**, 1547 (1963).
13. K. Kuriyama, T. Komeno and K. Takeda, *Tetrahedron* **22**, 1039 (1966).
14. A. Moscowitz, in I. Prigogine, Ed., *Advances in Chemical Physics*, Vol. IV. Interscience, New York, 1962, p. 67.
15. E. Gorin, J. Walter and H. Eyring, *J. Chem. Phys.* **6**, 824 (1938).
16. E. Gorin, W. Kauzmann and J. Walter, *J. Chem. Phys.* **7**, 327 (1939).
17. W. J. Kauzmann, J. E. Walter and H. Eyring, *Chem. Rev.* **26**, 339 (1940).
18. M. Wolfsberg and L. Helmholz, *J. Chem. Phys.* **20**, 837 (1952).
19. J. S. Rosenfield, Ph.D. Thesis, University of Minnesota, 1969; J. S. Rosenfield and A. Moscowitz, *J. Amer. Chem. Soc.* **94**, 4797 (1972).

Approaches to the Prediction of Cotton Effects: Organic Compounds

O. E. WEIGANG, Jr

Tulane University
New Orleans, U.S.A.

2.3.1 Introduction

One hopes, even expects, to find theoretical generalizations for predicting rotatory strengths (or Cotton effects) of molecular electronic transitions. Indeed, the approximate additivities and other regularities observed for a given transition in many different molecules seem to require that generalized models exist. We will define a number of such models and investigate their properties.

These models of course cannot replace more sophisticated and complete calculations, *ab initio* and otherwise. Indeed, applied indiscriminately, models can be misleading. On the other hand, one will find that models often give a basis for critical evaluation of more complete calculations.

For an overview, it is helpful to tabulate the different approaches available. Table 1 is mainly divided into nuclear equilibrium position (NEP) descriptions and nuclear motion (NM) descriptions of electronic transitions.

The NEP description is precisely the kind made in most quantum calculations of molecular electronic properties (e.g. state energies, molecular shape, transition

Table 1

Electronic Transition Cotton Effects

NUCLEAR EQUILIBRIUM POSITION (NEP) DESCRIPTIONS	NUCLEAR MOTON (NM) DESCRIPTIONS
Lowest-order Chromophore Inherently Dissymmetric	*Zeroth-Order (Q-independent Electronic Description)*
Dissymmetric Molecular Orbitals	NEP Description plus Franck–Condon Principle
Charge Transfer	*First, Second–, ..., nth Order (Q^n-dependent Electronic Description)*
. . . . .	
Lowest-order Chromophore Inherently Symmetric	Non-degenerate Electronic States—'Forbidden' Character
Static Coupling	Degenerate Electronic States—Dynamic Jahn–Teller Character
Dynamic Coupling	
. . . . .	

intensities). A repetition of the calculation at successive nuclear positions serves to trace out the classical energy well by which nuclei are constrained.

The NM description endows the nuclei with appreciable kinetic energies and yields the quantized levels which are often depicted as superposed on the classical potential well. Electronic spectra arise from transitions between such a level in the ground state and one in an excited state.

In many instances the NEP description is the electronic description incorporated in a more general NM zeroth-order treatment. In the so-called Case I,[1] this treatment is adequate for the ordinary absorption as well as the circular dichroism. We will return later to consideration of exceptions where the electronic description requires added terms for nuclear displacement yielding Cases II and III.[1-3]

The NEP descriptions have been meaningfully classified by Moscowitz[4-6] as those for inherently dissymmetric chromophores and those for inherently symmetric chromophores with dissymmetric environments. Most of the NEP models we discuss here will be concerned with the latter. Inherently symmetric will mean here that the lowest order (in these cases, zeroth-order) chromophores are symmetric.

2.3.2 Static Coupling

The first NEP model to be considered generates a transition rotatory strength by mixing in higher frequency transitions of the chromophore.[7-13] One usually accounts for this by inducing an admixture of two (or more) molecular orbitals. One is the molecular orbital to which the electron is promoted, another is a chromophore orbital which is mixed in under the influence of an environment that produces a dissymmetric static electric field. Crystal field theory has a similar approach.[10]

A model for such optical activity has a transition rotatory strength:[11]

$$R_{om} = \underbrace{\sum_k f(x, y, z)\, \varepsilon}_{\substack{\text{varies as} \\ \text{'repulsive'} \\ \text{or 'attractive'}}} \quad \underbrace{\theta^{xy}_{km}\, \boldsymbol{\mu}^z_{ok} \cdot i\boldsymbol{m}^z_{om}}_{\substack{\text{invariant for} \\ \text{a given } k}} \qquad [1]$$

for a symmetric chromophore whose transition $m \leftarrow o$ is electric dipole forbidden and magnetic dipole allowed ($m^z_{mo} \neq 0$). There is the familiar scalar product of electric and magnetic dipole transition vectors (bold face) with additional terms that represent the mix-inducing coupling of an electric quadrupole (θ^{xy}) with a dissymmetrically placed charge (ε).

This can be visualized (Fig. 1) for a transition upper state m resulting from an $n \rightarrow \pi^*$ orbital electron promotion in a ketone. The mixing is predominantly with a state k resulting from the $\pi \rightarrow \pi^*$ orbital promotion. Then the transition moments reduce to the molecular orbital matrix elements $\theta^{xy}_{n\pi}$, $\mu^z_{\pi\pi^*}$ and $m^z_{\pi^*n}$. If one knows enough about $\theta_{n\pi}$, the variation in sign and magnitude of the transition rotatory strength accompanying the $n \rightarrow \pi^*$ electron promotion can be deduced intuitively. The static charge ε interacting with the electric quadrupole $\theta_{n\pi}$ represents an attractive or repulsive configuration and determines the rotatory strength sign and magnitude.

To deduce the nature of the matrix element $\theta_{n\pi}^{xy}$ it is necessary to consider a 'transition charge density'. The 'transition charge density' is given by picking a point in space and determining the signed product of the two molecular orbital values for that point. The signs and magnitudes so obtained give a 'transition charge distribution'.

It should be clear from Fig. 1 that two p orbitals representing the main contributors from the n and π molecular orbitals would give the quadrupolar 'charge distribution' depicted on the right. That $\theta_{n\pi}$ must be the xy component of the quadrupole tensor could be anticipated for equation [1] by general group theory arguments.[10, 11]

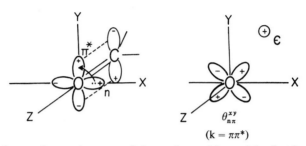

Fig. 1. The ketone chromophore n → π^* electronic transition and the electric quadrupole $\theta_{n\pi}^{xy}$. The quadrupole and the signed charge ε yield a sector rule for rotatory strength. It has been assumed the state k = $\pi\pi^*$ is mixed into the state m = $n\pi^*$ by the dissymmetrically placed charge.

In a similar way one can evaluate the 'transition charge density' given by the product of the complete two-centre π orbital with the two-centre π^* orbital. Taking the product values for one point in space at a time clearly generates a dipolar distribution of 'charge' with Z polarization. This is the electric dipole $\mu_{\pi\pi^*}^z$ mixed in to produce rotatory strength according to equation [1].

The magnetic dipole matrix element

$$m_{\pi^* n}^z = \frac{e}{2mc} (\pi^*|1_z|n)$$

can be appreciated by observing that

$$1_z|p_x) = i\hbar|p_y$$

The principal contributor to the matrix element becomes equivalent to a simple overlap integral, the net 'charge' of a 'product distribution' from two p_y orbitals on the oxygen. Taken altogether it can be verified that the sign for $i\theta_{km}^{xy}\mu_{ok}^z m_{mo}^z$ is real and invariant under any rephasing of the atomic orbitals. This confirms that the model has the necessary 'observable' properties for R_{om}. The sign of the geometrical factor $f(X, Y, Z)$ (X, Y, Z are the coordinates of the point charge) varies with the position in space such as to indicate the attractive or repulsive configuration of the signed static charge and the quadrupole. The result is a quadrant rule of ketone optical activity (cf. references 10 and 12).

One can alternatively consider the mixed-in state k to be the result of an n → d orbital electron promotion,[8, 12] a somewhat more complex case shown in Fig. 2. This calls for assessment of the 'transition charge distribution' of a molecular orbital

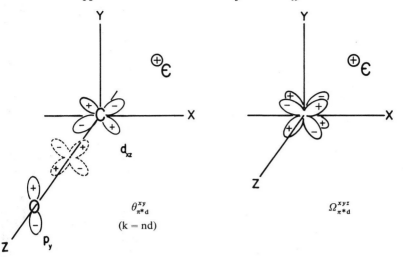

Fig. 2. Components of electric quadrupole $\theta_{\pi^*d}^{xy}$ (broken lines) and octupole $\Omega_{\pi^*d}^{xyz}$. The interaction of charge ε and the multipole components contribute to a ketone rotatory strength. The state m = nπ^* is mixed with a state k = nd.

product π^*d. A quadrupolar component of 'transition charge density' results from the product of a p_y orbital on one atom with a d_{xz} orbital on the other ketone chromophore atom. There are also octupolar (Ω^{xyz}) components of 'transition charge density' resulting from the product of these two atomic orbitals on the same centre.

The first component contributes quadrant rule behaviour, the second component, will additionally contribute octant rule behaviour. The relative magnitude of these two contributions will vary in a complex way depending on distance and orientation of the point charge from the various multipole centres. In a computational sense, the relative magnitudes will also vary with the consideration of overlap between chromophore atomic orbitals.

A difficulty with the static coupling model lies in summing properly over the contributions of all possible k states. Here one may introduce empirical observations on the effects charges have on ketone rotatory strength. These may be due to protonation, ionization, or introduction of static dipoles.

Some examples[14-16] are shown in Figs. 3 and 4. The data in parentheses are $\Delta\varepsilon$

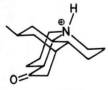

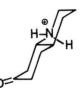

($\Delta\varepsilon_{289} = +4\cdot39$)   ($\Delta\varepsilon_{290} \approx -1\cdot02$)   ($\Delta\varepsilon_{288} = +0\cdot01$)

$\Delta\varepsilon_{285} = -0\cdot6$ $\Delta\varepsilon = -1\cdot26$ $\Delta\varepsilon_{294} = -0\cdot44$

Fig. 3. The values of $\Delta\varepsilon_{max}$ for free base (in parentheses) and protonated alkaloids. [From Ayer *et al.*[14] and Johnson *et al.*[15]]

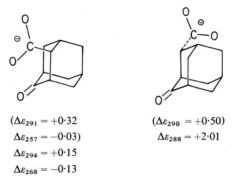

$$(\Delta\varepsilon_{291} = +0\cdot32 \qquad (\Delta\varepsilon_{290} = +0\cdot50)$$
$$\Delta\varepsilon_{257} = -0\cdot03) \qquad \Delta\varepsilon_{288} = +2\cdot01$$
$$\Delta\varepsilon_{294} = +0\cdot15$$
$$\Delta\varepsilon_{268} = -0\cdot13$$

Fig. 4. The values of $\Delta\varepsilon_{max}$ for free carboxylic acid (in parentheses) and carboxylate ion derivatives of adamantanone. [From Snatzke and Eckhardt.[16]]

values for the neutral species. Figure 3 shows in each case that the sign of the proton contribution is opposite to that for the ketone octant rule.[14] Figure 4 shows similar contributions for introduction of a proton. Such results raise serious questions as to the adequacy of incomplete-screening-of-nuclei perturbations used as bases for the ketone octant rule.

2.3.3 Dynamic Coupling

Another NEP model derives rotatory strength from mixing into the chromophore transition higher energy dipole transitions of a polarizable environment.[9, 11, 17, 18] When the symmetric chromophore transition is electric dipole forbidden and magnetic dipole allowed, such a model of rotatory strength gives the expression:[11]

$$R_{om} = \sum_{1} f(X,Y,Z)\,\underbrace{\mu^z_{o1}\,\mu^z_{o1}\,\theta^{xy}_{om}}_{\text{Varies to be 'attractive'}} \cdot \underbrace{im^z_{mo}}_{\text{Invariant}}$$

[2]

Again a scalar product of electric and magnetic dipole transition vectors (bold face) is evident.

In Fig. 5 it is assumed that state m results from a ketone chromophore $n \to \pi^*$ orbital promotion. The sum over perturber states l are absorbed in a polarizability. Then the $m \leftarrow o$ transition rotatory strength varies in sign and magnitude according to a dipole–quadrupole coupling. The dipole of the polarizable system dissymmetrically positioned about the quadrupole θ^{xy}_{om} is always induced in a sense that is 'attractive'. That is to say, the sign of the geometry factor $f(X, Y, Z)$ in equation [2] varies with position in space so as to correspond to μ^z_{o1} polarized in a sense attractive to $\theta^{xy}_{n\pi*}$. The scalar product of this dipole with $m^z_{mo}(= m^z_{\pi*n})$ results in an octant rule. It should be evident from our previous remarks that a rephasing of chromophore atomic orbitals can reverse the sense of polarization of μ^z_{o1} that is 'attractive'. But the polarization of $m^z_{\pi*n}$ will also be reversed maintaining the necessary invariance for the observable R_{om}.

The sign of $i\theta_{n\pi*}^{xy} \cdot m_{\pi*n}^{z}$ determines the absolute signs of the octant rule for this model. Assuming also that the state m has energy lower than all of the electronic states l of the environment, one finds that the signs predicted agree with the empirical ketone octant rule.

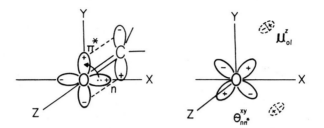

Fig. 5. The ketone chromophore n → π* electronic transition and its electric quadrupole $\theta_{n\pi*}^{xy}$. The interaction of the quadrupole and the dipole m_{ol}^{z} induced in a polarizable perturber contribute to a ketone rotatory strength. The perturber is shown in 2 position behind the *XY* plane.

Anticipating some consideration of lactone and lactam optical activity, we may use the long wavelength electronic transitions expected for a carboxylate ion chromophore as a further example. Two types of excited states resulting from n → π* orbital electron promotion are possible. In one the n orbital largely involves an antibonding pairing of oxygen p orbitals; in the other the pairing is bonding (Fig. 6). The π* orbital is the same for the two cases. These are shown in Fig. 6 as appropriate respectively to lactams and lactones when there is a subsequent substitution or modification of the carboxylate ion chromophore.

CARBOXYLATE ION

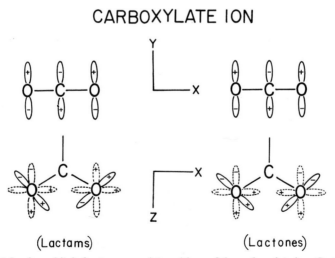

Fig. 6. Molecular orbitals for two n → π* transitions of the carboxylate ion. On the left are those assigned to the long-wavelength absorption when substitution yields a lactam, on the right when addition yields a lactone. Dotted-line orbitals are resolved components of the full-line orbital. [Ong, Cusachs and Weigang, in preparation.]

Though not generally the case, the magnetic transition dipole m_{mo} and electric quadrupole θ_{om} in this instance are each largely sums of two one-centre terms. It is further helpful to resolve the oxygen p orbitals into X and Z components with additive matrix elements. The methods outlined for evaluating matrix elements then show that the lactam transition will have a Z-polarized magnetic transition dipole and an XY component of quadrupole moment. The result is an octant rule with regular ketone octant rule signs (viewing the group in the negative Z direction with o-c-o in a horizontal XZ plane).

On the other hand, the transition specified for lactones has an X-polarized magnetic transition dipole, a YZ component of quadrupole moment, and an octant rule that has regular signs viewing down the X-axis, but therefore anti-octant viewing down the Z-axis. While the non-vanishing components of matrix elements can be deduced from group theory arguments, the sign of the matrix elements cannot be. Somewhat more detailed features of the molecular orbitals are required. This difference in lactam and lactone circular dichroism signs is actually observed.[19] Some detailed molecular orbital calculations indicate trends in molecular orbital energies on substitution that would justify these respective assignments for the long wavelength absorptions of lactams and lactones.[20]

2.3.4 Anisotropy Effects

The models we have considered generate sector rules. These are rules for predicting rotatory strength which require only the point of location of a dissymmetrically

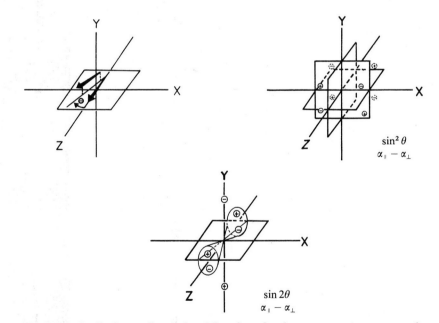

Fig. 7. Dipole–dipole coupling and nodal surfaces for the two-term rotatory strength. The trigonometric functions and polarizability anisotropy are additional factors that control the sign of rotatory strength. The signs shown are for perturber anisotropy $(\alpha_\parallel - \alpha_\perp) > 0$ and, for the conical surfaces, $0 < \theta < \pi/2$. [From Höhn and Weigang.[11]]

placed part of the chromophore environment. It appears that most attempts to develop rules on an empirical basis have been cast in such a form.[21]

A different kind of rule for rotatory strength calls for information about orientation relative to the chromophore of an anisotropic perturber. A rule of this kind develops from theory if the transition is electric dipole-allowed and couples with a dissymmetrically placed polarizable part of the environment. The coupling will then be at the dipole–dipole level. The rotatory strength is the sum of two contributions depicted by the nodal surfaces shown in Fig. 7.[11]

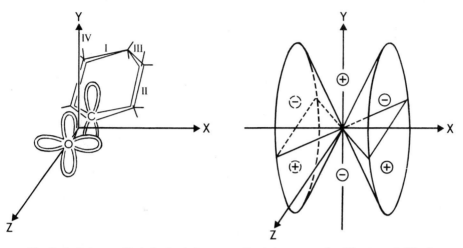

Fig. 8. Anisotropy effects in the ketone $n - \pi^*$ rotatory strengths. The types I–IV of perturber bonds in idealized cyclohexanone geometry are shown. The conical nodal surface is for bond type I with the factor $(\alpha_{\parallel} - \alpha_{\perp}) > 0$. For bond type III, the signs are reversed. For bond type II, the surfaces are rotated clockwise, for IV counter-clockwise by $\pi/2$ about the Z-axis.

It is always possible to orient a pair of dipoles, one at the coordinate origin along the Z axis, so that the second dipole is parallel to the XZ plane. The sector rule concept must be amended by two considerations. Firstly, the sign of anisotropy of polarizability, $\alpha_{\parallel} - \alpha_{\perp}$, may be positive or negative. Secondly, rotatory strength depends on the angle θ depicted in Fig. 7. The rule thus depends on a more detailed description of the dissymmetry than mere statement of perturber position.

The cone-shaped nodal surface defines a behaviour of rotatory strength which depends on the helicity of two dipoles, the one of the transition moment, the other along the axis of revolution (which defines $\alpha_{\parallel}$) of an ellipsoid of polarizability. With the angular dependence on $\sin 2\theta$, the phasing of the dipoles is irrelevant. The other set of nodal surfaces is made up of the familiar octant planes. Since the latter angular dependence here is on $\sin^2 \theta$, the behaviour appears to be much like a sector rule. However, one must remember the required orientation (parallel to the XZ plane) of the polarizability axis of the perturber. A varying dominance of these two types of contribution might accommodate the two kinds of rotatory strength rules for ethylene chromophores that have emerged in the literature.[22-25]

Anisotropy effects can also be expected for the electric-dipole-forbidden, quadrupole-allowed chromophore transitions considered above (Fig. 5). The electric dipole induced in an anisotropic perturber will not always be parallel to the chromophore magnetic dipole. This produces dynamic coupling contributions to rotatory strength in addition to those represented by equation [2]. Figure 8 shows the conical nodal surfaces for that kind of contribution.[11] It should be noted that the sign of the contribution depends on the orientation of the perturber polarizability ellipsoid as well as the sign of its anisotropy (i.e. whether the ellipsoid is oblate or prolate).

Hudec has collected circular dichroism data where nitrogen perturbs the ketone chromophore.[26] The $\Delta\varepsilon$ values show a strong dependence on the orientation of the lone-pair electrons relative to the ketone chromophore. In Fig. 9 these orientations are classified as if the lone pair defined a perturbing bond direction.

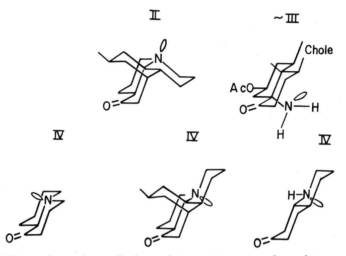

Fig. 9. Nitrogen lone-pair contributions to ketone rotatory strength as anisotropy effects. Roman numerals relate lone-pair orientations to bond types depicted in Fig. 8. [From Hudec.[26]]

The lower line of molecules all show a similar negative contribution to $\Delta\varepsilon$. The static dipole can be excluded as a cause since it is reversed, without reverse effect, between the first and second molecule of the line. On the other hand, a reversed (positive) contribution is observed for the first compound in the first line. This is as expected from anisotropy effects.

2.3.5 Degenerate Coupled Oscillators

The electron correlations which dynamic coupling represents become more pronounced as the virtual transition energies of the polarizable environment become more nearly equal to the transition energy of the chromophore. Whenever there is a degeneracy with the two transitions equal in energy (or at least very nearly so), the theory takes on a form not greatly different from the above.

Examples of this theory, involving the triple scalar product of transition moments and position vectors, are found in the rotatory strength rules associated with ring-substituted paracyclophanes (Fig. 10)[27-29] and dibenzoates.[30] The paracyclophanes afford an opportunity to observe the effects of rotating the transition moment of the substituted ring. Platt's theory of additive vector spectroscopic moments for substituted benzene transition dipoles can account for the turning as shown in Fig. 10. Thus, for the absolute configuration depicted, the theory predicts that a substituent with a positive spectroscopic moment will give a negative rotatory strength for the long-wavelength rotatory strength (the *negative* signs are applicable in the

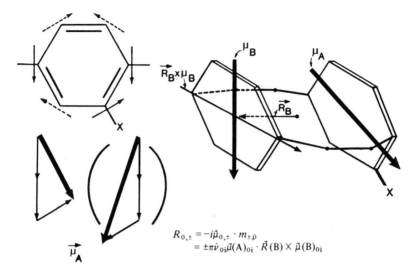

$$R_{0,\pm} = -i\vec{\mu}_{0,\pm} \cdot m_{\pm\rho}$$
$$= \pm\pi\bar{\nu}_{oi}\vec{\mu}(A)_{oi} \cdot \vec{R}(B) \times \vec{\mu}(B)_{oi}$$

Fig. 10. Vector constructions relating ring-substituted paracyclophane absolute configuration to rotatory strength. Substituent spectroscopic moments are shown on the left. They contribute to a benzene long-wavelength transition dipole moment $\vec{\mu}_A$ in a fashion that depends on location of the substituent (full arrows) and the magnitude and sign given to the spectroscopic moment. The net transition vector $\vec{\mu}_A$ is given for a positive (negative) substituent spectroscopic moment. The vector cross product on the right is then projected on $\vec{\mu}_A$ to yield rotatory strengths of a dimer transition couplet. The negative sign refers to the long-wavelength component. [From Weigang and Nugent.[27]]

equation). The work of Nugent *et al.*[28] and Falk *et al.*[30] summarized in Table 2 shows a large number of circular dichroisms that confirms this kind of electron correlation theory.

2.3.6 Low-symmetry Models

To this point our NEP descriptions of electronic transition rotatory strength have considered separately the static coupling (crystal field, one electron) mechanism and the dynamic coupling (electron correlation, coupled oscillator) mechanism. However, both of these models show that the noding of sector rules depends on the symmetry of the chromophore. The lower the symmetry of the chromophores, the less informative are the predictive rules that develop.

Double perturbation techniques can be used to follow the modification of a sector rule originally applying to a higher symmetry 'parent' chromophore. What results is a

O. E. Weigang, Jr

rather specific form of distortion of sector surfaces. The symmetry lowering of the chromophore is induced by a static coupling perturbation that induces no activity while the dissymmetric environment gives a dynamic coupling perturbation that

Table 2

Circular Dichroisms of Ring-Substituted Paracyclophanes

Paracyclophane ring substituent	Substituent spectroscopic moment	Sign of first CD band	$\Delta\varepsilon_{max}$
NH_2[a,b]	+38·4	−	−5·5
NHAc		−	−2·5
F	+20		
Cl[b]	+9·6	−	−1·0
Br[b]	+9·6		
C_2H_5	+7·2	−	−0·5
$(CH_2)_3CH_3$		−	−0·5
$(CH_2)_3CO_2H$		−	−0·5
$(CH_2)_4OH$		−	−0·5
CH_3[b]	+7	−	−0·8
CH_2OH[b]	−7	+	+0·8
CH_2Br[b]	−12	+	+2·1
C≡N	−17·6	+	+5·0
$COOCH_3$	−27·2	+	+4·0
$CONH_2$		+	+4·0
CON_3		+	+3·0
COOH[b]	−28	+	+5·0
CHO	−32		
$COCH_3$		+	+3·0
COC_3H_7		+	+5·5
$CO(CH_2)_2CO_2H$		+	+5·5

[a] Ref. 29. [b] Ref. 28.

produces the activity. Starting from the carboxylate ion description given above, 'substitution' to produce a lactam should give a distortion of the *YZ* nodal surface as shown in Fig. 11. A specification of the degree of such distortion probably must be obtained from empirical observations. But the direction of distortion can be predicted theoretically. The *XZ* and *XY* nodal surfaces remain planar in this model for isotropic perturbers.

Such a model recognizes that the electronic symmetry of a chromophore may be effectively higher than the nuclear symmetry. As the symmetry-lowering perturbation increases, the curved surface collapses in on itself to become a line in the −*X* direction. This limiting condition is a quadrant rule as might be expected considering the chromophore nuclear symmetry.

These techniques have been used with some success for the study of lactams.[19, 20] Some features of lactone optical activity are rationalized as well, but other problems are encountered. Perhaps such techniques can be useful for many more low-symmetry chromophores rigidly oriented with respect to their dissymmetric surroundings.

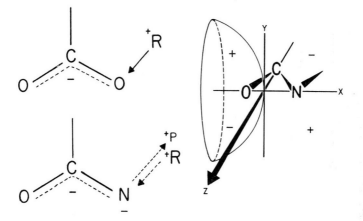

Fig. 11. A 'lowered-symmetry' sector rule for the lactam chromophore n → π* long-wavelength transition. The curved surface is a spherical distortion of the YZ surface of octant rule nodal planes. Other nodal surfaces remain planar. The signs refer to the back 'octants' and are those deduced from Fig. 6. [Ong, Cusachs and Weigang.[20]]

2.3.7 Inherently Dissymmetric Chromophores

The helicenes have been the subject of extensive experimental and theoretical investigation for their optical activity.[31-34] Few determinations of absolute configuration are available. Nevertheless, there has emerged so far one generalization[34] consistent with some theories of assignment in polynuclear aromatics and free-electron views on rotatory strength.

From a sizable body of experimental data, it appears that the absolute configuration of a helicene might be simply related to the rotatory strength sign of Clar's β band (^1B_b for hexahelicene[31, 33] in Platt's convention). A positive sign is associated with a right-handed helix. Platt's scheme characterizes this transition polarization as simple dipolar along the helix. Simple free-electron-on-a-helix models give positive rotatory strength for such simple dipolar transition polarizations on a right-handed helix.[35]

One should note that careful attention to the assignment of transitions is necessary as well as careful determination of rotatory strength sign. The reported determinations on hexahelicene have contradictory conclusions[31, 32].

2.3.8 Nuclear Motion Descriptions

In nuclear motion (NM) descriptions, an important property arises at the theoretical step where nuclear kinetic energy is introduced. The property is that, for levels higher than the zero-point level, the probability distribution favours the nuclei being found toward the extrema of a vibrational mode.[36] It is not surprising then that optical activity of transitions to such levels can be entirely different in sign and magnitude from the optical activity for transitions between zero-point levels.[2, 3] This is especially apparent if the vibrational mode in question is non-totally symmetric, thus in an extremum lowering the symmetry of the molecule or chromophore. The probability

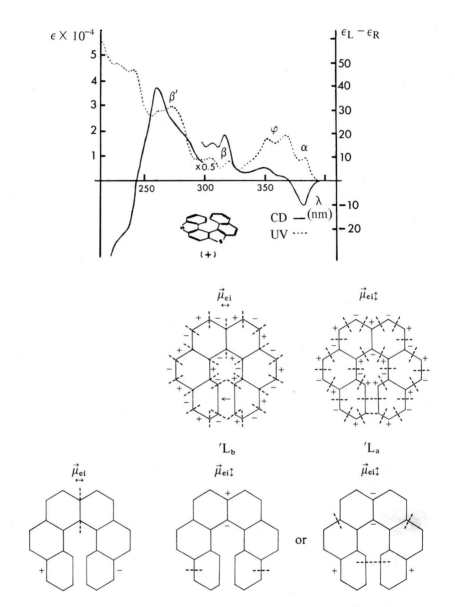

Fig. 12. The circular dichroism of a dithioheterohexahelicene. The Platt polarizations of hexahelicene are given showing the $^1B_b(\beta) \leftarrow {}^1A$ transition as simple dipolar along the helix. [From Groen and Wynberg,[34] and Weigang and Dodson.[33]]

distribution for a zero-point level, on the other hand, favours the nuclear equilibrium position.

The effect on transitions of vibrational modes participating in this manner depends on how sensitive the electronic symmetry is to nuclear symmetry-lowering. As recognized for low symmetry models, the electronic symmetry may remain effectively unchanged and produce 'allowed character' rotatory strength. To the extent the electronic symmetry is lowered, 'forbidden character' rotatory strength results.

The importance of such 'forbidden' intensity depends on its ability to compete with the NEP 'allowed' intensity. The fraction of total intensity from each intensity source will generally differ between the ordinary absorption and the circular dichroism modes of observation and so defines the limiting Case II or Case III.

Gaussian descriptions of circular dichroism bands[1, 4] can be extended to accommodate these vibronically coupled 'forbidden' components.[3] The mean frequency for example of a set of such Gaussian components, each with their own mean frequencies $\overline{\omega}_A^0$ or $\overline{\omega}_{F(\tau)}^0$ will be given by:[3]

$$\overline{\omega}_K^0 = g_A \overline{\omega}_A^0 + \sum_{\tau} g_{F(\tau)} \overline{\omega}_{F(\tau)}^0 \qquad [3]$$

where the corresponding fractions of total rotatory strength are g_A and $g_{F(\tau)}$. There is a similar expression for the ordinary absorption:[3]

$$\overline{\omega}_K = f_A \overline{\omega}_A + \sum_{\tau} f_{F(\tau)} \overline{\omega}_{F(\tau)} \qquad [4]$$

The various mean frequencies (and band widths as well) can be related to constants of the classical potential wells and changes in molecular equilibrium size or shape on electronic excitation.

Gross differences in the total band shapes of a circular dichroism and its corresponding ordinary absorption can be due to values of $f_{F(\tau)}$ that differ markedly from values of $g_{F(\tau)}$ for the same coupled τ mode. Indeed, the limiting Cases I–III, illustrations of the relation of ordinary absorption band contours to the corresponding circular dichroism band contours, can be defined through such weighting parameters.

Case I corresponds to $f_A = g_A = 1$. There is an exact correspondence in shape and position of the circular dichroism and ordinary absorption bands. Case III corresponds to both $f_{F(\tau)} \neq 0$ and $g_{F(\tau)} \neq 0$ for at least one τ mode. In a practical sense, Case III requires both $f_{F(\tau)}$ and $g_{F(\tau)}$ to have detectable magnitudes. Case II then corresponds to a limit of

$$\sum_{\tau} f_{F(\tau)} \approx 1$$

and $g_{F(\tau)} \approx 0$ for all τ modes within detectable degrees.

Significant differences of shape in circular dichroism from that in ordinary absorption for a given τ component can also contribute to total band-shape differences. These shape differences largely relate to coupling between the electronic description and the change in molecular equilibrium size or shape on electronic excitation.[3, 37]

It has been generalized that whenever a transition is strongly magnetic dipole allowed and electric dipole forbidden except for a dissymmetric molecular field, the fraction of forbidden character in the ordinary absorption will be significantly larger than the fraction of forbidden character in circular dichroism, i.e. that Case II is approached.[1] Nevertheless the projection of electric transition dipole induced by a dissymmetric environment on a large chromophore transition magnetic dipole may be small accidentally, i.e. not by symmetry. In one instance among others of interest which can be defined,[38] a molecular system may have a nearly symmetric electronic description in its equilibrium position. Dissymmetric modes of vibration from the chiral nuclear framework then create predominantly forbidden character circular dichroism.[38, 39]

The role of such vibronic coupling has been well documented for ordinary absorption. In the case of optical activity, studies have proceeded little beyond speculation (see also references 40–42). It is important, however, that definitive studies be carried out so that a firm basis for formulating theoretical expressions of sector rules can be established.

References

1. W. Moffitt and A. Moscowitz, *J. Chem. Phys.* **30**, 648 (1959).
2. O. E. Weigang, Jr, *J. Chem. Phys.* **43**, 3609 (1965).
3. S. E. Harnung, E. C. Ong and O. E. Weigang, Jr, *J. Chem. Phys.* **55**, 5711 (1971).
4. A. Moscowitz, in C. Djerassi, Ed., *Optical Rotary Dispersion: Applications to Organic Chemistry*. McGraw-Hill, New York, 1960, Chapter 12.
5. A. Moscowitz, *Tetrahedron* **13**, 48 (1961).
6. C. W. Deutsche, D. A. Lightner, R. W. Woody and A. Moscowitz, *Ann. Rev. Phys. Chem.* **20**, 436 (1969).
7. W. Kauzmann, J. Walter and H. Eyring, *Chem. Rev.* **26**, 339 (1940).
8. A. Moscowitz, *Advan. Chem. Phys.* **4**, 67 (1962).
9. I. Tinoco, Jr, *Advan. Chem. Phys.* **4**, 113 (1962).
10. J. A. Schellman, *J. Chem. Phys.* **44**, 55 (1966).
11. E. G. Höhn and O. E. Weigang, Jr, *J. Chem. Phys.* **48**, 1127 (1968).
12. T. D. Bouman and A. Moscowitz, *J. Chem. Phys.* **48**, 3115 (1968).
13. J. A. Schellman, *Accounts Chem. Res.* **1**, 144 (1968).
14. W. A. Ayer, B. Altenkirk, R. H. Burnell and M. Moinas, *Can. J. Chem.* **47**, 449 (1969).
15. R. A. Johnson, H. C. Murray, L. M. Reinecke and G. S. Fonken, *J. Org. Chem.* **33**, 3207 (1968).
16. G. Snatzke and G. Eckhardt, *Tetrahedron* **24**, 4543 (1968).
17. J. G. Kirkwood, *J. Chem. Phys.* **5**, 479 (1937).
18. M. P. Kruchek, *Opt. Spectrosc.* **17**, 294 (1964).
19. W. Klyne and P. M. Scopes. Private communication.
20. E. C. Ong, L. C. Cusachs and O. E. Weigang, Jr. In preparation.
21. See, for example, G. Snatzke, *et al.*, Section 3 of this book.
22. A. I. Scott and A. D. Wrixon, *Chem. Commun.* 1182, 1184 (1969).
23. M. Fetizon and I. Hanna, *Chem. Commun.* 462 (1970); 545 (1971).
24. A. Yogev and Y. Mazur, *Chem. Commun.* 552 (1965).
25. A. W. Burgstahler and R. C. Barkhurst, *J. Amer. Chem. Soc.* **92**, 7601 (1970).
26. J. Hudec, *Chem. Commun.* 829 (1970).
27. O. E. Weigang, Jr, and M. J. Nugent, *J. Amer. Chem. Soc.* **91**, 4555 (1969).
28. M. J. Nugent and O. E. Weigang, Jr, *J. Amer. Chem. Soc.* **91**, 4556 (1969); M. J. Nugent, A. Guest, P. Hoffman, W. Hocking. In preparation.
29. H. Falk, P. Reich-Rohrwig and K. Schloegel, *Tetrahedron* **26**, 511 (1969).
30. N. Harada and K. Nakanishi, *J. Amer. Chem. Soc.* **91**, 3989 (1969).
31. O. E. Weigang, Jr, J. A. Turner and P. A. Trouard, *J. Chem. Phys.* **45**, 1126 (1966).
32. S. F. Mason, W. S. Brickell, A. Brown and C. M. Kemp, *J. Chem. Soc. A.* 756 (1971).
33. O. E. Weigang, Jr, and P. T. Dodson, *J. Chem. Phys.* **49**, 4248 (1968).
34. M. B. Groen and H. Wynberg, *J. Amer. Chem. Soc.* **93**, 2968 (1971).
35. I. Tinoco and R. W. Woody, *J. Chem. Phys.* **40**, 160 (1964).

36. L. Pauling and E. B. Wilson, Jr, *Introduction to Quantum Mechanics*. McGraw-Hill, New York, 1935.
37. D. P. Craig and G. J. Small, *J. Chem. Phys.* **50**, 3827 (1969).
38. O. E. Weigang, Jr, *Abstracts, National Academy of Sciences Meeting*. Ann Arbor, October 1967.
39. R. T. Klingbiel and H. Eyring, *J. Phys. Chem.* **74**, 4543 (1970).
40. D. J. Caldwell, *J. Chem. Phys.* **51**, 984 (1969).
41. S. H. Lin, *J. Chem. Phys.* **54**, 1177 (1970).
42. See however: J. Horwitz, E. H. Strikland and C. J. Billups, *J. Amer. Chem. Soc.* **91**, 184 (1969).

Calculation of Circular Dichroism and Optical Rotatory Dispersion of Polymers

I. TINOCO, Jr

Department of Chemistry
University of California
Berkeley, California 94720, U.S.A.

2.4.1 Introduction

The main reason for measuring the circular dichroism or optical rotatory dispersion of a polymer is to learn about its conformation. What is the relative orientation of one monomer to the next? If the relative orientation is the same for each monomer unit, a linear polymer forms a helix (or a straight line, which is a special case of a helix). If the relative orientation is not constant, the polymer is usually characterized as a random coil. It should be obvious that most real polymers have structures in between these two extremes. The helix may have imperfections and the 'random coil' may have short helical regions. In fact the random coil could be thought of as just a combination of short helical regions. The shortest helical region would consist of only two monomers. A protein is then just a polypeptide with each residue in some helix geometry characterized by the angles it makes with its neighbours. In nucleic acids we have the additional structural feature of multistranded helices.

The optical properties of a polymer will depend on its conformation. The absorption can change slightly (10–30%) with change in conformation, but the CD and ORD can change by orders of magnitude. However, all these optical properties are sensitive mainly to local conformation. They will characterize the relative orientation of neighbouring monomers. In the succeeding sections we shall discuss in detail the information which can be obtained from CD and ORD. Simple empirical methods and more tedious theoretical methods will be described.

2.4.2 Empirical Methods

The easiest way to calculate the optical properties of a polymer is to use the measured properties of its monomers and oligomers. For any molecule a measured property can be thought of as a sum of sub-unit properties, plus interactions. Consider the very simple example shown in Fig. 1. The ORD per mole of monomer is given for the dinucleoside phosphate adenylyl-(3'-5')-adenosine, ApA, and is compared with the ORD of the monomer. We can write the measured ORD at each wavelength as

$$2[\text{ApA}] \equiv [\text{Ap}] + [\text{A}] + I_{\text{ApA}} \qquad [1]$$

The symbols [ApA], [Ap], etc. represent the measured rotation per mole of monomer at any wavelength. The interaction term I_{ApA} is defined by this equation; if its value is generally large it indicates that there is large interaction between the monomer units. From Fig. 1 we see that this is indeed true for the adenines in ApA at pH 7 in water. Heating the solution decreases the ORD of ApA much more than that of the monomers; the effect is reversible. This tells us that the interaction is fairly weak, but it is not due to hydrophobic interactions which would increase at higher temperatures. In fact the enthalpy of interaction has been estimated to be about 7 kcal from

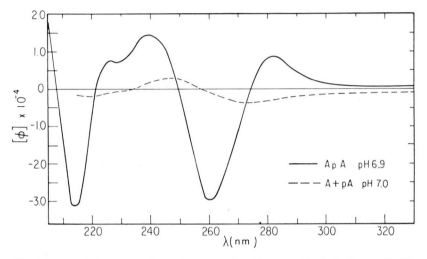

Fig. 1. The optical rotatory dispersion per mole of base at pH 7 of adenylyl-(3′-5′)-adenosine compared with the sum of its monomers: adenosine and 5′-adenylic acid. [Data from Warshaw and Tinoco, *J. Mol. Biol.* **13**, 54 (1965).]

the temperature dependence of the ORD.[1] Adding alcohol or lowering the pH also decreases the interaction. In uridylyl-(3′-5′)-uridine the interaction is much less, as illustrated in Fig. 2.

We have thus learned about the conformations of dimers and how they change with temperature, solvent and pH simply by comparing their ORD with that of the monomers.

What about the dependence of the interaction on distance? We can answer that question empirically by comparing trimers with dimers.

$$3[ApGpU] \equiv 2[ApG] + 2[GpU] - [Gp] + I_{ApGpU} \qquad [2]$$

A next nearest-neighbour interaction term is defined by this equation. Figure 3 shows a comparison between measured ORD for some trinucleoside diphosphates and the right-hand side of equation [2] with I set equal to zero. One sees from the good agreement that next nearest-neighbour interactions are small in these trimers,[2] although this is not true for all trimers.[3] For ApUpG, for example, the interaction (as measured by ORD) between the adenine and guanine is quite large.

Another test of longer range interactions is provided by homopolymers. If one sets all interactions except those of nearest neighbours equal to zero, a simple equation results.

$$[\text{poly X}] = 2[\text{XpX}] - [\text{X}] \qquad [3]$$

Figure 4 shows this comparison[4] for polyadenylic acid, polycytidylic acid and polyuridylic acid. The differences in the curves are a measure of all non-nearest-neighbour interactions.

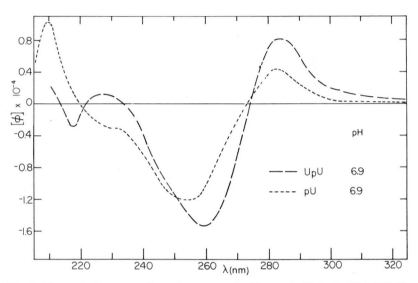

Fig. 2. The optical rotatory dispersion per mole of base at pH 7 of uridylyl-(3′-5′)-uridine compared with 5′-uridylic acid. [Data from Warshaw and Tinoco, *J. Mol. Biol.* **13**, 54 (1965).]

We conclude from all these data that the assumption that only nearest-neighbour interactions are significant is a fair first approximation for single-strand poly-nucleotides. Furthermore, the conformation of monomers in the polymer is similar to that in the dimers. This allows one to estimate the ORD or CD of any single-strand polynucleotide from the measured properties of 16 dinucleoside phosphates and 4 mononucleosides.[4] For a polymer of N bases with n_i nearest neighbours of type i and m_j nucleotides of type j (omitting the two end bases)

$$N[\text{polymer}] = \sum_{i=1}^{16} n_i[XY]_i - \sum_{j=1}^{4} m_j[X_j] \qquad [4]$$

As N becomes large, end effects can be neglected; then n_i/N and m_j/N can be replaced by the corresponding mole fractions. The calculated curve is expected to have approximately the correct shape and magnitude. Comparison with experimental curves can be used to test the identity of the polymer and to ensure that it is actually single stranded. Figure 5 shows calculated CD curves for single-strand polymers

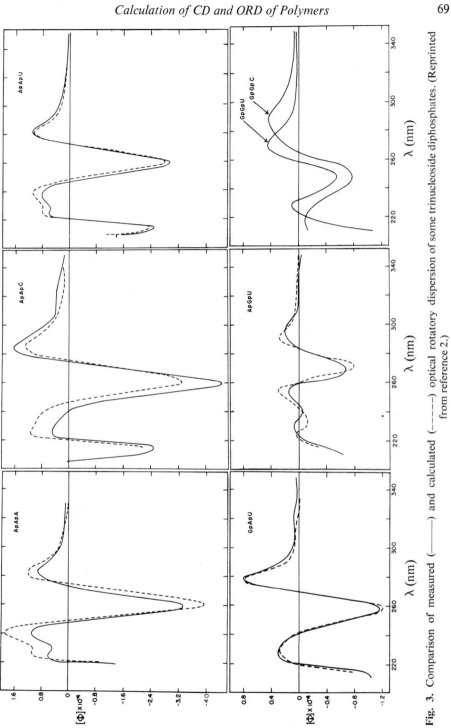

Fig. 3. Comparison of measured (———) and calculated (———) optical rotatory dispersion of some trinucleoside diphosphates. (Reprinted from reference 2.)

with a random sequence of bases containing different amounts of adenine plus uracil. The single-strand polymer is not constrained to have adenine=uracil and guanine=cytosine, but the calculations were done with this constraint for later

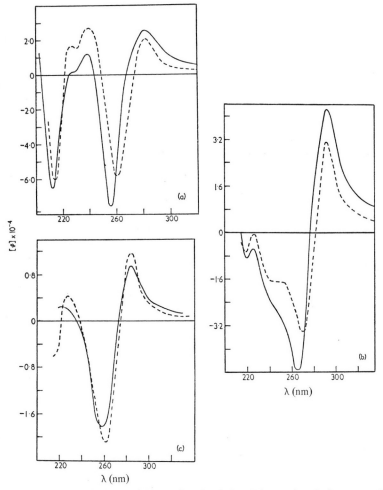

Fig. 4. Comparison of measured (————) and calculated (––––) optical rotatory dispersion for (a) polyadenylic acid, (b) polycytidylic acid, and (c) polyuridylic acid. (Reprinted from reference 4.)

comparison with double-stranded polymers. The calculated curves are also sensitive to the sequence of bases in the polymer.

If we deduced that it was necessary to include next-nearest-neighbour interactions in our calculations, we could write the CD or ORD of a polymer in terms of the measured properties of 64 trimers and 16 dimers. For example

$$4[ABCD] = 3[ABC] + 3[BCD] - 2[BC] \qquad [5]$$

For double-stranded DNA or RNA we can use the same principle, but we do not have appropriate sub-units. Base-paired mononucleosides, such as A:U, and base-paired dinucleoside phosphates, such as

$$ApG$$
$$\ddot{U}p\ddot{C}$$

are not stable in aqueous solution. We must use oligomers or polymers from which the contributions of the sub-units can be obtained.

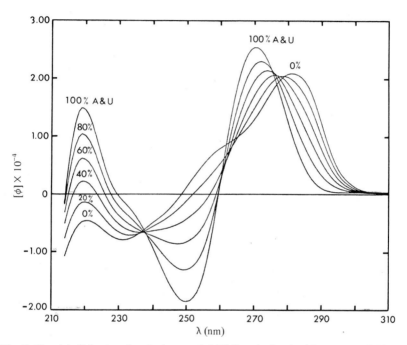

Fig. 5. Circular dichroism for single-stranded RNA calculated with nearest-neighbour approximation from measured data on mononucleosides and dinucleoside phosphates of Warshaw and Cantor, *Biopolymers* **9**, 1079 (1970). The molar ellipticity is calculated for a random sequence of bases with A = U and C = G. (See reference 9.)

For DNA double-stranded polymers the nearest-neighbour contributions can be obtained from polymers of simple repeating sequence and from natural DNAs of known nearest-neighbour frequencies. Although there are 16 possible nearest neighbours for 4 bases, one can show that only 8 polymers of measured properties are needed.[5] That is, with the nearest neighbour approximation, the CD of any DNA can be calculated in terms of 8 known CDs. Of course, all the DNAs must have the same conformation. Comparison of calculated and observed CD for various DNAs[6] indicates that the nearest-neighbour approximation is a useful one. Figure 6 shows the calculated CD for random-sequence double-stranded DNA as a function of percent A + T. The data for the calculation came from DNA molecules which are presumably in the B-form. Note the similarities between these curves for double-stranded B-form DNA and Fig. 5 for single-stranded RNA. What about 0 and 100% A + T? The measured curves for poly A : poly T and poly G : poly C are very different from those calculated. The obvious conclusion is that these polymers are not in B-form conformation. Langridge[7] and Wells et al.[8] have suggested that double-stranded DNAs of the structure polypurine:polypyrimidine do not necessarily have B-form geometry.

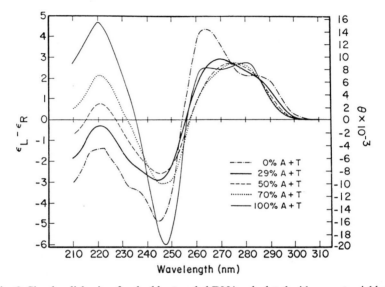

Fig. 6. Circular dichroism for double-stranded DNA calculated with nearest-neighbour approximation from measured data on DNAs of known nearest-neighbour frequencies. (Reprinted from reference 6 by permission of John Wiley and Sons Inc.)

The same method can be applied to RNA double-stranded polymers. We do not as yet have data on the CD of 8 independent RNA double strands of known nearest-neighbour frequencies. However, with further approximations Blum[9] has calculated curves for random-sequence double-stranded RNA as a function of percent A + U (Fig. 7). These calculated curves are very different in shape from either DNA or single-stranded RNA. This is consistent with the different geometry in double-stranded RNA compared to DNA. Double-stranded RNA is known to have its bases tilted similar to A-form DNA.[10] However, single-stranded RNA apparently has the bases in a conformation like B-form DNA.

Other useful model compounds for RNA double strands are of the following type: A_nXYU_n and $A_n\overline{YX}U_n$.[11] The symbols X and Y represent any two bases; $\overline{X}$ and $\overline{Y}$ are their complementary pairs. The adenine and uracil bases on either side provide the necessary stability for the formation of Watson–Crick double-stranded structures. There are not yet enough data available on these molecules to compare with the nearest-neighbour contributions obtained from the RNA polymers.

Although all the examples discussed here have been polynucleotides, it should be clear that these general methods can be applied to any polymer. One simply compares the appropriate sum of monomer, dimer or trimer spectra with that of the polymer.

With simple polymers there is hope that less empirical methods, such as those described in the following sections, can give more information. However, for large aggregates and complexes, probably only empirical methods will be available for a

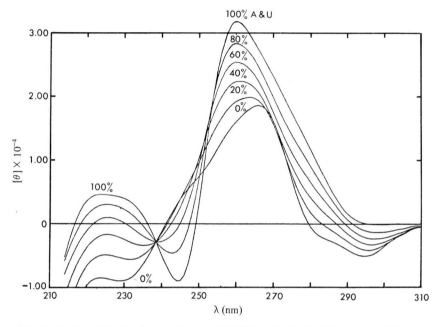

Fig. 7. Circular dichroism for double-stranded RNA calculated with nearest-neighbour approximation from measured data shown in Fig. 9. (See reference 9.)

long time. At present all we can do for these aggregates is to ask if the CD or ORD of the aggregate is different from the sum of the parts. This is essentially a zero-neighbour approximation with the 'monomer' equal to a macromolecule. ORD measurements of T-even bacteriophage[12] have shown that the DNA is not in the B-form inside the virus. The RNA in ribosomes has the same ORD as that free in solution.[13] These are the sorts of conclusions which can be drawn about nucleic acids and proteins in membranes, chromosomes, etc.

2.4.3 Theoretical Methods

We have discussed how to use CD simply to follow changes in conformation. Now we will see if we can actually determine an absolute conformation for a polymer from its measured CD or ORD. It is important to define what we mean by determining a conformation. The optical measurements do not have enough information in them to determine more than a few parameters. Therefore, we will usually be satisfied to choose among a few possible conformations, or to determine a range of structures which are consistent with the data. The method then consists of using known monomer properties plus an assumed geometry to calculate the polymer CD. Figure 8 shows measured CD spectra of Warshaw and Cantor[14] for 4 dinucleoside phosphates containing only adenine and guanine as chromophores. The very different CD must be due in large part to different conformations for each dimer. From space-filling models one could decide on reasonable geometries to try.

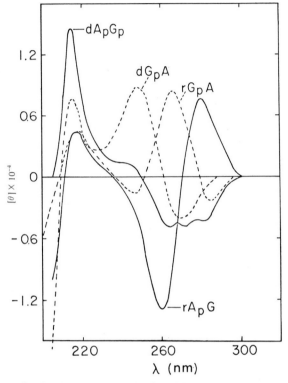

Fig. 8. Measured molar ellipticity (per mole of base) for two deoxydinucleoside phosphates and two ribodinucleoside phosphates. (Reprinted from reference 14 by permission of John Wiley & Sons Inc.)

Figure 9 shows measured [15] CD curves for different double-stranded RNA molecules. Here the obvious geometry to try first would be the one deduced from X-ray diffraction of fibres.[16] The equations linking the geometry to the polymer CD will be discussed in the following paragraphs.

A. Quantum-mechanical Perturbation Methods

The circular dichroism $\varepsilon_L - \varepsilon_R(v)$ can be related to electronic transitions in a molecule through the rotational strength of each transition, R_i, and the shape factor, $(v - v_i)$, for the transition.

$$\frac{\varepsilon_L - \varepsilon_R(v)}{v} = \sum_i R_i f(v - v_i) \tag{6}$$

To determine rotational strengths experimentally, the measured CD curve must be resolved into components and then integrated.

$$R_i = \int_i \frac{\varepsilon_L - \varepsilon_R(v).\,dv}{v} \qquad [7]$$

The resolution of a measured CD curve into meaningful components is very difficult, because there may be much cancellation from positive and negative contributions

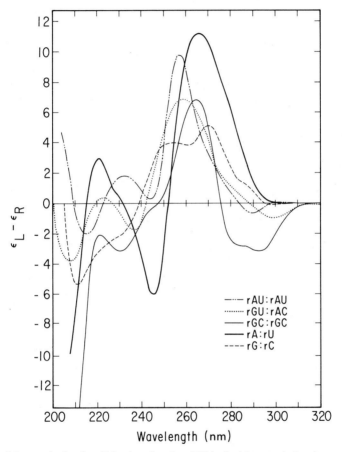

Fig. 9. Measured circular dichroism for five RNA double-stranded polymers. (Unpublished data from D. M. Gray.)

to the CD. The experimental rotational strengths are therefore somewhat arbitrary. For the methods discussed in this section only rotational strengths are calculated; no attempt is made to predict band shapes.

The rotational strength is defined in the usual way in terms of polymer electronic wave functions, ψ, and the electric (μ) and magnetic (m) dipole operators.[17]

$$R_i \equiv R_{OA} = \mathrm{Im}\,\boldsymbol{\mu}_{OA}.\boldsymbol{m}_{AO}$$

$$\boldsymbol{\mu}_{OA} = \int \psi_O^* \boldsymbol{\mu} \psi_A \, d\tau$$

$$\boldsymbol{m}_{AO} = \int \psi_A^* \boldsymbol{m} \psi_O d\tau \qquad\qquad\qquad [8]$$

ψ_O = electronic ground state wave function for polymer

ψ_A = electronic excited state wave function for polymer

The problem is, as usual, to obtain useful wave functions. The key to the solution is to divide the polymer into sub-units which do not have significant exchange of electrons between them. A working definition of a polymer for our purposes could then be a molecule in which such sub-units can be found. This general method was first applied by Kirkwood[18] to small molecules in which the sub-units were methyls, ethyls, etc. Moffitt[19] extended the method to consider explicitly polymers of identical groups. Many other workers have since contributed to the development of this method.[20]

A1. First-order perturbation. We will illustrate the method with the simplest molecule which leads to all the terms found in a general polymer; that is, a dimer of identical monomers. For each transition in the monomer, two transitions will occur in the polymer. The intensity and position of each band will depend on the geometry of the dimer and the electronic properties of the monomers. As the distance between the monomers increases, the splitting will become smaller with the frequency of each band approaching the monomer frequency. The monomer electronic properties, which we need to know in principle to calculate rotational strengths, include electric and magnetic transition dipole moments between all states, and permanent electric dipole moments for all states. Often only the dominant terms are included. For electrically allowed transitions this means that all magnetic transition moments are neglected (although they are not necessarily equal to zero). The important point is that an explicit equation can be obtained linking the polymer CD to monomer properties and polymer geometry.

Consider a monomer with only three electronic states: a ground state and two excited states with wave functions ϕ_o, ϕ_a, ϕ_b. The transition frequencies for the monomers are ν_{oa} and ν_{ob}. The zero-order wave functions for the dimer are:

$$\psi_O^0 = \phi_{10}\phi_{20} \qquad\qquad \text{ground state} \qquad\qquad [9]$$

$$\psi_{A+}^0 = \frac{1}{\sqrt{2}}(\phi_{10}\phi_{2a} + \phi_{1a}\phi_{20})$$

$$\psi_{A-}^0 = \frac{1}{\sqrt{2}}(\phi_{10}\phi_{2a} - \phi_{1a}\phi_{20})$$

$$\psi_{B+}^0 = \frac{1}{\sqrt{2}}(\phi_{10}\phi_{2b} + \phi_{1b}\phi_{20})$$

$$\psi_{B-}^0 = \frac{1}{\sqrt{2}}(\phi_{10}\phi_{2b} - \phi_{1b}\phi_{20})$$

singly excited states   [10]

$$\left.\begin{array}{l} \psi_{AA}^{0} = \phi_{1a}\,\phi_{2a} \\[4pt] \psi_{BB}^{0} = \phi_{1b}\,\phi_{2b} \\[4pt] \psi_{AB+}^{0} = \dfrac{1}{\sqrt{2}}(\phi_{1a}\,\phi_{2b} + \phi_{1b}\,\phi_{2a}) \\[8pt] \psi_{AB-}^{0} = \dfrac{1}{\sqrt{2}}(\phi_{1a}\,\phi_{2b} - \phi_{1b}\,\phi_{2a}) \end{array}\right\} \text{ doubly excited states} \qquad [11]$$

The interaction potential between monomers (V_{12}) mixes in all other wave functions into each first-order wave function. The first-order ground state becomes:

$$\psi_{O}^{1} = \phi_{10}\phi_{20} - \frac{2V_{10a;\,200}\,\phi_{1a}\phi_{20}}{v_{oa}} - \frac{2V_{10b;\,200}\,\phi_{1b}\phi_{20}}{v_{ob}}$$

$$- \frac{V_{10a;\,20a}\,\phi_{1a}\phi_{2a}}{v_{oa}} - \frac{V_{10b;\,20b}\,\phi_{1b}\phi_{2b}}{v_{ob}} \qquad [12]$$

$$- \frac{2V_{10a;\,20b}\,\phi_{1a}\phi_{2b}}{v_{oa} + v_{ob}}$$

$$V_{10a;\,200} = \int \phi_{10}\phi_{20}\,V_{12}\,\phi_{1a}\phi_{20}\,d\tau \qquad [13]$$

The units for V_{12} and v are cm^{-1}. Similar equations can be written for the other V_{12} terms and for the first-order wave functions for the excited states.

To first order, the dimer transitions will have frequencies

$$v_{OA\pm} = v_{oa} \pm V_{10a;\,20a} + V_{1aa;\,200} - V_{100;\,200} \qquad [14]$$

The monomer frequency is thus split by the interaction between transition moments ($V_{10a;\,20a}$). It is also shifted by the difference in interaction between ground state permanent moments and excited state permanent moments ($V_{10a;\,200} - V_{100;\,200}$).

The rotational strengths are obtained by substituting wave functions into equation [8] with

$$\boldsymbol{\mu} = \boldsymbol{\mu}_1 + \boldsymbol{\mu}_2$$

$$\boldsymbol{m} = \frac{e}{2mc}[\boldsymbol{R}_1 \times \boldsymbol{p}_1 + \boldsymbol{R}_2 \times \boldsymbol{p}_2] + \boldsymbol{m}_1 + \boldsymbol{m}_2 \qquad [15]$$

The magnetic moment operator depends on an (arbitrary) choice of origin for the polymer. Thus this operator has contributions from the angular momentum of the electrons in each group about the origin, and also from magnetic moment operators $\boldsymbol{m}_1$ and $\boldsymbol{m}_2$ relative to origins in each monomer. $\boldsymbol{R}_1$ and $\boldsymbol{R}_2$ are constant vectors from the polymer origin to each monomer origin. $\boldsymbol{p}_1$ and $\boldsymbol{p}_2$ are linear momentum operators for each monomer.

The results to first order for the two rotational strengths are

$$R_{OA\pm} = \mp \frac{\pi v_{oa}}{2} R_{12} \cdot \mu_{10a} \times \mu_{20a} \tag{16a}$$

$$+ 2\pi V_{10a;\,20b} R_{12} \cdot \mu_{10a} \times \mu_{20b} \frac{v_{oa} v_{ob}}{v_{ob}^2 - v_{oa}^2} \tag{16b}$$

$$+ \operatorname{Im}(\mu_{10a} \cdot m_{1ao} \pm \mu_{10a} \cdot m_{2ao}) \tag{16c}$$

$$- 2 \operatorname{Im} \frac{V_{10a;\,20b}}{v_{ob}^2 - v_{oa}^2} (v_{oa} \mu_{10a} \cdot m_{2bo} + v_{ob} \mu_{10b} \cdot m_{2ao}) \tag{16d}$$

$$- \operatorname{Im} \frac{V_{1ab;\,200}}{v_{ob} - v_{oa}} (\mu_{10a} \cdot m_{1bo} + \mu_{10b} \cdot m_{1ao}) \tag{16e}$$

$$- \operatorname{Im} \frac{V_{10b;\,200}}{v_{ob}} (\mu_{10a} \cdot m_{1ab} + \mu_{1ab} \cdot m_{1ao}) \tag{16f}$$

$$- \operatorname{Im} \frac{V_{10a;\,200}}{v_{oa}} (\mu_{iaa} - \mu_{ioo}) \cdot m_{iao} \tag{16g}$$

$$R_{12} = R_2 - R_1$$

Equation [16a] gives the conservative[21] CD for a dimer with exciton splitting; the CD of the dinucleoside phosphate, adenylyl (3'-5')-phosphate, can be characterized by this term.[22] Equation [16b] represents contributions of all other transitions to the $O \rightarrow A\pm$ transition; it leads to non-conservative CD curves.[21] The remaining terms [16c–16g] involve magnetic dipole transitions. Equation [16c] contains the intrinsic CD of each monomer and [16d] shows the mixing of transition electric and magnetic dipoles from different monomers. The last three terms [16e–16g] all contain permanent electric moments. They are usually neglected unless the $O \rightarrow a$ monomer transition is electrically forbidden (as in an $n \rightarrow \pi^*$ transition), then they contain the dominant terms.

A2. Variation method (all order in V_{12}).[20e, 20f] The first-order perturbation equations (equation [16]) can be easily improved by using wave functions which include V_{12} to all orders. The zero-order wave functions (equations [9–11]) are used as a basis set for diagonalizing the Hamiltonian ($\mathscr{H}_1 + \mathscr{H}_2 + V_{12}$). This gives energies and through the secular equations one obtains all-order wave functions which are linear combinations of the zero-order ones. These wave functions are used with the operators in equation [15] to obtain all-order rotational strengths.

A3. Applications. In order to use these equations it is necessary to know the appropriate monomer properties. Accurate monomer wave functions would give all the required information. However, it is good to test and adjust the monomer molecular orbitals so that they reproduce measured monomer properties such as absorption spectra. The directions and magnitudes of electric dipole transition moments from the ground state can thus be obtained experimentally. Measurement of permanent dipole moments is also useful.

Calculations have been done for polypeptides[23] and polynucleotides;[24] some of the work has been reviewed recently.[25] We will very briefly mention some of the pertinent results.

Figure 10 shows calculated and observed results for the α-helix of poly-L-alanine by Woody.[23c] Agreement is very good and indicates that in this wavelength region knowledge of the amide spectrum is sufficient for this type of calculation. Pysh[23a, b]

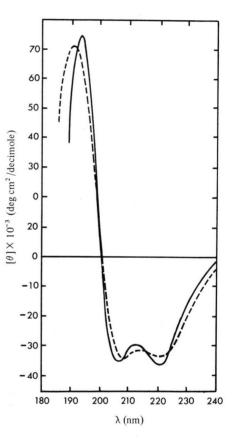

Fig. 10. Measured (-----) and calculated (———) molar ellipticity for helical poly-L-alanine. The calculation was done for an α-helix with an extension of the quantum mechanical method illustrated by equation [16]. (Reprinted from reference 23c.)

and Woody have thus been able to make useful conclusions about polypeptides in other conformations such as β-structures and polyproline. Cassim and Yang[26] first deduced, by comparing Kronig–Kramers transforms of ORD with CD, that the CD below 185 nm did not agree with Woody's calculations.[23c] Figure 11 shows the CD measured to 165 nm,[27] which confirms their deduction. There seems to be a new CD band at about 175 nm. A band at this wavelength was not assumed in the amide spectrum used by Woody, therefore no such band would appear in the calculated polypeptide spectrum. This illustrates how important it is to have a thorough knowledge of the monomer spectrum. A recalculation is in progress, but the results above 190 nm should not be changed too much.

Calculations for dinucleoside phosphates as a function of conformation have been made.[24b] An example of calculated and measured results is shown in Fig. 12. One can conclude as expected that dinucleoside phosphates are generally in DNA-like

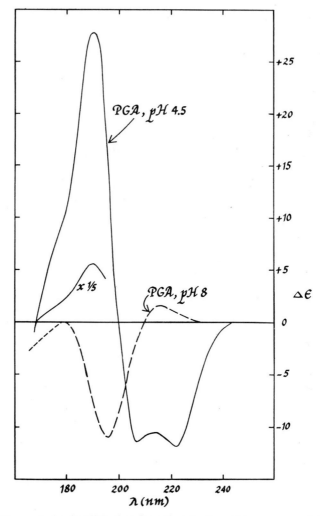

Fig. 11. Measured circular dichroism for polyglutamic acid in aqueous solution. The conformation at pH 4.5 is the α-helix, at pH 8 it is a coil. Note the new band below 180 nm. (From reference 27.)

geometry. However, a new result is that base-stacked conformations very different from the optimum lead to very different shapes for calculated CD curves. While unstacked conformations lead to curves which have similar shape, but decreased magnitude. This means that the decreased magnitude of the CD found with increasing temperature must be interpreted as an unstacking. This conclusion invalidates an earlier suggestion that the temperature dependence of the CD could be explained in terms of a wiping motion of the bases without unstacking.[28]

B. Classical Theory

A very different-seeming theory which is actually similar to the all-order variational method discussed earlier is the classical theory of DeVoe.[29] It is essentially a

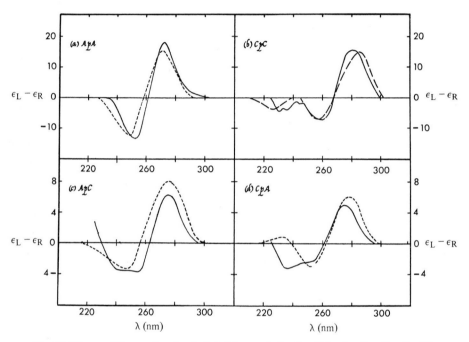

Fig. 12. Measured (————) and calculated (————) circular dichroism for dinucleoside phosphates. The calculation was done as a function of conformation with a variational quantum mechanical method. (From reference 24b by permission of John Wiley & Sons Inc.)

phenomenological theory in that one calculates the polarization (dipole moment induced per unit volume) in the sample at each frequency and the CD or ORD follows from it. The dipole moment induced (μ) in a molecule by an electromagnetic field can be written as

$$\mu = \alpha \cdot E - (\beta/c) \cdot \frac{\mathrm{d}H}{\mathrm{d}t} \qquad [17]$$

The α is the usual electrical polarizability tensor; it depends on frequency and is a complex quantity. β is an analogous parameter linking the electric dipole induced and the time-dependent magnetic field and E and H are the electric and magnetic vectors of the incident light. A polymer is treated as a collection of point-polarizable groups. The dipole induced in each group depends on the incident light and on the dipoles induced in every other group. Summing all the induced dipoles leads to the polymer induced dipole and thus the polymer CD. The effects of static electric fields can be included by considering that the polarizabilities are not those of the isolated monomers, but are polarizabilities for the monomer in the static field of the polymer.

The equations can be illustrated by considering a dimer. The dipoles induced in each monomer at any frequency are

$$\boldsymbol{\mu}_1(v) = \boldsymbol{\alpha}_1(v) \cdot \boldsymbol{E} - \alpha_1(v) \cdot \boldsymbol{T}_{12} \cdot \boldsymbol{\mu}_2(v) - (\boldsymbol{\beta}_1/c) \cdot (\mathrm{d}H/\mathrm{d}T)$$

The general equations for a polymer[29] can best be understood if we consider a dimer of identical monomers with simple properties. In general each monomer must be characterized by a complex polarizability tensor whose components and principal axes are frequency dependent. However, for a single absorption band the polarizability tensor can be written

$$\boldsymbol{\alpha}(v) = \alpha(v)\,\boldsymbol{ee}$$
$$\alpha(v) = \mathrm{Re}\,\alpha(v) + \mathrm{i}\,\mathrm{Im}\alpha(v) \tag{18}$$

The direction of the electric transition moment is along unit vector $\boldsymbol{e}$. The magnitude of the imaginary polarizability is directly proportional to the molar extinction coefficient, $\varepsilon(v)$.

$$\mathrm{Im}\,\alpha(v) = -\frac{6909}{8\pi^2 v N_0}\varepsilon(v) \tag{19}$$

The real part of the polarizability can be obtained from a Kronig–Kramers transform.

$$\mathrm{Re}\,\alpha(v) = \frac{-2}{\pi}\int_0^\infty \frac{v'\,\mathrm{Im}\alpha(v')\,\mathrm{d}v'}{(v')^2 - v^2} \tag{20}$$

The magnetic parameter $\boldsymbol{\beta}$ is assumed to be directly proportional to $\boldsymbol{\alpha}$.

$$\boldsymbol{\beta}(v) = b\alpha(v)\,\boldsymbol{ee}' \tag{21}$$

The unit vector $\boldsymbol{e}'$ is along the magnetic transition moment and b is a real constant. The value of b and the direction of $\boldsymbol{e}'$ can be obtained from the CD of the monomer.

$$\varepsilon_\mathrm{L} - \varepsilon_\mathrm{R}(v) = \frac{-96\pi^2 v^2 N_0 b\boldsymbol{e}\cdot\boldsymbol{e}'}{3298}\,\mathrm{Im}\alpha(v) \tag{22}$$

The molar CD of the dimer is

$$\varepsilon_\mathrm{L} - \varepsilon_\mathrm{R}(v) = \frac{-48\pi^2 v^2 N_0}{3298}\,\mathrm{Im}\left[\frac{\alpha^2\,G_{12}\,\boldsymbol{R}_{12}\cdot\boldsymbol{e}_1\times\boldsymbol{e}_2}{1 - G_{12}^2\alpha^2}\right] \tag{23a}$$

$$+ \frac{192\pi^2 v^2 N_0 b}{3298}\,\mathrm{Im}\left[\frac{\alpha^2\,G_{12}\,\boldsymbol{e}_1\cdot\boldsymbol{e}_2' - \alpha\boldsymbol{e}_1\cdot\boldsymbol{e}_1'}{1 - G_{12}^2\alpha_2}\right] \tag{23b}$$

$$G_{12} = \frac{1}{R_{12}^3}\left[\boldsymbol{e}_1\cdot\boldsymbol{e}_2 - \frac{3\boldsymbol{R}_{12}\cdot\boldsymbol{e}_1\,\boldsymbol{R}_{12}\cdot\boldsymbol{e}_2}{R_{12}^2}\right]$$

The units are: cm^{-1} for v, cm for b and R_{12}, and cm^3 for α. Equation [23a] is equivalent to [16a] + [16b], but it is correct to all orders in the interaction, G_{12}. Similarly, equation [23b] is equivalent to [16c] + [16d]. The interaction G_{12} is written as a point-dipole interaction, but it can be replaced by any better approximation. The main advantage of equation [23] is that it gives the molar CD directly instead of the rotational strength. A rotational strength could, of course, be calculated by appropriate integration.

$$R_{OA} = \int_{\text{band A}} \frac{\varepsilon_L - \varepsilon_R(v)\,dv}{v} \qquad [24]$$

These equations have not been tested yet on polymers. However, analogous equations for polymer absorption have given useful results for hypochromicity in DNA.[30]

C. Helices

Moffitt[19] was the first to consider explicitly the absorption and rotation of a polymer with helical symmetry. Although the equations presented earlier, equation [16] and equation [23], apply to helices when they are generalized from dimers to polymers, the calculations become impractical as the number of monomer units becomes very large. In principle there is no problem. With the generalized equation [16] one must calculate N rotational strengths for each monomer transition in an N-mer. With the generalized equation [23] one must diagonalize an N by N matrix to get the desired CD. We will only consider the extension of equation [16], the first-order perturbation equation, at this time.

We can divide the contributions to the polymer CD into two parts: one comes from interaction among identical transitions in the monomers, the other from interactions among different transitions. The interactions among different transitions present no new concepts and can be obtained by replacing G_{12} in equations [16b–16g] by a sum over G_{ij}. They will not be discussed further. The interaction among identical groups, the generalization of equation [16a], is of interest. The results can be most easily understood if we consider oriented helices. It also follows that more thorough deductions about conformations can be made if experiments are done on oriented helices. The qualitative conclusions[19, 20a, 31] are that for light incident parallel to the helix axis a single absorption band is seen for each monomer band. It is a doubly degenerate, perpendicular polarized band centred at $v_\perp$. The CD for light incident parallel to the helix axis has its cross-over at $v_\perp$ and has the shape of the derivative of the absorption band. The rotational strength of this band is zero when the integration is carried over both positive and negative lobes of the CD. For light incident perpendicular to the helix axis two absorption bands are seen. One is polarized perpendicular to the helix axis and occurs at $v_\perp$ as before. The other is polarized parallel to the helix axis and occurs at $v_\parallel$. The ratio of intensities of the parallel and perpendicular absorption bands depends on the direction each monomer transition moment makes with the helix axis. Equal and opposite CD bands occur at $v_\parallel$ and $v_\perp$. For an unoriented sample, the average of all these bands is seen.

For light incident perpendicular to the helix axis quantitative results can be obtained using re-entrant boundary conditions.[19] The zero-order wave functions are

$$\text{Ground state:} \quad \psi_O = \prod_{i=1}^{N} \phi_{i0} \qquad [25]$$

$$\text{Excited state:}\quad \psi_K = \frac{1}{\sqrt{N}} \sum_{n=1}^{N} e^{2\pi i n K/N}\, \psi_n\,(K=1,2,\ldots,N) \qquad [26]$$

$$\psi_n = \frac{\phi_{na}}{\phi_{n0}}\, \psi_O$$

The excited-state wave functions show that any of the N monomers can be excited to the a state and that the correct wave functions are linear combinations of these singly excited states. These wave functions can be used to calculate the N transition frequencies, ν_K, the N rotational strengths, R_K, and the N dipole strengths, D_K, for the helix. Most of the D_K and R_K are zero or negligible for N large; the non-zero ones lead to the selection rules.[31]

Light incident perpendicular to helix axis:

$$D_\perp = (3/2)\, N\mu_\perp^2$$

$$R_\perp = -(3/2)\, N\pi a\nu_{oa}\, \mu_\parallel\, \mu_t \qquad [27]$$

$$\nu_\perp - \nu_{oa} = 2 \sum_{j=1} V_j \cos\,(2\pi j/P)$$

$$D_\parallel = 3N\mu_\parallel^2$$

$$R_\parallel = (3/2)\, N\pi a\nu_{oa}\, \mu_\parallel\, \mu_t \qquad [28]$$

$$\nu_\parallel - \nu_{oa} = 2 \sum_{j=1} V_j$$

The components of the monomer transition are $\mu_\perp$ (perpendicular to helix axis), $\mu_\parallel$ (parallel to helix axis) and μ_t (tangent to helix). The radius of the helix is a and the number of monomers per turn is P. The interaction energy between monomer first neighbours is V_1, second neighbours V_2, etc. If the interaction among identical monomers is the dominant one, then equations [27] and [28] can be used to obtain the parameters of the helix.

For light incident parallel to the helix axis, re-entrant boundary conditions do not lead to the correct CD.[20a] The problem is that some rotational strengths depend on N^2 and thus diverge as N becomes very large. However, the CD from the sum of all rotational strengths remains finite. The CD is calculated from a Taylor expansion of equation [6] around $\nu_\perp$

$$\frac{\varepsilon_L - \varepsilon_R(\nu)}{\nu} = f(\nu - \nu_\perp) \sum_{K=1}^{N} R_K$$

$$+ \left.\frac{\partial f(\nu - \nu_K)}{\partial \nu_K}\right|_{\nu_\perp} \sum_{K=1}^{N} R_K(\nu_K - \nu_\perp) \qquad [29]$$

The first term is zero because the sum of all rotational strengths over K is zero. The second term can be evaluated without any assumption about the wave functions.[31]

$$\sum_{K=1}^{N} R_K(\nu_K - \nu_\perp) = 6\pi z\mu_\perp^2 \sum_j j V_j \sin\,(2\pi j/P) \qquad [30]$$

The parameter z is the axial distance between monomer units in the helix. It is interesting to note that for a monomer transition moment perpendicular to the helix axis, the only CD comes from equation [30]. Very similar equations can be written for double-strand helices;[31] the double-strand analogue of equation [30] seems to be the explanation of the 260 nm CD band of *B*-form DNA. This conclusion is strengthened by measurements of the CD of oriented DNA by Holzwarth.[32]

The above discussion of the CD of helices has been in the context of the original definition of rotational strengths.[17] It has recently been pointed out[33] that re-entrant boundary wave functions (equation [26]) can be used, if the usual rotational strength is abandoned. The probability of a transition to state K in the presence of light of frequency v_{0K} is proportional to

$$\int \psi_0 e^{2\pi i z v 0K} p_x \psi_K \, d\tau \qquad [31]$$

The light is incident along z and polarized along x. The linear momentum operator along x is p_x. Usually the dimensions of the molecule are such that $z v_{0K}$ is small enough that the exponential can be approximated by 1. This leads to the dipole strength for absorption and the usual rotational strength for CD. Use of the transition probability, equation [31], leads to a deeper understanding of the optical properties of helices. The selection rules now include conservation of linear and angular momentum for the light and the polymer. There is a slight splitting of the perpendicular band. However, the resulting equations for interaction among identical monomers are the same as equations [27], [28] and [30]. The one advance from the new derivation[33] is that a theoretical reason for restricting the sum over j to small j in the equations replaces the intuitive reasons. Of course the transition probability equations are more correct in general and should be used, if practical.

2.4.4 Conclusions

There are probably enough correct published theories to interpret the CD, ORD, and absorption of polymers. However, there has, as yet, been mostly qualitative discussion of optical properties. Very few new deductions about conformation have been published. In my opinion the most important information needed to allow significant, new conclusions is a better understanding of monomer properties. With known monomer properties the only unknown in the calculation of polymer optical properties is the polymer geometry. Measurements of optical properties for oriented polymers will provide the best data for comparison with calculations. An assumed geometry which gives agreement for many monomer bands for both parallel and perpendicular incidence of light will probably be unique and correct.

This work was partly supported by NIH grant GM 10840. I wish to thank Dr. Arlene Blum and Dr. Marcos Maestre for helpful discussions.

References

1. R. C. Davis and I. Tinoco, Jr, *Biopolymers* **6**, 223 (1968).
2. C. R. Cantor and I. Tinoco, Jr, *J. Mol. Biol.* **13**, 65 (1965).
3. (a) Y. Inoue, S. Aoyagi and K. Nakanishi, *J. Amer. Chem. Soc.* **89**, 5701 (1967). (b) D. M. Gray, University of California, Berkeley. Unpublished work.

4. C. R. Cantor, S. R. Jaskunas and I. Tinoco, Jr, *J. Mol. Biol.* **20**, 39 (1966).
5. D. M. Gray and I. Tinoco, Jr, *Biopolymers* **9**, 223 (1970).
6. F. S. Allen, D. M. Gray, G. P. Roberts and I. Tinoco, Jr, *Biopolymers* **11**, 853 (1972).
7. R. Langridge, *Abstracts Seventh International Congress of Biochemistry* **1**, 57 (1967).
8. R. D. Wells, J. E. Larson, R. C. Grant, B. E. Shortle and C. R. Cantor, *J. Mol. Biol.* **54**, 465 (1970).
9. A. D. Blum, Ph.D. Thesis, University of California, Berkeley, 1971.
10. S. Arnott, M. H. F. Wilkins, W. Fuller and R. Langridge, *J. Mol. Biol.* **27**, 535 (1967).
11. (*a*) F. H. Martin, O. C. Uhlenbeck and P. Doty, *J. Mol. Biol.* **57**, 201 (1971). (*b*) O. C. Uhlenbeck, F. H. Martin and P. Doty, *J. Mol. Biol.* **57**, 217 (1971).
12. M. F. Maestre and I. Tinoco, Jr, *J. Mol. Biol.* **23**, 323 (1967).
13. (*a*) A. Blake and A. R. Peacocke, *Nature* **208**, 1319 (1965). (*b*) P. K. Sarkar, J. T. Yang and P. Doty, *Biopolymers* **5**, 1 (1967). (*c*) P. M. McPhie and W. B. Gratzer, *Biochemistry* **5**, 1310 (1966).
14. M. M. Warshaw and C. R. Cantor, *Biopolymers* **9**, 1079 (1970).
15. D. M. Gray. Unpublished work.
16. S. Arnott, *Progr. Biophys. Mol. Biol.* **21**, 265 (1970).
17. L. Rosenfeld, *Z. Phys.* **52**, 161 (1928).
18. J. G. Kirkwood, *J. Chem. Phys.* **5**, 479 (1937).
19. W. Moffitt, *J. Chem. Phys.* **25**, 467 (1956).
20. (*a*) W. Moffitt, D. D. Fitts and J. G. Kirkwood, *Proc. Natl. Acad. Sci., U.S.A.* **43**, 723 (1957). (*b*) I. Tinoco, Jr, *Advan. Chem. Phys.* **4**, 113 (1962). (*c*) J. A. Schellman and P. Oriel, *J. Chem. Phys.* **37**, 2114 (1962). (*d*) I. Tinoco, Jr, R. W. Woody and D. F. Bradley, *J. Chem. Phys.* **38**, 1317 (1963). (*e*) P. M. Bayley, E. B. Nielsen and J. A. Schellman, *J. Phys. Chem.* **73**, 228 (1969). (*f*) W. C. Johnson, Jr, and I. Tinoco, Jr, *Biopolymers* **8**, 715 (1969).
21. C. A. Bush and J. Brahms, *J. Chem. Phys.* **46**, 79 (1967).
22. C. A. Bush and I. Tinoco, Jr, *J. Mol. Biol.* **23**, 601 (1967).
23. (*a*) E. S. Pysh, *Proc. Natl. Acad. Sci. U.S.A.* **56**, 825 (1966). (*b*) E. S. Pysh, *J. Mol. Biol.* **23**, 587 (1967). (*c*) R. W. Woody, *J. Chem. Phys.* **49**, 4797 (1968). (*d*) V. Madison and J. Schellman, *Biopolymers* **9**, 569 (1970).
24. (*a*) W. C. Johnson, Jr, and I. Tinoco, Jr, *Biopolymers* **7**, 727 (1969). (*b*) W. C. Johnson, Jr, M. S. Itzkowitz and I. Tinoco, Jr, *Biopolymers* **11**, 225 (1972).
25. (*a*) C. W. Deutsche, D. A. Lightner, R. W. Woody and A. Moscowitz, *Ann. Rev. Phys. Chem.* **20**, 407 (1969). (*b*) I. Tinoco, Jr, and C. R. Cantor, *Methods Biochem. Anal.* **18**, 81 (1970).
26. J. Y. Cassim and J. T. Yang, *Biopolymers* **9**, 1475 (1970).
27. W. C. Johnson, Jr, and I. Tinoco, Jr, *J. Amer. Chem. Soc.* **94**, 4389 (1972).
28. D. Glaubiger, D. A. Lloyd and I. Tinoco, Jr, *Biopolymers* **6**, 409 (1968).
29. H. DeVoe, *J. Chem. Phys.* **43**, 3199 (1965).
30. H. DeVoe, *Ann. N. Y. Acad. Sci.* **158**, 298 (1969).
31. I. Tinoco, Jr, R. W. Woody and D. F. Bradley, *J. Chem. Phys.* **38**, 1317 (1963).
32. S. Y. Wooley and G. Holzwarth, *J. Amer. Chem. Soc.* **93**, 4066 (1971).
33. (*a*) F. M. Loxsom, *J. Chem. Phys.* **51**, 4899 (1969). (*b*) C. W. Deutsche, *J. Chem. Phys.* **52**, 3703 (1970).

Relationship of Chiroptical Properties (ORD and CD) with Structure

The Carbonyl Chromophore, Saturated Ketones

W. KLYNE and D. N. KIRK

Westfield College
London NW3 7ST, U.K.

3.1.1 Introduction

This is the first chapter in this book on applications of the chiroptical techniques to small molecules, and it is therefore appropriate to review in a general way the nature of these applications, and also the relations between theory and empiricism in this field.

Principal references for all topics up to 1970 are given by Crabbé,[1] and full references up to 1966 are given by the same author.[2] See also recent *Annual Reports of the Chemical Society*.[3]

A. Applications

1. Determination of absolute configuration (chirality).
2. Determination of relative configuration.
3. Determination of position of a chromophore.
4. Conformational problems.
5. Solvation.
6. Quantitative analysis.
7. Spectroscopic studies.

The most important application hitherto has been in the determination of absolute configuration (chirality). Today the use of the chiroptical techniques, which provide a sensitive, as well as a chiral, molecular probe, is of growing importance in studying the nature of electronic transitions in molecules. Information given by the two chiroptical techniques (ORD and CD) for many structural and stereochemical problems is of equal value; for most purposes the two techniques may be regarded as interchangeable. Preferences in the past have been determined very largely by the availability and reliability of equipment. Now that good CD equipment is available, the theoretical advantages which this technique has always had over ORD will make it the preferred technique in nearly all circumstances.

However, where older ORD data are available, they can very often be 'translated' approximately into CD results by using the simple relationship $a = 40\Delta\varepsilon$. In this paper, we refer to CD throughout.

B. *Theory and Empiricism*

The mathematical complexity of all theoretical treatments of the chiroptical techniques is such that, even with computer help, their application to extensive ranges of compounds is hardly feasible and perhaps not yet appropriate, in view of continuing uncertainties regarding the correct theoretical approach. In this situation, it is our belief that the empirical analysis of data for large groups of closely related compounds offers the best hope of providing the theoretician with guidance. The development of the 'Octant Rule' in its original form[4] depended partly upon work done by Djerassi and his co-workers[1, 2] in the preparation of simple decalones and hexahydroindanones as test-series. Recent important developments, both for carbonyl CD (Hudec[5]) and for other groups (e.g. olefins[6]), indicate that much more work of this kind will be necessary. A close collaboration between the experimental organic chemist and the theoretician, in designing suitable series of compounds for study and then interpreting the data, should lead to a better eventual understanding of chiroptical phenomena.

The empirical worker using chiroptical techniques, as in many other fields of organic chemistry, argues by analogies, and the correctness of his conclusions depends entirely upon their soundness. The literature is scattered with examples of errors due to bad analogies. Arguments from close analogy however, while usually safe, add little to our fundamental understanding of the chiroptical phenomena. They may nonetheless be very valuable in tackling structural problems, e.g. for hexahydroindan-2-ones of the type shown by formulae I and II. Provided that no unusual substituents were present in the neighbourhood of the carbonyl group, the sign of the CD for an unknown compound would indicate without any doubt whether the absolute configuration was of type I or II.

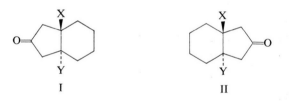

In such work, the study of molecules with rigid conformations must always precede applications to flexible molecules. The initial choice of decalones was the logical one, because cyclohexanone rings, when *trans*-fused, provide almost perfect tetrahedral arrays of atoms and bonds, the symmetry of which greatly simplifies both empirical and theoretical treatments.

It is now realized that Djerassi's original choice of the n → π* absorption band (at *c*. 290 nm) of the carbonyl group for the first extensive studies with modern ORD equipment was a stroke of genius for another reason, viz. that this absorption band is so far removed from the next band of higher energy (at about 190 nm) that there is no danger of confusion from overlap with other bands. Recent experience with other functional groups, e.g. the olefin chromophore,[6] shows a less happy state of affairs, because there is undoubtedly overlap between two, if not three, absorption bands close together.

C. *Importance of Pair-wise Comparisons*

Many of our arguments concerning structures depend on the comparison of an unknown compound X with three other known compounds (A, B, C) of character such that X is related to A as B is related to C. Collections of data for interpretation are frequently dependent on simple comparisons of two compounds—one containing a particular substituent and one without it—as for example in the recent important publications by Hudec.[5] It is generally true to say that the chiroptical techniques will answer only one question at a time. The careful ORD/CD worker will be guided in his applications of the techniques in this way. For example, given the relative configuration of a compound X, CD may be able to tell us the absolute configuration; *vice versa*, given the absolute configuration, CD may be able to tell us the conformation. It will rarely be safe to deduce *both* absolute configuration and conformation, or *both* absolute configuration of a skeleton and relative configuration of substituents from one single CD curve.

3.1.2 Carbonyl Group: General Considerations

All considerations of the chiroptical properties of the saturated carbonyl group ($>C{=}O$) must be based on the symmetry properties of the group itself (C_{2v}); the two mirror-planes of this group are two essential pieces of the framework, in terms of which we consider the positions relative to carbonyl of dissymmetrically placed atoms or bonds. All 'Rules', empirical or otherwise, must therefore be of a 'Quadrant' type, or else of a character involving further sub-division of space, such as the initial 'Octant Rule' (Moffitt *et al.*;[4] Höhn and Weigang[7]).

Nearly all published work so far has dealt with the n → π* transition of the carbonyl group at *c.* 290 nm, and all of this review refers to this transition (except for Section 3.1.7).

3.1.3 Theoretical Treatments

The applications of various theoretical ideas to interpret and modify the original Octant Rule have been concisely tabulated by Crabbé (reference 1, pp. 13–14). More recent communications to be noted are those of Hudec[5] on orbital interactions, and of Coulombeau and Rassat[8] regarding the shape of the Sector boundaries. All these theoretical treatments, in our opinion, need much more thorough testing with data for compounds of known stereochemistry, high purity—and, incidentally, data of higher precision than have often been available in the past.

One of the most important ideas which has been developed over the last two or three years is that of considering the dissymmetry of a compound in terms of bonding patterns, rather than simply the distribution of matter in space. Dr. J. Hudec of Southampton, in several brief published papers,[5] has put forward general ideas which seem to be very significant. We ourselves have been applying these and similar ideas, more particularly to compounds without hetero-substituents, and are firmly convinced of the great significance of *anti*-periplanar zig-zag patterns of carbon–carbon bonds in arrays of cyclohexane rings.

References have been made to many of these matters in Chapters 2.1–2.3. The division between this chapter and the succeeding one (Chapter 3.2) on unsaturated ketones appears increasingly artificial.

3.1.4   Factors for Consideration in Assembling Data

A. Rotational Strengths and Dissymmetry Factors

The calculation of rotational strength (R) from the area under a CD band gives a theoretically more desirable measure of the ellipticity than does the maximum alone ($\Delta\varepsilon$ or θ). However, few schools have yet made the integration of the band areas a matter of routine; we cannot yet say whether the extra labour involved in integration is justified as a standard procedure. Professor G. Snatzke pointed out in discussion that calculation of rotational strength is much more important in cases where some compounds show fine structure and others do not. The use of capital gamma (Γ) by some French schools (e.g. Levisalles[9]) as a measure of half-band width is worth noting. The use of Kuhn's dissymmetry factor (g; the ratio of $\Delta\varepsilon/\varepsilon$) to characterize transitions is well known (see for example Mason[10]). There has, however, been little, if any, significant use of g in comparing compounds within a single series containing the same chromophore, such as carbonyl.

B. Dipole Strengths

Even less common are integrations of the areas under ketone UV absorption bands to give dipole strengths (D); resolution of bands might be necessary because of overlap with bands of shorter wavelength.

The simple calculation of the ratio of rotational strength to dipole strength (R/D) has also been relatively unpopular.

C. Curves with Branches of Opposite Sign; Fine Structure

The 'ideal' picture of a simple Gaussian CD curve corresponding to a simple absorption band is very commonly observed for the n → π* transition of ketones. Those compounds which display fine structure in their CD curves (usually in non-polar solvents) often show spacing of the sub-bands which corresponds, as expected, to the spacing of vibrational levels (cf. infrared frequencies[11]). It has long been known that fine structure shows up in non-polar solvents such as hexane, but not in polar solvents such as methanol. There has, however, been, so far as we know, no systematic consideration of the fact that some compounds show marked fine structure in hexane and others show little or none. We ought to be asking ourselves the questions 'What structural types give rise to fine structure?' and 'What neighbouring groups give rise to fine structure?' Figure 1 shows an interesting comparison of two A-nor-steroids which we recently measured for Professor Romeo of Rome; the A-nor-2-ketone, which shows beautiful fine structure, has a local C_2 axis of symmetry; the A-nor-3-ketone, which merely shows shoulders on either side of its principal maximum, is a compound having no local symmetry around the chromophore. Clearly this is a subject where collection of many data is required, and we are proceeding slowly with this.

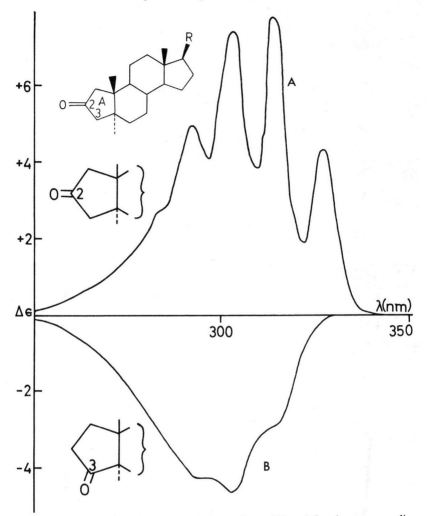

Fig. 1. Curves for 5-methyl-A-nor-5α-cholestan-2-one (A) and for the corresponding 3-one (B), in hexane. Compounds provided by Professor A. Romeo, Rome.

Fine structure, provided that all the sub-bands are of the same sign, hardly complicates the interpretation of CD curves for structural purposes. However, a significant proportion of experimental curves show, in the region corresponding to the n → π* transition, two branches of opposite sign. Such 'two-branched' or 'double-humped' curves—for which the term *bisignate* is now proposed—have been ascribed to the following possible causes:

- (i) existence of a compound in two different conformations (Djerassi *et al.*[12]);
- (ii) existence of solvated and unsolvated molecules (Coulombeau and Rassat[8]);
- (iii) allowed and forbidden branches of the absorption band (Weigang[11]); vibronic coupling (Severn and Kosower[13]).

Cause (i) can be excluded for compounds of rigid conformation; cause (ii) can be largely discounted by working in non-associating solvents. Hydrocarbon solvents are to be preferred for fundamental work here, if the compounds are soluble, because they are essentially of non-associating character. (This is supported by some work on CD of rigid ketones in the vapour phase; vapour-phase[14] and hexane solution give for fairly rigid compounds essentially the same CD curves. This is, however, not the case for some flexible compounds; see studies on *S*-4-methylhexan-3-one by Lardicci

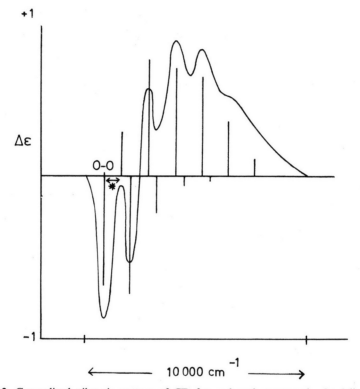

Fig. 2. Generalized vibronic pattern of CD for carbonyl compounds. An 'allowed' progression of the carbonyl stretching frequency (shown in this example as negative) is complemented by a 'forbidden' band system (shown here as positive). All intervals are 1200 cm⁻¹ except that marked * which is 900 cm⁻¹. (Based on Weigang.[11])

et al.[14a]) Even if these two causes are set aside with good reason, however, the constitutional features which give rise to bisignate curves appear to be largely unexplored.

Weigang[11] in an important paper on vibrational structuring has developed a general equation for the CD of compounds in which both electric and magnetic moments are considered to have significant components arising from molecular vibration. The general pattern presented by Weigang consists of an allowed progression of one sign complemented by a forbidden progression of the opposite sign (Fig. 2); these ideas were applied to a very scattered range of individual compounds.

The questions which we need to ask are: (1) 'Why do we sometimes see only one sign and sometimes two signs, i.e. a bisignate curve?' (2) 'If we do have a bisignate curve, which branch ought to obey the Octant Rule?' Again we shall obtain an answer which is meaningful for the organic chemist only if we study carefully chosen series of ketones of related structural types.

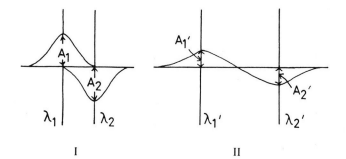

Fig. 3. Superposition of CD curves, *not* to scale (based on Wellman *et al.*[15]) I represents two separate curves of opposite signs; $\Delta\varepsilon_{max}$ A_1 and A_2 at wavelengths λ_1 and λ_2. II represents the resultant curve with *observed* $\Delta\varepsilon_{max}$ A_1' and A_2' at wavelengths λ_1' and λ_2'. Example: I λ_1 300; λ_2 302 nm. A_1, A_2 ±1. II λ_1' 287; λ_2' 315 nm. A_1', A_2' ±0·09.

The *patterns* to which overlapping bands give rise, whatever their origin may be, were fully discussed by Wellman *et al.*[15] (Fig. 3). It should be possible to make some progress in resolving complex or bisignate curves into their components by means of a curve-resolver; however, it is not clear at the moment whether (or how) one can reach a unique solution.

D. Temperature Dependence

Although measurements of temperature dependence of CD were first made some years ago[16] and commercial accessories are now available, the bulk of published work is as yet small. The instrument-time necessary for extensive studies is such as to suggest that these will be made only on a small proportion of promising examples. Professor Legrand, in Chapter 4.1, deals with certain factors which influence the temperature-dependence of curves, including conformational changes, solvation and vibrational changes.

3.1.5 Present State of Empirical Knowledge and Possible Future Trends

There is no published catalogue of all the chiroptical data on saturated ketones, the number of which must now be many thousands. The data are of varying reliability and precision, and repetition of much early work with newer equipment is necessary. The most extensive of the lists of references is that of Crabbé[2] (about 1000 references). Some of the main collections of data and certain recent references are given in Table 1.

Table 1

Some Recent Collections of Data on Carbonyl n → π* Transition CD and ORD

This list contains only a selection of the more accessible papers. References included in the main text are shown as 1, 2, 3, etc. and are listed at the end of the review; references occurring only in this table are shown as 1/1, 1/2, 1/3, etc. and are shown at the foot of the Table.

Group of compounds	References
Extended decalones	1/1, 34
Extended decalones, with contributions of substituents and front octant effects	1/2, 8
Extended steroids; 3-oxo steroids of abnormal configuration	20, 31
Various A-ring oxosteroids	1/3
Simple decalones	1/4
Adamantanones	17
Effects of 'α', 'β', 'γ', 'δ' substituents; halogens and others	5, 18
Cyclopentanones (simple)	1/5
Extended hexahydroindanones (steroid D-ring ketones and A-nor-ketones)	1/6, 1/7
Cycloheptanones, extended; A-homosteroid ketones	1/8, 9
Bornanones; bicyclo-(2,2,1)-heptanones	5, 8, 19, 23
Steroid side-chain ketones (pregnan-20-ones)	1/9

References

1/1. C. Djerassi and W. Klyne, *J. Chem. Soc.* 4929 (1962).

1/2. C. Djerassi and W. Klyne, *J. Chem. Soc.* 2390 (1963).

1/3. J. Levisalles and others, *Bull. Soc. Chim. Fr.* 3166–3194 (six papers) (1969).

1/4. L. Mion, A. Casadevall and E. Casadevall, *C.R.H. Acad. Sci.* **269**C, 653 (1969).

1/5. C. Ouannes and J. Jacques, *Bull. Soc. Chim. Fr.* 3601 and 3611 (1965).

1/6. M. J. Brienne, A. Heymes, J. Jacques, G. Snatzke, W. Klyne, and S. R. Wallis *J. Chem. Soc. C* 423 (1970).

1/7. J. C. Jacquesy, J. Levisalles, and J. Wagnon, *Bull. Soc. Chim. Fr.* 670 (1970).

1/8. J. B. Jones, J. M. Zander, and P. Price, *J. Amer. Chem. Soc.* **89**, 94 (1967); J. B. Jones and J. M. Zander, *Can. J. Chem.* **47**, 3501 (1969).

1/9. H. Mitsuhashi, T. Nomura and M. Fukuoka, *Steroids* **4**, 483 (1964).

A. Test Series of Compounds

The development of more detailed theoretical and semitheoretical treatments now demands the preparation of further series of compounds of high purity. Among the test-series which have been, are being, or should be considered, we may note the following:

(i) *The adamantanones* (Snatzke[17])—very valuable for β-substituents.

(ii) *Camphor derivatives*—many examples by Hudec, Beckett *et al.*;[18] joint work between this laboratory and Professor Erdtman's group in Stockholm.[19]

(iii) *Many ordinary steroids*—these are extremely valuable as being fairly rigid, and readily available as starting materials. We may note the important paper by Jacobs of Leiden.[20]

(iv) D-*homosteroid ketones* (general structure III)—work from the authors' laboratory;[21] nearly all positions have now been covered. These compounds have the great advantage of providing an unstrained and completely regular *trans–anti–trans* system. In other words, we are doing what Nature really ought to have done in her design for the steroid molecule; it would have been far more convenient for the organic chemist if the D-ring were six-membered in natural products!

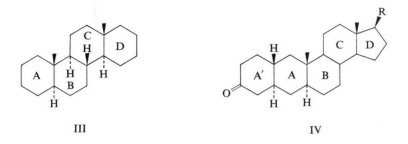

III   IV

(v) *Perhydroanthracene-ketones*—this is virtually unexplored territory; the only examples which we know at present are some steroids carrying an additional A′ ring (IV) which include the perhydroanthracene nucleus (Bloch and Ourisson[22]; see also reference 22a).

In this work, high precision of measurements is needed, care must be taken as to choice of solvent (or solvents), and compounds studied must as far as possible be free from remote substituents (e.g. 17-substituents on a 6-oxo-steroid), which would previously have been disregarded as insignificant. Cross-checks between instruments of different types and different laboratories are very necessary.

B. Bonding Patterns

In its earliest form, the Octant Rule[4] considered the disposition of *atoms* around the carbonyl chromophore, treating them as partially screened nuclei in well-defined positions—with perhaps too little consideration of the polarizability of the groups.

The ideas of bond character and bonding pattern, which have been recently developed by the Southampton school,[5, 18, 23] are certainly going to give us a more refined octant (or perhaps quadrant) rule in due course. Much earlier work needs to be re-interpreted, probably after experimental refinement, in the light of these ideas.

Some striking examples are provided by amino-ketones.[5] According to Hudec, one of the lobes of the carbonyl π^* orbital may interact through σ bonds with the lone-pair on a nitrogen atom in two different ways. (a) If the chain of bonds (and lobes) is formed entirely of *anti*-periplanar links (W-arrangement), as in V, the nitrogen substituent has an 'octant' effect, i.e. an effect of the *same* sign as an alkyl group in the same position. (b) If the chain of bonds (and lobes) includes one or more *syn*-clinal links, as in VI, the nitrogen has an 'anti-octant' effect—i.e. an effect of the *opposite* sign to an alkyl group in the same position.

Nitrogen-substituents (Hudec, 1970[5])

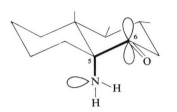
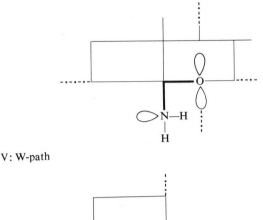

V: W-path

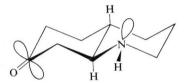
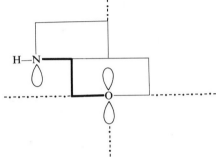

VI: Skew path

When the lone-pair on nitrogen is protonated, the octant behaviour of case (a) above (V) is changed to anti-octant, and the anti-octant behaviour of case (b) is increased. Examples are shown in Table 2.

The term 'anti-octant' is, of course, a relative one, referring in the present context to the observed effect of replacing a hydrogen atom by a particular substituent group, in those cases where the resulting change in the value of $\Delta\varepsilon$ is opposite in sign to that indicated by the octant rule in its simplest form.[4]

Table 2

Effect of Nitrogen Substituents on CD of Carbonyl Groups (Hudec[5])

V has lone-pair of nitrogen in 'W-path' relationship to carbonyl; the reference compound has —CH₃ in place of —NH₂; nitrogen has 'octant' effect. VI has lone-pair of nitrogen in 'skew-path' relationship with carbonyl; the reference compound has CH₂ in place of NH; nitrogen has 'anti-octant' effect.

		$\Delta\varepsilon$	λ (nm)	Solvent
V W-path	5α-NH₂, 6-CO-steroid	−7·0	310	Dioxan
	cf. 5α-CH₃, 6-CO-steroid	−3·9	288	MeOH
VI Skew-path	*trans*-Decahydroquinolin-7-one	0	288	MeOH
	ditto, HCl	−0·4	294	CHCl₃
	cf. *trans*-2-decalone	+1·4		MeOH

It is convenient to regard hydrogen as providing an arbitrary 'zero', that is, a dividing line between octant and anti-octant behaviour. We cannot at present conceive an experimental means for evaluating the contribution of a particular group or atom (e.g. hydrogen) *relative to nothing* in the same location.

C. Oxygen Functions

Several groups of workers have recently studied the effects of hydroxyl and acetoxyl groups 'α' to carbonyl. Enslin and colleagues[24] have provided a good series in the

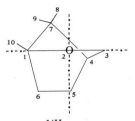 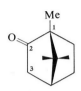

VII

A and B rings of steroids. Work done in our own laboratories[19] covers a series of hydroxy- and acetoxy-camphors (VII) with Professor Erdtman and Dr. Thoren of Stockholm. All of these groups, which are in bisectional positions (Table 3), give

Table 3

CD of Bornanone Derivatives: Summary of $\Delta\varepsilon$ Values and Differences ($\Delta\Delta\varepsilon$) (From Bartlett *et al.*[19])

Solvent: hexane. Principal CD maxima only are shown. Signs for $\Delta\Delta\varepsilon$ are 'anti-octant' in every case.

	λ (nm)	$\Delta\lambda$ (nm)	$\Delta\varepsilon$	$\Delta\Delta\varepsilon$
Hydroxy-groups				
Bornan-2-one	303	—	+1·50	—
endo-3-OH	320[a]	+17	+0·31[a]	−1·19
exo-3-OH	304	+1	+1·85	+0·35
Bornan-3-one	306	—	−1·46	—
endo-2-OH	317[b]	+11	−0·76[b]	+0·70
exo-2-OH	304	−2	−2·07	−0·61
Acetoxy-groups				
Bornan-2-one	303	—	+1·50	—
endo-3-OAc	325[c]	+22	+0·36[c]	−1·14
exo-3-OAc	304	+1	+2·18	+0·68
Bornan-3-one	306	—	−1·46	—
endo-2-OAc	327[d]	+21	−0·23[d]	+1·23
exo-2-OAc	308	+2	−2·34	−0·88

[a]–[d] Additional maxima of opposite sign at shorter wavelength, as follows:

	a	b	c	d
$\Delta\varepsilon$	−0·20	+0·16	−0·09	+0·35
λ (nm)	288	283	283	292

anti-octant effects; a few give bisignate curves. '*α*'-Alkoxy ketones available are too few in number to permit generalizations.

D. Halogens

The effects of '*α*'-axial halogen atoms on carbonyl groups were discovered very early in the pioneer studies of Djerassi;[25] it was early realized that fluorine gave effects of sign *opposite* to those for chlorine, bromine and iodine. Extensive studies have been made by Hudec[5] in this field, with collections of his own and published data. A very brief summary of the effects of halogens in '*α*', '*β*', '*γ*' and '*δ*' positions is given in Table 4 (formulae VIII–XI).

Table 4

Representative Values for CD Contributions of Halogen Atoms in Positions '*α*', '*β*', '*γ*' and '*δ*' to Carbonyl, see Formulae VIII to XI (Based on Data Collected by Hudec[5] and Snatzke.[17])

Examples for '*α*', '*β*' and '*δ*' are in cyclohexanone or *trans*-decalone systems; examples for '*γ*' are in camphor derivatives. W-paths joining carbonyl to halogens are shown in heavy lines. All data are $\Delta\Delta\varepsilon$ values.

Halogen position	Formula and symbol		F	Cl	Br	I
'*α*' eq.	VIII	W	−0·3	−0·2	−0·1	+0·2
'*α*' ax.	VIII	X	−1	+2·5	+4	+
'*β*' eq.	IX	Y	+0·2	−4	−8	−14
'*β*' ax.	IX	Z	0	+0·4	+0·5	+0·8
'*γ*' W-path	X	P	+0·8	−1·6	−4	−8
'*δ*' eq.	XI	Q	−0·6	+0·3	+1·0	+2·4
'*δ*' ax.	XI	R	−0·3	−0·5	−0·4	−0·2

These ideas on interactions through bonds are likely to be particularly fruitful, because they may allow us to link the chiroptical properties with other conformationally-sensitive physical properties such as NMR coupling constants[26] and with chemical reactivities, as measured, for example, by Hammett constants.[27]

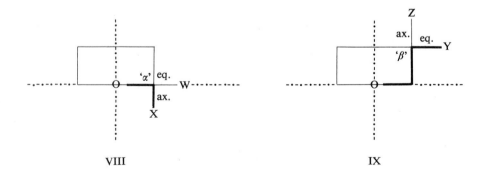

VIII   IX

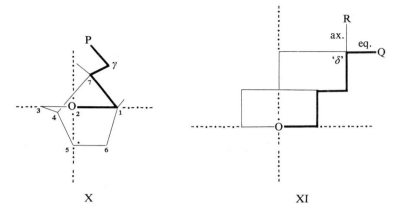

X   XI

E. Effects of Alkyl Substituents

Hudec[5] has dealt very ably with extensive series of hetero-substituents varying from nitrogen carrying a positive charge, through uncharged nitrogen, oxygen, and halogens to sulphur carrying a negative charge. One of us (D.N.K.), has been trying to rationalize the contributions of alkyl groups and rings in terms of *anti*-periplanar zig-zag paths as having the dominant contributions. Here the D-homosteroid ketones[21] are particularly valuable in providing strain-free reference compounds.

F. Wavelength Changes Caused by Substituents

From the early days of Djerassi's work,[25] it has been realized that hetero-atoms in 'α'-axial positions give a very striking change in the wavelengths of the CD maxima. These run parallel, as expected, with those of the unpolarized UV absorption. Since the UV maxima are often not very prominent, studies of the positions of the CD maxima might be valuable, even in problems where the chirality of the chromophore and its surroundings are not in question. The wavelength effects of alkyl substituents and other rings are generally small, and have been little investigated.

G. Octant versus Quadrant Rules

There is a long-standing argument regarding the nature of the regional rule for the carbonyl group; Octant *versus* Quadrant. Whatever the theoretical arguments may be (see reference 1, pp. 13–14) we feel that the experimental evidence is now slightly in favour of an Octant Rule, with front octants having contributions of *opposite* signs to those of the groups in rear octants (as originally proposed by Moffitt[4]).We have recently been able[28] to compare CD data for two 7-oxo steroids which provide a clear instance of 'front octant' effects. The des-D-5α-androstan-7-one (XII) provides a reference value ($\Delta\varepsilon$, $-0\cdot48$ in hexane) for a compound with the front octant regions unoccupied. Comparison with D-homo-5α-androstan-7-one (XIII) ($\Delta\varepsilon$, $+0\cdot17$) reveals a positive increment due to $C_{(15)}$ (and possibly also more remote parts of the ring D) lying in a front 'positive' octant.

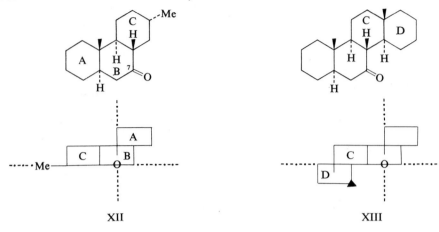

XII   XIII

The reality of front octant effects is supported by earlier published data for the 1-oxo-5α-steroid (XV) and the corresponding *trans*-1-decalone (XIV). A detailed mapping of front octant regions will clearly require studies on many more carefully selected compounds.

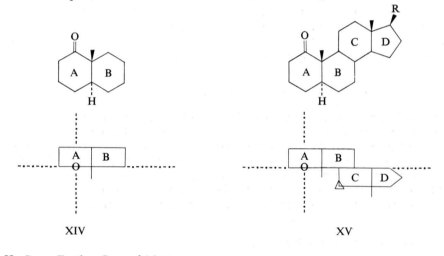

XIV   XV

H. Some Further General Matters

Before discussing applications, a few further points should be made. The complexity of theoretical treatments has been emphasized by Professor Weigang in Chapter 2.3. We need to ask our theoretical colleagues: 'What are the ranges of application of the various treatments?' or (to put the same question in a slightly different form) 'For which types of structure is each of the relevant factors dominant?'

Any treatment of a physical property for structural purposes in organic chemistry must involve dividing the structures into units or fragments which have characteristic values, at least until theoreticians are able to extend precise mathematical treatments to give a full description of the structures of complex molecules. If division into structural units cannot be done, or if the values are not reasonably additive, then the physical technique cannot be of general value to the structural organic chemist—

although it may well be fascinating for the physical chemist. This raises the question: 'What *are* the appropriate structural fragments?', and here ideas tend to change as knowledge of the subject accumulates.

3.1.6 Examples Illustrating Applications

Applications have been listed in the Introduction (3.1.1)

1–3. Applications of the chiroptical techniques to the *determination of absolute configuration* or *relative configuration* of a compound, or of the *position of a chromophore*, are now commonplace. Good examples from earlier work were given in a previous review (Klyne[29]), which formed part of the report of the 1965 NATO Summer School in Bonn. A few recent examples are the following:

(+)-Twistan-4-one; absolute configuration; Adachi *et al.*; Tichy and Sicher; Snatzke[30]
Coleone B (nor-diterpene); absolute configuration; Ribi *et al.*[30a]
3-Oxosteroids of 'abnormal' configuration; relative configurations; Bucourt *et al.*[31]
Zeorin (triterpene); relative configuration of side chain; Yosioka *et al.*[32]
Derivatives of steroidal saponin, ginsenoside Rg_1; position of carbonyl group; Nagai *et al.*[33]

4. Applications to *conformational problems* are discussed by Legrand in Chapter 4.1.

5. *Solvation*—Only a small proportion of the many thousand ketones examined have been studied in a range of solvents.

A study was made of a large number of ketones in this Department with Dr. S. R. Wallis several years ago.[34] Whatever the nature of interactions between solvent and chromophore, the diagram (Fig. 4) helps us to visualize the topography of the situation. For a wide range of substituents, or additional rings (except for the α-axial methyl group), the percentage difference

$$\frac{\Delta\varepsilon(\text{methanol}) - \Delta\varepsilon(\text{hexane})}{\Delta\varepsilon(\text{hexane})}$$

is approximately constant (20–25 %). For the 'α'-axial methyl (and methylene) groups the solvent effect is very much smaller. We have suggested that the different behaviour of 'α'-axial groups in this respect may result from their close proximity to the chromophore, whereas more remote groups, exerting their effect over greater distances, may be more dependent upon solvent character. This suggestion, however, avoids any assumption concerning the mechanism of interaction.

A better understanding of the interactions *within* molecules responsible for the chiroptical effects may lead to a new insight into solvent–solute interactions involving the carbonyl chromophore.

6. *Quantitative analysis*—References in the literature to the use of chiroptical measurements to determine concentrations—and hence e.g. equilibria or reaction rates—are few. The greatly improved precision of recent instruments may make such applications increasingly useful.

Several classical examples are in the literature;[35] a recent excellent example (not in the carbonyl field) is that of the plant-growth hormone abscisic acid, which can be measured in μg quantities thanks to its very high specific rotation at certain wavelengths.[36] Crabbé and co-workers have recently reported a quantitative study of the formation of acetals from steroid ketones and various alcohols.[37]

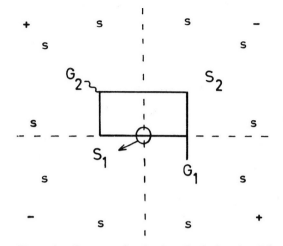

Fig. 4. Diagram illustrating dissymmetric solvation of substituted cyclohexanones; signs refer to rear octants (from Kirk *et al.*[34]). $G_1 G_2$, substituent groups; $S_1 S_2$, solvent molecules in positions 'enantiomeric' to $G_1 G_2$; s, other solvent molecules.

7. *Spectroscopic studies*—The great sensitivity of the chiroptical effects to small changes in molecular structure and geometry renders them a delicate tool for studies of the electronic transitions which give rise to these effects.

'Ordinary' (i.e. unpolarized) UV absorption curves of non-conjugated chromophores such as carbonyl do not as a rule yield much detailed information on the structure of a compound. For almost every new ketone, however similar it may be to known compounds, some IR and NMR data are given as a matter of course; however, the UV absorption is usually either not mentioned, or given as λ_{max} and ε_{max}; the reader usually cannot tell what is the shape of the curve (Gaussian character; half-width of band; presence or absence of fine structure; overlap with 'tails' of absorption bands at shorter wavelength).

Comparison of CD and UV curves in many laboratories has shown that, even if they are considered only as 'empirical patterns', the CD curves show much more marked differences between related compounds than do the (unpolarized) UV curves (Table 5).

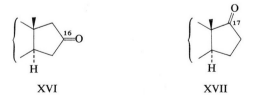

Table 5

Comparison of UV and CD Data for Two Types
of *trans*-Hexahydroindanones (Steroid 16- and
17-Ketones) (Based on Mason[10])

Position of CO group		Formula	
		XVI	XVII
UV			
λ		300	294 nm
$10^{-3}\ \nu$		33·3	34·0 cm^{-1}
ε		34	40
10^{40} D		575	520 c.g.s.
CD			
$\Delta\varepsilon$		−6	+3
10^{40} R		−17	+8 c.g.s.
g-Factor			
$\Delta\varepsilon/\varepsilon$		−0·18	+0·08

3.1.7 The Short Wavelength Band: 185–195 nm: Preliminary Comments

This has been attributed to the allowed n → σ* transition of the carbonyl group,[38] although the π → π* band, considered to occur at slightly shorter wavelength, may also be involved. This region of the spectrum has only recently become accessible for CD measurements, and UV spectra are virtually unknown except for simple ketones. CD measurements in the short wavelength region have recently been reported for (+)-3-methylcyclopentanone[14] (down to 165 nm) and for (*S*)-4-methyl-hexan-3-one[14a] (to 185 nm).

During 1970, Dr. E. Otto of Professor Snatzke's Department came and studied a series of about 50 ketones (mainly steroids) on our Jouan 185 Dichrograph; subsequently, some of these have been re-run on the Cary 60, which has enabled us to measure the curves to shorter wavelengths and given peaks in nearly all cases[39] (Table 6).

We now provisionally suggest that for six-membered ring ketones (except for the 1-, 7- and 11-oxosteroids where 'front octant' effects may occur) the results may be rationalized in terms of a normal 'octant' pattern as shown in Fig. 5A, with *large* contributions for 2-axial and 3-axial substituents, but only relatively *small* contributions for 2-equatorial or 3-equatorial substituents.

In *trans*-hexahydroindanones, *quasi*-axial substituents at the 2- or 3- positions again make large octant contributions, but the cyclopentanone ring makes its own contribution, as it does for the better known n → π* transition (Fig. 5B). Initial results indicate, however, that the *sign* of the cyclopentanone contribution at short wavelength is opposite to that in the n → π* transition. We suggest tentatively that the sign at short wavelength may be dominated by the *quasi*-axial 'α' hydrogen atoms, exerting an octant effect.

Many compounds show a preliminary weak band above 200 nm; no structural regularities are yet apparent.

Table 6

CD of Steroid Ketones at 185–195 nm

Values are for hexane solution. Figures in parentheses indicate the number of compounds examined. 'Predictions' are based upon dominant 'octant' contributions from 'α'- and 'β'- axial methyl groups.[39]

	$\Delta\varepsilon$	
Class of compound	Found	Predicted sign
Steroidal analogues of trans-decalones		
5α-1-one (1)	+3·7	(+)
19-nor-5α-2-one (1)	c. 0	Small
5α-2-one (2)	+3·7 to +5·2	(+)
5α-3-one (7)	c. 0 to +0·5	Small
5β,9β,10α-3-one (1)	c. 0	Small
5α-4-one (3)	−4·8 to −5·6	(−)
19-nor-5α-6-one (1)	−3·7	Small
5α-6-one (4)	+4·4 to +5·5	(+)
5α-7-one (2)	c. 0 to −2·6	a
D-homo-5α-7-one (1)	−4·3	a
11-one (7)	+3·6 to +5·6	a
12-one (4)	+4·3 to +10·5	(+)
D-homo-17a-one (2)	−5·3 to −6·1	(−)
Steroidal analogues of trans-hexahydroindanones		
A-nor-19-nor-5α-2-one (1)	−5·6	(−)
A-nor-5α-2-one (1)	c. 0	Small
5-Methyl-A-nor-5α-2-one (1)	+2·8	(+)
16-one (1)	c. 0	Small
17-one (2)	−7·5 to −9·4	(−)

a No prediction possible at present; may include 'front octant' contribution.

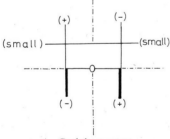

A. Cyclohexanones

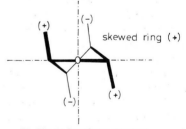

skewed ring (+)

B. Skewed cyclopentanones

Fig. 5. Octant-type projections for short-wavelength (n $\rightarrow$ σ*) band of ketones; signs for methyl and methylene groups in rear octants only.

3.1.8 Conclusion

For the organic chemist's most likely application of chiroptical techniques—the solution of a specific stereochemical problem concerning a ketone—our advice is to follow the octant rule in its original form, or one of the more sophisticated forms, and to use good analogies.

Our ultimate objective must be to reach as full an understanding of the chiroptical phenomena as possible, on the one hand for purely intellectual satisfaction, on the other hand because a deeper understanding, even of a highly complicated situation, ultimately reduces both the effort and the uncertainty in using the technique. Only when we arrive at an all-embracing rule, or set of rules, can we cease to feel encumbered by awkward doubts and exceptions as at present.

However, if the deeper understanding is not yet accessible, our standpoint is that of the family doctor—the 'General Practitioner'—as distinct from the medical specialist. Those of us whose interests range widely in the field of the chiroptical properties are presented with problems from colleagues which cover almost the whole range of organic chemistry, and especially natural products. We have to do our best to help them, with whatever tools and data are at present available.

The theoretical worker may perhaps be likened to the specialist in some branch of medicine, who restricts his attention to a particular organ. By careful study he may gain an intricate knowledge within his special field, but he should never ignore the fact that 'his' speciality, however important, is truly significant only as an integral part of the living organism, i.e. the patient.

In our case the living organism is organic chemistry, and it is essential that the specialist and the 'general practitioner' should cooperate to the full in the study and applications of chiroptical properties, for the benefit of organic chemistry as a whole.

Our thanks are due to Dr. P. M. Scopes, who has been in charge of the ORD/CD section of this Department for the last 11 years, and to the succession of research students and assistants who have done all the experimental work. Our thanks are equally due to the people in many laboratories all over the world who have made compounds and kindly put them at our disposal; this free exchange of materials and information is still one of the gratifying features of international science. We are indebted to the Science Research Council and the Medical Research Council for continuing support.

References

1. P. Crabbé, *An Introduction to the Chiroptical Methods in Chemistry*. Mexico, 1971. This work gives principal references for all topics.
2. P. Crabbé, *Applications de la Dispersion Rotatoire Optique et du Dichroïsme Circulaire Optique en Chimie Organique*. Gauthier Villars, Paris, 1968. This work gives full references for all topics.
3. P. M. Scopes, *Ann. Rep. Chem. Soc.* **66B**, 34 (1969); **67B**, 36 (1970); **68B**, 102 (1971).
4. W. Moffitt, R. B. Woodward, A. Moscowitz, W. Klyne and C. Djerassi, *J. Amer. Chem. Soc.* **83**, 4013 (1961).
5. J. Hudec, *Chem. Commun.* 829 (1970); M. T. Hughes and J. Hudec, *Chem. Commun.* 805 (1971); G. P. Powell and J. Hudec, *Chem. Commun.* 806 (1971).
6. A. I. Scott and A. D. Wrixon, *Tetrahedron* **27**, 4787 (1971); M. Fétizon, I. Hanna, A. I. Scott, A. D. Wrixon and T. K. Devon, *Chem. Commun.* 545 (1971); J. K. Gawronski and M. A. Kielczewski, *Tetrahedron Lett.* 2493 (1971); A. W. Burgstahler and R. C. Barkhurst, *J. Amer. Chem. Soc.* **92**, 7601 (1970).
7. E. G. Höhn and O. E. Weigang, Jr, *J. Chem. Phys.* **48**, 1127 (1968).

8. C. Coulombeau and A. Rassat, *Bull. Soc. Chim. Fr.* 516 (1971).
9. J. Levisalles and G. Teutsch, *Bull. Soc. Chim. Fr.* 263 (1971) and many previous papers.
10. S. F. Mason, *Quart. Rev. Chem. Soc.* **17**, 20 (1963).
11. O. E. Weigang, Jr, *J. Chem. Phys.* **43**, 3609 (1965).
12. A. Moscowitz, K. M. Wellman and C. Djerassi, *Proc. Natl. Acad. Sci. U.S.A.* **50**, 799 (1963).
13. D. J. Severn and E. M. Kosower, *J. Amer. Chem. Soc.* **91**, 1710 (1969).
14. G. Horsman and C. A. Emeis, *Tetrahedron* **22**, 167 (1966); S. Feinleib and F. A. Bovey, *Chem. Commun.* 978 (1968); O. Schnepp, E. F. Pearson and E. Sharman, *Chem. Commun.* 545 (1970).
14(a). L. Lardicci, P. Salvadori, C. Botteghi and P. Pino, *Chem. Commun.* 381 (1968).
15. K. M. Wellman, P. H. A. Laur, W. S. Briggs, A. Moscowitz and C. Djerassi, *J. Amer. Chem. Soc.* **87**, 66 (1965).
16. K. M. Wellman, E. Bunnenberg and C. Djerassi, *J. Amer. Chem. Soc.* **85**, 1870 (1963).
17. G. Snatzke and G. Eckhardt, *Tetrahedron* **24**, 4543 (1968); **26**, 1143 (1970).
18. A. H. Beckett, A. Q. Khokhar, G. P. Powell and J. Hudec, *Chem. Commun.* 326 (1971).
19. L. Bartlett, D. N. Kirk, W. Klyne, S. R. Wallis, H. Erdtman and S. Thorén, *J. Chem. Soc. C* 2678 (1970).
20. H. J. C. Jacobs and E. Havinga, *Tetrahedron* **28**, 135 (1972).
21. D. N. Kirk, W. Klyne, C. M. Peach and M. A. Wilson, *J. Chem. Soc. C* 1454 (1970); D. N. Kirk and M. A. Wilson, *J. Chem. Soc. C* 414 (1971); N. M. Jones, D. N. Kirk and W. Klyne. In preparation.
22. J. C. Bloch and G. Ourisson, *Bull. Soc. Chim. Fr.* 3011, 3018 (1964).
22(a). A simple optically active perhydroanthracene ketone has recently been prepared; F. Fernandez and D. N. Kirk, unpublished results.
23. D. E. Bays, G. W. Cannon and R. C. Cookson, *J. Chem. Soc. B* 885 (1966).
24. J. R. Bull and P. R. Enslin, *Tetrahedron* **26**, 1525 (1970).
25. C. Djerassi, J. Osiecki, R. Riniker and B. Riniker, *J. Amer. Chem. Soc.* **80**, 1216 (1958).
26. L. M. Jackman and S. Sternhell, *Applications of NMR Spectroscopy in Organic Chemistry*. Pergamon, London, 1969, p. 312.
27. J. Shorter, *Quart. Rev. Chem. Soc.* **24**, 433 (1970).
28. D. N. Kirk, W. Klyne and W. P. Mose, *Tetrahedron Lett.* 1315 (1972).
29. W. Klyne, in G. Snatzke, Ed., *Optical Rotatory Dispersion and Circular Dichroism in Organic Chemistry*. Heyden, London, 1967, p. 139.
30. K. Adachi, K. Naemura and M. Nakazaki, *Tetrahedron Lett.* 5467 (1968); M. Tichy and J. Sicher *Tetrahedron Lett.* 4609 (1969); G. Snatzke and F. Werner-Zamojska, *Tetrahedron Lett.* 4275 (1972).
30(a). M. Ribi, A. Chang Sin-Ren, H. P. Küng and C. H. Eugster, *Helv. Chim. Acta* **52**, 1685 (1969).
31. R. Bucourt, D. Hainaut, J. C. Gasc and G. Nominé, *Bull. Soc. Chim. Fr.* 1920 (1969).
32. I. Yosioka, T. Nakanishi, H. Yamauchi and I. Kitagawa, *Tetrahedron Lett.* 1161 (1971).
33. Y. Nagai, O. Tanaka and S. Shibata, *Tetrahedron* **27**, 881 (1971).
34. D. N. Kirk, W. Klyne and S. R. Wallis, *J. Chem. Soc. (C)* 350 (1970).
35. See e.g. N. L. Allinger, R. B. Hermann and C. Djerassi, *J. Org. Chem.* **25**, 922 (1960).
36. J. W. Cornforth, B. V. Milborrow and G. Ryback, *Nature* **210**, 627 (1966).
37. L. H. Zalkow, R. Hale, K. French and P. Crabbé, *Tetrahedron*, **26**, 4947 (1970).
38. H. L. McMurry, *J. Chem. Phys.* **9**, 231 and 241 (1941); P. G. Wilkinson, *J. Mol. Spectrosc.* **2**, 387 (1958).
39. D. N. Kirk, W. Klyne, W. P. Mose and E. Otto, *Chem. Commun.* 35 (1972).

CHAPTER **3.2**

The Carbonyl Chromophore: Unsaturated
Ketones and Lactones

G. SNATZKE

University of Bonn (F.R.G.)

and

F. SNATZKE (formerly WERNER-ZAMOJSKA)

Polish Academy of Sciences
Warsaw (PL)

3.2.1 Introduction

The chiroptical properties of simple saturated ketones can be explained on the basis
of the Octant rule,[1] either in its original form, or in a slightly modified one (twisted
cycloalkanones,[2] α-axial haloketones,[3] cf. Chapter 3.1[4]). It can not, however,
be applied to other types of ketones, for which different 'local' rules have had to be
developed. In order to understand these, a hypothesis has been put forward[5, 6]
which can be applied not only to ketones, but also to acid derivatives,[7] nitro compounds,[8] benzene derivatives,[9] etc. The molecule is divided into 'spheres' (Fig. 1);

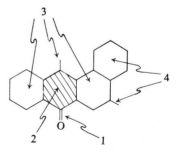

Fig. 1. Schematic representation of the different spheres
of a ketone.

the atoms of all spheres contribute to the Cotton effect within any absorption band,
but these contributions are not simply additive. That chiral sphere which is nearest
to the chromophore determines in most cases the sign and to a great extent even the
magnitude of the rotational strength.

3.2.2 The R-Band Cotton Effect

The first and second spheres are achiral in a cyclohexanone in the chair (or C_s-boat) conformation, and thus the distribution of atoms in the third (fourth, . . .) sphere determines the Cotton effect according to the Octant rule[1, 4] (A, Fig. 2).

Crossed conjugated cyclohexadienones have also C_s-symmetry of the ring and a Quadrant or Octant rule should, therefore, be applicable to this chromophore,

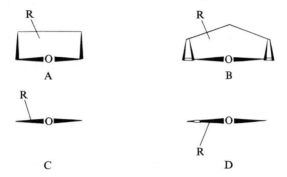

A

B

C

D

Fig. 2. Rules for R-band CD of oxo compounds with achiral first and achiral second sphere (all for positive CD).

    A: Octant rule for cyclohexanones in chair conformation.
    B: Crossed conjugated cyclohexadienones.
    C: Open-chain saturated oxo compounds.
    D: Open-chain conjugated oxo compounds with coplanar C=C—C=O grouping.

too, though the sign pattern need not necessarily be the same as in the common octant rule.[1] The negative CD of santonin (I) or $\Delta^{1,4}$-cholestadien-3-one (II) at about 350 nm supports the original sign distribution of the octant rule (B, Fig. 2).

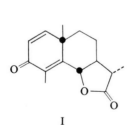

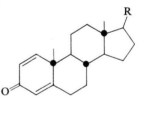

I   II

In the case of the missing second sphere (open-chain compounds), the usual octant rule[1] (C, Fig. 2) can be used to determine the third- (fourth-, . . .) sphere contributions to the n → π* CD, the signs are, however, inverted if a coplanar conjugated enone (D, Fig. 2) is involved.[10]

In a cycloalkanone in the twist conformation (with the C=O at the 'point' of the twist) the second sphere is chiral (C_2 symmetry) and this helicity of the second sphere determines the sign of the Cotton effect[2, 4] (E, Fig. 3). If an intermediate conformation is present, it is again the chirality of the ring which determines the CD (F, Fig. 3). It is not necessary to assume that all σ-bonds of the ring are of importance and the ring as such is responsible for the large Cotton effect caused by a chiral

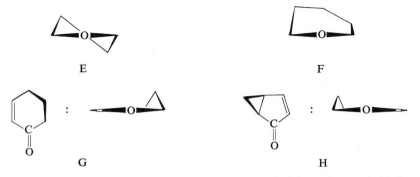

Fig. 3. Rules for R-band CD of oxo compounds with achiral first sphere and chiral second sphere (all for positive CD).

E: Twisted cycloalkanones (C=O coinciding with C_2 axis).
F: Twisted cycloalkanones (C=O not coinciding with C_2 axis).
G: Cyclohexenones with coplanar C=C—C=O grouping.
H: Bicyclo[3,1,0]hexenones,

second sphere, because we can interpret this situation in another, equivalent way. We can describe the CD of a ketone by taking into account the contributions from the β-, γ-, δ-, etc. atom (the α-atom cannot give any contribution because it lies in a nodal plane). If in a first approximation we take into consideration only the nearest atom which gives a contribution to the Cotton effect, i.e. the β-C-atom, then according to Fig. 4 we can say that a negative torsion angle (*I*) leads to a positive and a positive (*J*) one to a negative CD. The magnitude of this contribution will vary

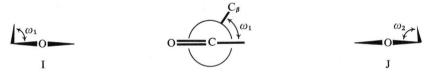

Fig. 4. Newman projection along C(=O)—C_α of a ketone and partial structures with negative (*I*) and positive (*J*) torsion angles ω leading to positive (*I*) and negative (*J*) Cotton effects (other interpretation of rules E and F).

with the torsion angle and is zero at least for $\omega = 0°$ and $\omega = 180°$. In a ring with C_s-symmetry as in a chair conformation the two contributions from the two sides of the ketone group compensate each other exactly and there remain only contributions from the 'third sphere'. In case E (Fig. 3) the two contributions have the same sign, whereas for F (Fig. 3) they compensate each other in part only. The torsion angle around the C(=O)—C_α- bond is, therefore, an equivalent description for the chirality of the second sphere, and indeed we have already used this view successfully in discussing the CD of nitro steroids.[8] The relatively strong CD of a 20-keto steroid[12] may also be explained on this basis.

Other examples for ketones with a chiral second sphere are cyclohexenones with a coplanar enone grouping[5] (G, Fig. 3) as e.g. steroids of type III or VII, and α',β'-methano-α,β-cyclopentenones (H, Fig. 3)[13] of the umbellulone type, as e.g. lumisantonin (VIII). Experiments show that the correlation between the sign

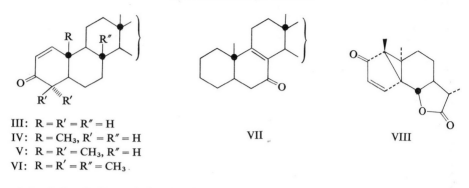

III: R = R′ = R″ = H
IV: R = CH₃, R′ = R″ = H
V: R = R′ = CH₃, R″ = H
VI: R = R′ = R″ = CH₃.

VII

VIII

of the R-band CD and the absolute configuration is that given in Fig. 3H. This observed sign inversion for homochiral saturated (F) *vs.* conjugated ketones (G) is in agreement with Kuriyama's[10] theory for the corresponding open-chain compounds.

In a molecule with noncoplanar enone grouping the π^*-orbital is inherently chiral, furthermore there will be a different electrostatic interaction between the (localized) π-orbitals of the C=C-bond and the n-orbital. One can thus expect that the chirality of the enone grouping (first sphere) will determine the sign of the R-band Cotton effect, and for transoid enones Whalley[14] has indeed found such a correlation (K, Fig. 5). We[5] have collected many more examples and have also

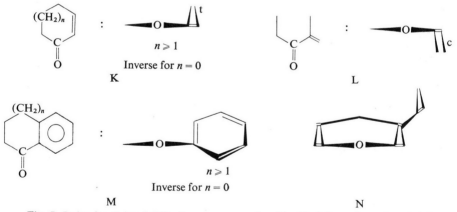

Fig. 5. Rules for R-band CD of oxo compounds with chiral first sphere, Part I (all for positive CD).

    K: Transoid noncoplanar enones.
    L: Cisoid noncoplanar enones.
    M: Acetophenone chromophore (C=O noncoplanar with benzene ring).
    N: Crossed conjugated trienones.

given a similar rule for cisoid noncoplanar enones (L, Fig. 5) as well as for the acetophenone type chromophore (M, Fig. 5). Formally, the latter follows the rule for the corresponding transoid (K, Fig. 5) and cisoid (L, Fig. 5) enones, but we should not like to see more than a mnemotechnic help to nature in this fact. The shape of the ring is not of great importance, only the torsion angle of the enone grouping. If it is really the chirality (helicity) of this first sphere, which determines the sign of the R-band Cotton effect then the rotational strength must increase with increasing torsion angle. This was indeed found experimentally[5] and is shown by a comparison of the CD of the Δ^1-en-3-ones III–VI. By increasing the steric repulsion between the axial methyl groups, the C=C—C=O grouping is more and more twisted and the respective $\Delta\varepsilon_{max}$ -values are[5] −0·81 (III), about −1 (average for several compounds of partial structure IV), −1·8 (V), and −3·2 to −3·7 (VI). Instead of repeating many examples[5] which illustrate these rules we shall give only three newer ones.

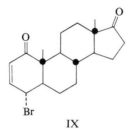

IX

An X-ray analysis[15] of the bromo diketone IX showed a conformation in the crystalline state with negative torsion angle within the ring around the $(C_{\alpha'})C(=O)$—C_α-bond.* If in solution the same conformer is preferred, the helicity rule (K, Fig. 5) gives the right result (negative R-band CD).[15] The bromine atom is thus without essential influence, as is the 'conjugated' N-atom in the enone multi-florine (X)[16]; though being a vinylogous lactam it follows the usual rule. The difference of $\Delta\varepsilon$-values for 5α- (+1·44 at 341 nm) and 5β-steroids (+2·56 at 333 nm) with 14α-hydroxy-Δ^7-en-6-one partial structure (XI) has frequently been used in the ecdyson series to determine the ring junction of rings A/B.[17]

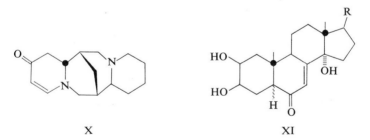

X   XI

The case of Δ^4-en-3-ones (XII–XXV) must be described in more detail. Three conformations have been discussed[18] for ring A (Fig. 6), two halfchairs a and b and one halfboat c. The first leads to a negative, the last two to a positive R-band CD. The change of sign from negative in the unsubstituted compound XII to positive

---

* For the isolated C(=O)—C=C moiety this corresponds to a *positive* torsion angle around the same bond. Viewed along the C_2 axis, this skewed system forms a left-handed screw (M-helix). A description of this situation as 'right-handed chirality' is meaningless if the mode of projection is not defined exactly.

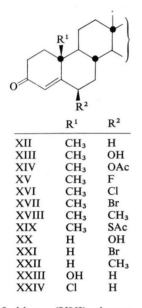

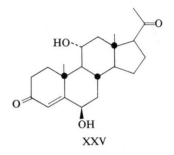

	R¹	R²
XII	CH₃	H
XIII	CH₃	OH
XIV	CH₃	OAc
XV	CH₃	F
XVI	CH₃	Cl
XVII	CH₃	Br
XVIII	CH₃	CH₃
XIX	CH₃	SAc
XX	H	OH
XXI	H	Br
XXII	H	CH₃
XXIII	OH	H
XXIV	Cl	H

XXV

for 6β-chloro- (XVI), -bromo- (XVII), -methyl- (XVIII), or -acetylthio-derivative (XIX) was interpreted originally [5, 14, 19] as being due only to steric interactions between the 19-methyl group and the bulky 6β-substituent, since the 6β-methyl-19-nor-steroid XXII, all 6α-substituted derivatives and those 6β-substituted ones, which have a small group in this position, like OH (XIII), OAc (XIV) or F (XV), do not show this sign inversion. The finding that the 6β-bromo-19-nor-steroid XXI also gives a positive R-band CD[20] led to another interpretation, viz. that such a γ-axial substituent of greater polarizability can also interact electronically, and a parallelism to the geometry of long-range NMR coupling has been proposed.[21]

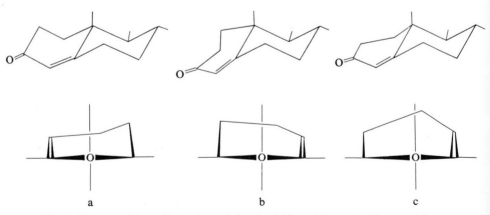

Fig. 6. Three possible conformations of ring A of Δ⁴-ene-3-keto steroids. a and b are halfchair conformations, c is a halfboat conformation.

The fact that 10-hydroxy- (XXIII) or 10-chloro-19-nor-testosterone (XXIV) give 'normal' negative Cotton effects shows that these abnormalities are indeed very sensitive to constitution and stereochemistry. Obviously in such cases the chromophore not only consists of the orbitals of the C=C—C=O moiety but also includes the σ-bond to the 6β-substituent. Steric and electronic effects are acting at the same time and the latter are most probably only of importance for groups with large polarizabilities (e.g. Br). Further support for the action of steric forces comes from the fact that neither a 6β-OH (XIII) nor an 11α-OH alone inverts the sign of the Cotton effect, though both influence the equilibrium between a, b, and c (Fig. 6), because $\Delta\varepsilon_{max}$ decreases in each case. Both actions together (XXV) suffice, however,

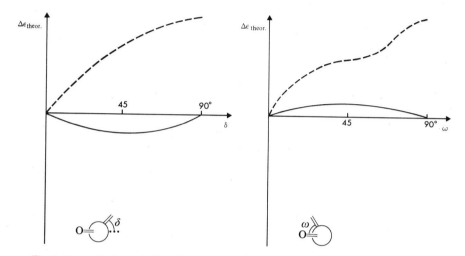

Fig. 7. Theoretical correlation of R- and K-band CD with chirality of the C=C—C=O moiety. δ is the angle describing the deviation from coplanarity of transoid enones, ω the torsion angle along C(=C)—C(=O) of cisoid enones. ———— R-band CD; - - - - - - - K-band CD.

to change the preferred conformation from a to b, as the CD of XXV is positive.[5] A substitution (even with polar groups) at the C=C double bond does not appreciably change the Cotton effects.[22]

The many examples investigated hitherto only very seldom show an exception to the rule (K, Fig. 5) and this can fairly safely be used for establishing the absolute conformation of the transoid noncoplanar C=C—C=O system. It has also been found to be applicable to cycloheptenones; with 5-membered rings, however, sign inversion takes place for transoid enones[5] (K, Fig. 5) as well as for 1-indanones (M, Fig. 5).[23] A theoretical calculation[24] of the correlation between the deviation from coplanarity of an (isolated) C=C—C=O 'chromophore' and the signs and magnitudes of R- and K-band CDs gave the result (Fig. 7) that for transoid as for cisoid enones that part of the n → π* band CD which comes from first-sphere chirality is greatest for a deviation of 45° from coplanarity, and goes to zero for the (chiral!) perpendicular arrangement of C=C to C=O. The calculated signs are in agreement with the experimentally found ones (K, L, Fig. 5). By calculating the

CD of real molecules Hug and Wagnière[24] found that due to other geometry of nodal surfaces a sign inversion is indeed expected for a chiral cyclopentenone. At

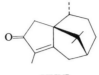

XXVI

present it is difficult for the chemist to predict the sign of the R-band CD of a cyclopentenone as e.g. cyperotundone (XXVI) with higher ring strain follows the 'cyclohexenone rule'.[25] Also, polar groups in the vicinity of the enone system can obviously

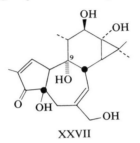

XXVII

influence the exact position of these nodal surfaces. Thus homochiral derivatives of phorbol (XXVII) give positive or negative Cotton effects depending on e.g. the acetylation of the OH at C-9.[26]

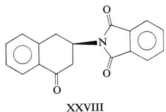

XXVIII

Examples for the acetophenone chromophore are taken from the flavanone series.[27-30] Compound XXVIII[28] whose absolute configuration is known without any doubt serves as a reference compound and shows a negative CD (−3·11) at 325 nm. (−)-Naringenin glucoside (XXIX), taxifoline (XXX) and astilbin (XXXI) belong to the heterochiral series and all give positive CDs in this wavelength range.

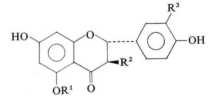

XXIX: R^1 = Glucose, R^2 = R^3 = H
XXX: R^1 = H, R^2 = R^3 = OH
XXXI: R^1 = H, R^2 = O-Rhamnose, R^3 = OH

As their configuration is known, too, the CD proves that the ring conformation is not strongly influenced by substitution even in the vicinity of the keto group. As in such keto compounds the nonaromatic ring may adopt three conformations,[27] viz. halfchair, sofa and deformed sofa, and the last two give opposite CD signs to the first one, within the R-band a prediction of the Cotton effect from models is not always unequivocal, especially for 2-substituted tetralones-1. The negative CD of

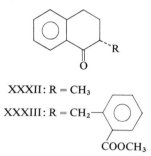

XXXII: R = CH₃

XXXIII: R = CH₂—

ĊOOCH₃

XXXII* and XXXIII[23] allows by mere comparison of the CD spectra the assignment of the absolute configuration at the chiral centre next to the carbonyl group of (−)-XXXIV[31] to be *R*. At room temperature the CD of (4*S*)-methyl tetralone-1

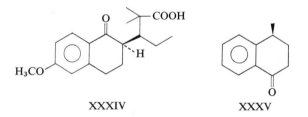

XXXIV   XXXV

(XXXV) is very weak with several positive and negative partial bands (Fig. 8), indicating in this case a conformational equilibrium, as at low temperature only a negative Cotton effect (with pronounced finestructure) is found.[27] Assuming an equatorial conformation for the side chain of indanones-1 like XXXVI, the 'inverse' rule M (Fig. 5) follows as for cyclopentenones.[23]

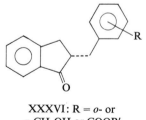

XXXVI: R = *o*- or
p-CH₂OH or COOR′

---

* In reference 27, a positive CD has been cited for (*S*)-XXXII, but repetition of this work has shown that it is in fact negative: private communication from Professor Kagan, Paris.

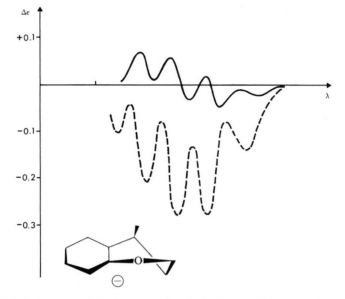

Fig. 8. CD of XXXV at +20°C (————) and −170°C (-----) in EPA solvent (5:5:2).

For linear dienones the conformation of the α,β-double bond determines the sign of the CD, its magnitude depends, however, also on the chirality of the C=C—C=C system.[5] The rule for crossed conjugated trienones (N, Fig. 5) is a logical extrapolation of the rule for enones (K, Fig. 5).[5]

β,γ-unsaturated ketones can give relative large dipole strengths within the n → π^* band if geometry allows for interaction between the respective orbitals and the same holds for the rotational strength.[32] According to Labhart and Wagnière[33] the n → π^* transition borrows intensity from the allowed π → π^* transition and the mechanism has been assumed to be either charge-transfer[34] or interaction of localized orbitals.[35] With optimal geometry (O, Fig. 9) $\Delta\varepsilon_{max}$-values up to 36 may be observed

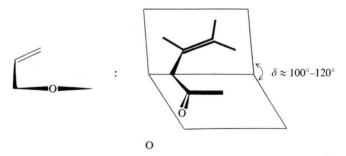

O

Fig. 9. Rules for R-band CD of oxo compounds with chiral first sphere, Part II (for positive CD).

O: β,γ-unsaturated oxo compounds.

(e.g. for santonide (XXXVII)[36]). The double bond may be replaced by a phenyl ring (e.g. XXXVIII, a = +303)[37] and the keto group by an aldehyde (e.g. laurolenal

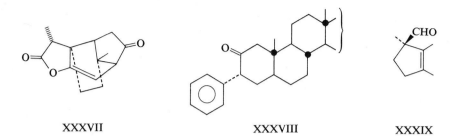

| XXXVII | XXXVIII | XXXIX |

XXXIX, $\Delta\varepsilon_{max} = +10\cdot30$).[38] This rule (O, Fig. 9) has sometimes been called the 'generalized octant rule'[32] though it is not yet proved whether in this case it is a quadrant rather than an octant rule.

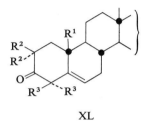

XL

For differently substituted Δ^5-en-3-ones (XL, R^1, R^2, R^3 being H or CH$_3$) $\Delta\varepsilon_{max}$-values of +0·6 to +1·9 have been described in the literature. Such small values do not justify the assumption of intensity borrowing,[33] and they can just be taken as a disproof of the conformation of Fig. 9 but not as a proof of absolute configuration.

A weaker interaction with the orbital system of the C=C group is exerted by 'conjugation' with a cyclopropane or an epoxy ring (P, Q, Fig. 10), but one can still speak of a chirality of the first sphere.[13, 39, 40] In most cases the rules of Fig. 10 are observed, but some exceptions[41, 42] are found if the chirality of the second

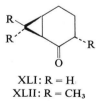

XLI: R = H
XLII: R = CH$_3$

sphere is much larger than that of the first and its CD is of opposite sign to that of the latter. Thus the difference in signs for homochiral α,β-methano-cyclohexanone (XLI)[42] and (+)-carone (XLII) are easily explained (cf. Fig. 11). Some β,γ-cyclopropyl ketones have been investigated by Lightner and Beavers.[43]

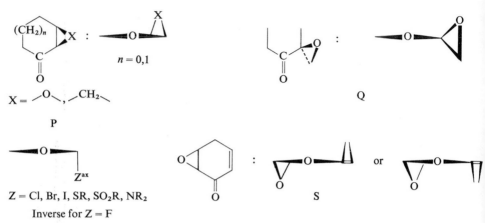

P: O, CH₂

Q

Z^{ax}

$Z = Cl, Br, I, SR, SO_2R, NR_2$

Inverse for Z = F

R

S

Fig. 10. Rules for R-band CD of oxo compounds with chiral first sphere, Part III (all for positive CD).

    P: Transoid cyclopropyl ketones and epoxy ketones.
    Q: Cisoid epoxy ketones.
    R: α-axially substituted ketones.
    S: Oxabicyclo[4,1,0] heptenones.

Only a very few examples exist of the chromophore of type Q (Fig. 10);[40, 44] α-axially substituted ketones of type R (Fig. 10), which are compounds containing a chiral first sphere, are the subject of Chapter 3.1.[4]

The simultaneous presence of an epoxide ring and a conjugated double bond create a new chromophore. If the larger ring is five-membered, rule H (O instead of

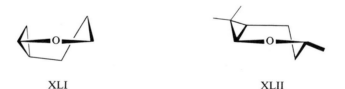

XLI   XLII

Fig. 11. Projection from O to C of carbonyl group of homochiral bicyclo(-4,1,0-)heptanone (XLI) and (+)-carone (XLII). For XLI, first-sphere chirality is weakly negative, and second-sphere chirality strongly negative; for XLII: first-sphere chirality negative and second-sphere chirality strongly positive.

CH_2) holds,[13] for six-membered rings (S, Fig. 10) experiment shows that formally the 'epoxide rule' (P, Fig. 10) is superior to the 'enone rule' (K, Fig. 5).[45] With the help of this rule the absolute configuration of panepoxydone (XLIII) could be established.[45] It is interesting to note that no sign inversion takes place for homochiral epoxide ketones by going from cyclopentanones to cyclohexanones.[46]

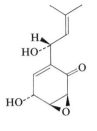

XLIII

The chiroptical properties of lactones etc. are the subject of another chapter of this book (3.3).[47] Here we shall mention only briefly those which contain a chiral first sphere; they can be treated in a similar way to the corresponding ketones,

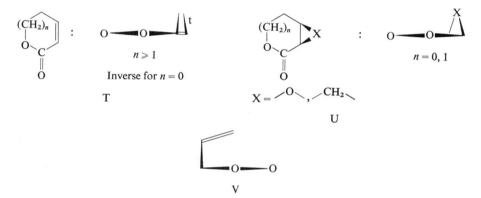

Fig. 12. Rules for R-band CD of acid derivatives with chiral first sphere (all for positive CD).

T: Transoid conjugated lactones with noncoplanar C(=O)—C(=C) moiety.
U: Cyclopropyl and epoxy lactones.
V: β,γ-unsaturated acid derivatives.

and the rules summarized in Fig. 12 (T, U, V) have also been established experimentally.[7, 48, 49]

3.2.3 The K-Band Cotton Effect

The chiral first sphere of noncoplanar transoid (W, Fig. 13) and cisoid (X, Fig. 13) conjugated enones has been treated as an 'inherently chiral chromophore'[50] by several authors[24, 51, 52] and it has been assumed that the helicity of the C=C—C=O moiety unequivocally determines the sign of the K-band ($\pi \to \pi^*$) Cotton effect (W, X, Fig. 13). Several exceptions have, however, been noticed[53] and it has been proposed that this helicity rule be replaced by an 'allylic axial chirality contribution rule'[53] (W', Fig. 13). The allylic axial substituents (hydrogen included) which are indicated in the partial formula contribute positively, the other three negatively to the Cotton effect, which would seem to be a violation of our general principles.

But these allylic axial bonds must obviously be included in the chromophore, so
that it extends over the whole grouping

$$\begin{array}{c} R'' \\ {>} \\ R' \end{array} C{=}C({-}R){-}C{=}O$$

which becomes the first sphere, and the chirality of that part with $(\pi - \sigma)$-conjugation
overcomes in general that of the part with $(\pi - \pi)$-conjugation. The two rules (K,

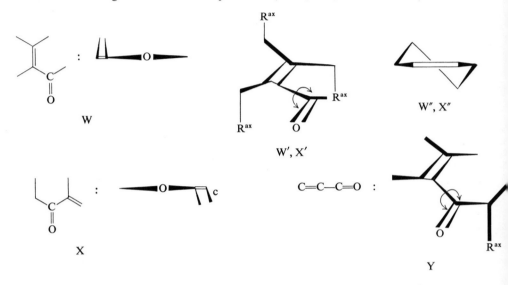

Fig. 13. Rules for short-wavelength CD bands of oxo compounds with chiral first sphere
(all for positive CD).

W: Transoid noncoplanar enones: enone helicity rule for K-band CD.
X: Cisoid noncoplanar enones: enone helicity rule for K-band CD.
W', X':   Allylic axial chirality contribution for K-band CD.
W", X";   Cycloalkene helicity rule for K-band CD.
Y: α'-axial chirality contribution to 210 nm CD band.

Fig. 5; W, or W', Fig. 13) can thus be generalized as follows. The R-band Cotton
effect is more sensitive to the conformation of the C=C—C=O system, and the
K-band CD more to the configuration around the same chromophore, because a

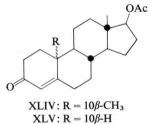

XLIV: R = 10β-CH₃
XLV: R = 10β-H
XLVI: R = 10α-CH₃

change from small positive to small negative torsion angles in the ring will not change appreciably the relative orientation of the allylic axial bonds. This situation is exemplified by the CD curves of the three testosterone derivatives XLIV–XLVI (Fig. 14).[54] The nearly equal magnitudes of the K-band CDs for XLIV and XLV suggests that either the 'cisoid' allylic group is less important than the 'transoid' one, or that a hydrogen atom and a methyl group give the same contribution to this Cotton effect. The published data can also be explained by a third rule (W″, X″, Fig. 13) which takes into account the helicity or chirality of the ring(s) containing the C=C-double bond only.

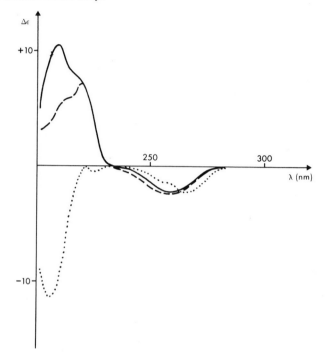

Fig. 14. CD curves of XLIV (———), XLV (-----) and XLVI (····). (Reprinted from F. Korte, Ed., *Methodicum chimicum*, vol. 1, chap. 5.7, Fig. 15, G. Thieme, Stuttgart, 1973, with permission.)

For conjugated cyclopentenones the situation is not yet fully understood because of lack of data; the CDs of both bands may either have opposite signs to each other, or the same signs (cf. e.g. reference 26).

Velluz, Legrand and Viennet[54] have shown that conjugated ketones do not only give two, but three Cotton effects; the one at shortest wavelengths (around 210 nm) coincides with a minimum in the corresponding UV-absorption curve and must thus be due to a forbidden transition (second n → π*?). Burgstahler and Barkhurst[53] have proposed that the sign of this Cotton effect may be governed by the axially disposed substituent (including H) in α'-position to the C=O group (Y, Fig. 13). The positive sign of this band for XLIV and XLV is thus compatible with conformation a (Fig. 6) as has been deduced from the R-band CD.

A special case of the enones is that of the cyclopropenones, as e.g. XLVII in which the first and second sphere must be achiral. A medium strong UV-absorption at 259 nm is optically active ($\Delta\varepsilon_{max} = -0.7$) and a second, positive, CD ($+0.2$) appears at 227 nm.[55]

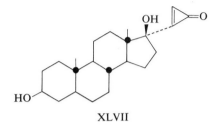

XLVII

Crossed conjugated dienones as I or II give three additional CD bands[54] besides that within the R-band absorption, no rules have however until new been suggested for this type of chromophore within the mentioned three bands.

Finally it should be mentioned that the K-band CD of some other ketones with a chiral first sphere has also been investigated; it has the same sign as the R-band CD for epoxido ketones,[41] but opposite for cyclopropyl ketones,[41] α-axial halogeno ketones,[56] and β,γ-unsaturated ketones.[57]

References

1. W. Moffitt, R. B. Woodward, A. Moscowitz, W. Klyne and C. Djerassi, *J. Amer. Chem. Soc.* **83**, 4013 (1961).
2. C. Djerassi and W. Klyne, *Proc. Natl. Acad. Sci. U.S.A.*, **48**, 1093 (1962).
3. C. Djerassi and W. Klyne, *J. Amer. Chem. Soc.* **79**, 1506 (1957).
4. This book, p. 89.
5. G. Snatzke, *Tetrahedron* **21**, 413, 421, 439 (1965); G. Snatzke, ed., *Optical Rotatory Dispersion and Circular Dichroism in Organic Chemistry*. Heyden, London, 1967, p. 208.
6. Cf. also Chapter 3.5 of this book, p. 173.
7. G. Snatzke, H. Schwang and P. Welzel, in R. Bonnett and J. G. Davis, eds., *Some Newer Physical Methods in Structural Chemistry*. United Trade Press, 1967, p. 159.
8. G. Snatzke, *J. Chem. Soc.* (*London*) 5002 (1965).
9. Chapter 3.4 of this book, p. 148.
10. K. Kuriyama, footnote on p. 461 of ref. 11.
11. W. Nagata and Y. Hayase, *J. Chem. Soc.* (*London*) C, 460 (1969).
12. K. M. Wellman and C. Djerassi, *J. Amer. Chem. Soc.* **87**, 60 (1965).
13. K. Schaffner and G. Snatzke, *Helv. Chim. Acta* **48**, 347 (1965).
14. W. B. Whalley, *Chemistry and Industry* 1024 (1962).
15. J. R. Hanson, T. D. Organ, G. A. Sim and D. N. J. White, *J. Chem. Soc.* C, 2111 (1970).
16. S. J. Goldberg and R. F. Moates, *J. Org. Chem.* **32**, 1832 (1967).
17. K. Nakanishi, M. Koreeda, S. Sasaki, M. L. Chang and H. Y. Hsu, *Chem. Commun.* 3191 (1967); M. Koreeda and K. Nakanishi, *ibid.*, 351 (1970).
18. K. Kuriyama, E. Kondo and K. Tori, *Tetrahedron Lett.* 1485 (1963).
19. R. Villotti, C. Djerassi and H. J. Ringold, *J. Amer. Chem. Soc.* **81**, 4566 (1959).
20. K. Kuriyama, M. Moriyama, T. Iwata and K. Tori, *Tetrahedron Lett.* 1661 (1968).
21. R. N. Totty and J. Hudec, *Chem. Commun.* 785 (1971).
22. J.-C. Bloch and S. R. Wallis, *J. Chem. Soc.* **B**, 1177 (1966).
23. M. J. Luche, A. Marquet and G. Snatzke, *Tetrahedron* **28**, 1677 (1972).
24. R. Hug and G. Wagnière, *Helv. Chim. Acta* **54**, 633 (1971).

25. H. Hikino, K. Aoto and T. Takemoto, *Chem. Pharm. Bull.* (*Tokyo*) **13**, 626 (1965), and own measurements.
26. E. Hecker *et al.* In preparation.
27. J. Barry, H.-B. Kagan and G. Snatzke, *Tetrahedron* **27**, 4737 (1971).
28. E. Dornhege and G. Snatzke, *Tetrahedron* **26**, 3059 (1970).
29. K. R. Monkham and T. J. Mabry, *Tetrahedron* **24**, 823 (1968).
30. W. Gaffield, *Tetrahedron* **26**, 4093 (1970).
31. J. C. Dubois, A. Horeau and H. B. Kagan, *Bull. Soc. Chim. Fr.* 1827 (1967).
32. K. Mislow, M. A. W. Glass, R. E. O'Brian, P. Rutkin, D. H. Steinberg, J. Weiss and C. Djerassi, *J. Amer. Chem. Soc.* **84**, 1455 (1962).
33. H. Labhart and G. Wagnière, *Helv. Chim. Acta* **42**, 2219 (1959).
34. R. C. Cookson, *Proc. Roy. Soc.* **A297**, 27 (1967).
35. A. Moscowitz, A. E. Hansen, L. S. Forster and K. Rosenheck, *Biopolymers*, Symposia No. 1, 75 (1964).
36. R. E. Ballard, S. F. Mason and G. W. Vane, *Trans. Faraday Soc.* **59**, 775 (1963).
37. R. C. Cookson and J. Hudec, *J. Chem. Soc.* 429 (1962).
38. G. Snatzke and K. Schaffner, *Helv. Chim. Acta* **51**, 986 (1968).
39. M. Legrand, R. Viennet and J. Caumartin, *C.R.H. Acad. Sci.* **252**, 2378 (1966).
40. C. Djerassi, W. Klyne, T. Norin, G. Ohloff and E. Klein, *Tetrahedron* **27**, 163 (1965).
41. K. Kuriyama, H. Tada, Y. K. Sawa, S. Itô and I. Itôh, *Tetrahedron Lett.* 2539 (1968).
42. R. K. Hill and J. W. Morgan, *J. Org. Chem.* **33**, 927 (1968).
43. D. A. Lightner and W. A. Beavers, *J. Amer. Chem. Soc.* **93**, 2677 (1971).
44. T. M. Feeley and N. K. Hargreaves, *J. Chem. Soc.* C, 1745 (1970).
45. Z. Kis, A. Closse, H. P. Sigg, L. Hruban and G. Snatzke, *Helv. Chim. Acta* **53**, 1577 (1970).
46. G. Snatzke, L.Lábler and Ch. Tamm, *Helv. Chim. Acta* **55**, 886 (1972).
47. W. Klyne, Chapter 3.3 of this book, p. 126.
48. G. Snatzke and E. Otto, *Tetrahedron* **25**, 2041 (1969).
49. W. Stoecklin, T. G. Waddell and A. Geissman, *Tetrahedron* **26**, 2397 (1970).
50. A. Moscowitz, K. Mislow, M. A. W. Glass and C. Djerassi, *J. Amer. Chem. Soc.* **84**, 1945 (1962).
51. C. Djerassi, R. Records, E. Bunnenberg, K. Mislow and A. Moscowitz, *J. Amer. Chem. Soc.* **84**, 870 (1962).
52. Cf. also E. Charney, H. Ziffer and U. Weiss, *Tetrahedron* **21**, 3121 (1965).
53. A. W. Burgstahler and R. C. Barkhurst, *J. Amer. Chem. Soc.* **92**, 7601 (1970).
54. L. Velluz, M. Legrand and R. Viennet, *C.R.H. Acad. Sci.* **261**, 1687 (1965).
55. P. Crabbé, *Proc. Natl. Acad. Sci., U.S.A.* **66**, 232 (1970).
56. K. Kuriyama, T. Iwata, M. Moriyama, M. Ishikawa, H. Minato and K. Takeda, *J. Chem. Soc.* C, 420 (1967).
57. Cf. e.g. D. E. Bays, R. C. Cookson and S. McKenzie, *J. Chem. Soc.* B, 215 (1967); D. E. Bays and R. C. Cookson, *ibid.*, 226 (1967).

The Carboxyl and Related Chromophores

W. KLYNE and P. M. SCOPES

Westfield College
London NW3 7ST, U.K.

3.3.1 Introduction

A previous chapter (3.1) dealt with the saturated carbonyl group, which is not only well explored experimentally, but is a functional group for which the theoretical knowledge of the transition involved in the absorption and CD bands is essentially adequate. For the groups which form the subject of the present chapter, this is unfortunately not the case; however, many references will be found in the collected data in the literature.[1-3]

The chromophores include carboxyl itself, the carboxylate anion, the ester group, and the ester group in cyclic form, i.e. the lactone group. In parallel with these we have the corresponding functions in which one oxygen atom is replaced by nitrogen, i.e. the amide, substituted amide and lactam groups. The related peptide group will be dealt with mainly in later chapters about polymers. Other less common variants in this class include the acid anhydride and imide.

Amides (UV)

$n_0 \rightarrow \pi^*$ 220 nm

$\pi_1 \rightarrow \pi^*$ 190 nm

	λ (nm)	$10^{-3}.\varepsilon$
$R \cdot CONH_2$	185	
$Me \cdot CONHMe$	187	8·8
$Me \cdot CONMe_2$	195	9·4

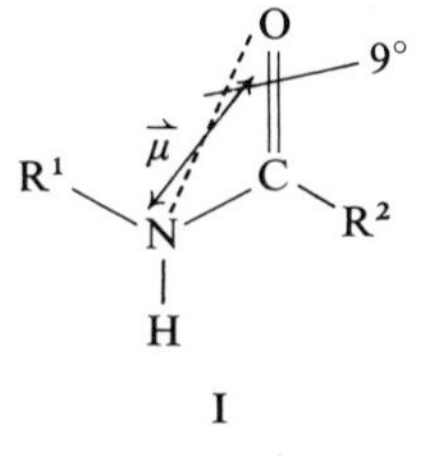

I

The available data, which are considerable but still inadequate, will be summarized here. The tentative regional rules also will be presented, in order to provide guide lines for further work. The incompleteness of the picture does not of course invalidate any simple arguments based on close analogy.

Recent literature suggests that the transitions involved in the absorption of carboxyl and lactone groups in the region of 190–220 nm are not well understood.

Table 1

Ultraviolet Absorption of Compounds Containing Carboxyl, Amide and Related Groups
Solvents: E, ethanol; HC, hydrocarbon (hexane, isooctane or cyclohexane); M, methanol; W, water.

Type and individual compound	Solvent	λ_{max} (nm)	ε	Ref.
A. *Carboxylic acids*				
Acetic acid	W	204	38	b
2-Chloropropanoic acid	M	220	90	24
2-Bromopropanoic acid	M	230	260	24
B. *Salts (carboxylate anions)*				
Acetate anion	W	No maximum		b
C. *Esters*				
Ethyl acetate	W	204	60	b
	HC	211	58	c
Methyl acetate	HC	210	57 ⎫	
	E	207	57 ⎬	c
	W	203	61 ⎭	
Methyl hexanoate	HC	212	63 ⎫	d
	M	209	66 ⎭	
D. *Lactones*				
1. *γ-Lactones; five-membered rings*				
Butanolide (butyrolactone)	HC	214	25 ⎫	c
	M	208	40 ⎭	
α-Campholide	HC	220	70	e
D-Ribono-γ-lactone	W	217	79	18
2. *δ-Lactones; six-membered rings*				
Pentanolide (valerolactone)	HC	222	40	f
	M	214	55	d
5-Decanolide	HC	221	50	29
Diterpene lactone (13 → 8)	HC	223	48 ⎫	f
	E	213	59 ⎭	
Lactide	M	207	115ᵃ	g
E. *Amides*				
Acetamide	W	182	7600	h
N-Methylacetamide	W	187	8800	i
N,N-Dimethylacetamide	W	195	9360	i
	HC	196	6850	h
N-Acetylpyrrolidine	W	197	9100 ⎫	h
	HC	200	7100 ⎭	
Pyrrolidin-2-one	W	190	7400 ⎫	h
	HC	185	6250 ⎭	

Table 1—*continued*

Type and individual compound	Solvent	λ_{max} (nm)	ε	Ref.
F. *Imides*				
Glutarimide	W	250 sh	—	b
		230 sh	—	
		201	18,000	
Succinimide	W	238	87	b
		193	19,400	
N-Methylsuccinimide	W	235	125	b
		201	17,400	

References

[a] For *each* of two lactone groups.
[b] H. H. Perkampus *et al*. Eds., *The DMS U.V. Atlas of Organic Compounds*, Vol. I. Butterworths–Verlag Chemie, 1971. [c] W. D. Closson and P. Haug, *J. Amer. Chem. Soc.* **86**, 2384 (1964). [d] W. D. Closson, P. J. Orenski and B. M. Goldschmidt, *J. Org. Chem.* **32**, 3160 (1967). [e] A. F. Beecham and R. R. Sauers, *Tetrahedron Lett.* 4763 (1970). [f] G. Lindsay, Ph.D. Thesis, Glasgow, 1970. [g] R. C. Schulz and J. Schwaab *Makromol. Chem.* **87**, 90 (1965). [h] E. B. Nielsen and J. A. Schellman, *J. Phys. Chem.* **71**, 2297 (1967). [i] W. B. Gratzer, W. Rhodes and G. D. Fasman, *Biopolymers*, **1**, 319 (1963).

Some UV absorption data for typical carboxyl compounds and derivatives are presented in Table 1. A better picture is perhaps available of the amide (I, $R^1 = H$) or peptide (I, $R^1 = $ alkyl) groups in terms of an $n \rightarrow \pi^*$ band near 220 nm and a $\pi \rightarrow \pi^*$ band near 190 nm (split in polymers) as discussed by Gratzer[4, 5] (see Fig. 1). Here the work on simple compounds has been greatly aided by extensive studies on regular polymers.

When we turn to the carboxyl and related groups containing two oxygen atoms, we have no sound theoretical backing and as yet rather scanty empirical knowledge to help us to interpret the CD curves. There is even less systematic work on the unpolarized absorption spectra of carboxyl compounds than on those of ketones. One significant recent paper on the absorption spectra of acids and related compounds is that of Basch *et al*.[6] Here, and in our own specialized sphere of chiroptical measurements, we are restricted by the fact that the absorption and CD bands of carboxyl and related groups are rather near to the lower limit of penetration even of modern instruments.

A further important factor which complicates the situation is the lack of firm knowledge about the preferred conformations even of six-membered lactone groups in solution. The data available from X-ray measurements indicate that some six-membered lactone groups approximate to a half-chair form, and others to a half-boat—and there is no clear rule by which one can decide which conformation will be preferred;[7–10] some references are given in Table 2. Various intermediate forms are also possible; furthermore we are all aware of the fact that the conformation of a flexible molecule in solution is not necessarily the same as that in the crystal—although this does not mean to say that it is necessarily different—and it is convenient to think initially with reservations, in terms of the crystal structure.

Professor H. Wolf has emphasized the generalization, suggested by him in 1966, viz. that for six-membered lactones the half-boat was the preferred conformation

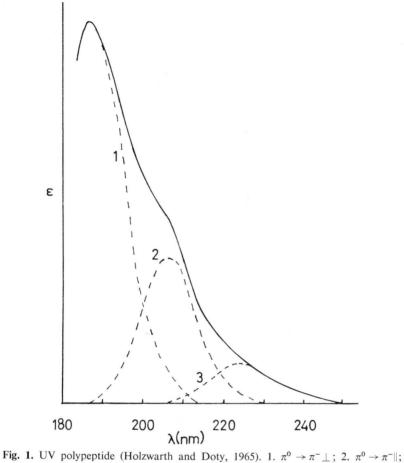

Fig. 1. UV polypeptide (Holzwarth and Doty, 1965). 1. $\pi^0 \to \pi^- \perp$; 2. $\pi^0 \to \pi^- \|$; 3. $n_1 \to \pi^-$.

Table 2

Suggested Conformations of δ-Lactones

Preferred conformation	Evidence	Date	Reference
Half-boat	X-ray	1963	Mathieson[8]
Half-boat (unless 'flag-pole' substituent present)	ORD/CD	1965–6	Wolf[16]
Half-chair (half-boat in special cases)	X-ray and IR	1965	Cheung, Overton and Sim[7a]
Half-chair (flattened)	NMR, chemical (and IR)	1968	Sheppard and Turner[7b]
Detailed survey of 6 natural products (comment on non-planar lactone groups)	X-ray	1970	McKechnie, Kubina and Paul[9]
Half-boat	X-ray (also CD)	1970	Meier[10]

except when this conformation would put a substituent in a flag-pole position; in such cases the half-chair conformation is preferred (cf. reference 16). It seems to us that although this statement may perhaps be generally valid, there is at present insufficient evidence to show that it is always true.

This lack of a firm basis for empirical correlations has been a major hindrance to progress. Whatever arguments we may have about the nature of the interaction between surroundings and chromophore, and whatever form we may give to a Quadrant or Octant Rule for the carbonyl group, its basic symmetry is known (C_{2v}). Furthermore, we know from many other physical and chemical properties that we can approximate the true conformation of a very large proportion of cyclohexanones by something which is close to a perfect chair.

With the lactone, lactam and derived functions the situation is very different. The only symmetry element is a plane (Schellman[11]) and the disposition of the immediate surroundings (corresponding to the cyclohexanone ring for ketones) does not follow any simple or consistent pattern. We must therefore proceed, perhaps for some time, by amassing data and evolving empirical rules, before we can hope to develop a general treatment for those groups. (We expressed very similar views in 1965 at the Bonn meeting,[12] and the lack of better generalizations today is perhaps disappointing. No major proposals were offered in the discussions after this paper).

3.3.2   Rules for Lactones, Acids and Related Chromophores and their Fields of Application

A. Sector Rule (Klyne and Scopes)

This approach[13] was based on ideas developed by Moscowitz from the octant rule for ketones. It has been widely applied for lactones,[13] esters and free carboxylic acids,[14] but lacks a definite basis for sector boundaries. The disadvantage of this approach is its over-emphasis on the partial double-bond character of the (O:)C—O bond, by treating it as an alternative 'carbonyl' for the octant rule, see Figs. 2 and 3.

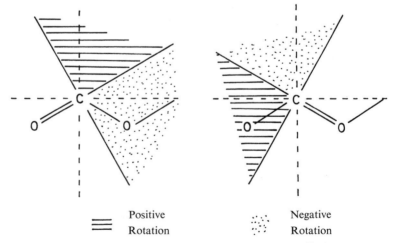

	Positive		Negative
═	Rotation	⋰⋰	Rotation

Fig. 2. Derivation of Sector Rule (Jennings *et al.*[13]).

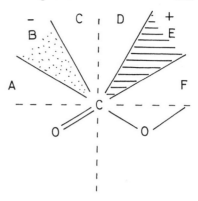

Fig. 3. Sector Rule (Jennings *et al.*[13]).

The Sector Rule has served well, but there is an undoubted need for a synthesis of this and other concepts, to give a broader picture.

B. *Alternative Sector Rule ('Comet' Rule: Snatzke)*

This takes an alternative view of the lactone chromophore, which it treats as a perturbed carbonyl group,[15] thereby under-estimating the partial double-bond character of the bond between carbon and the alkoxy oxygen (see Fig. 4). For most compounds this rule gives the same predictions as the previously mentioned Sector Rule.

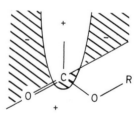

Fig. 4. Sector (Comet) Rule: Signs for upper
sectors (Snatzke *et al.*[15]).

C. *Ring Chirality Rules (Wolf; Legrand; Beecham)*

In most five- and six-membered lactone rings the ring itself is chiral, and three groups of workers have proposed rules[16–18] according to which the chirality of the ring, or in other words the position of one or two key atoms with reference to the chromophore, determines the sign of the lactone Cotton effect, see Fig. 5. This qualitative statement is broadly true—but to give a quantitative picture more than this is needed. We may note for further study: (i) the significant $\Delta\varepsilon$ values of some five-ring lactones which are rigidly fused to other rings and which must be almost planar; (ii) the not inconsiderable contributions of substituents in the lactone ring. In terms of Snatzke's 'Doctrine of Spheres', we may say that the first sphere (the chiral lactone-ring) dominates the picture, but that the second and third spheres cannot be neglected.

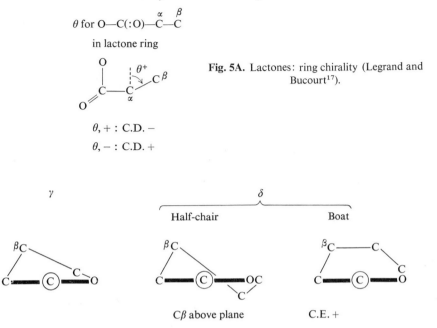

$$\theta \text{ for } O—C(:O)—\overset{\alpha}{C}—\overset{\beta}{C}$$

in lactone ring

$\theta, + : \text{C.D. } -$

$\theta, - : \text{C.D. } +$

Fig. 5A. Lactones: ring chirality (Legrand and Bucourt[17]).

γ

δ

Half-chair   Boat

$C\beta$ above plane   C.E. +

Fig. 5B. Lactones: ring chirality (Wolf; Legrand; Beecham[16-18]).

The Doctrine of Spheres is just one way of saying that the nature and position of atoms or bonds nearest to the chromophore have the greatest influence on the observed circular dichroism; sector rules (with whatever quantitative detail can be added) are another way of saying the same thing. Because of the conformational problems, these additional quantitative details are vastly more difficult to assess in the carboxyl–lactone field than in the ketone field.

It may be that, after a further period of exploration, methods of thinking based on bond-character (as for ketones, see Chapter 3.1) will provide the overall view required.

D. New Sector Rules for Lactams and Lactones

Professor O. E. Weigang has discussed in Chapter 2.3 a new Sector Rule for lactams, the pattern of which is illustrated in Fig. 6. This figure shows the sector boundaries for the lactam chromophore, and signs for alkyl group contributions to the Cotton effect in upper sectors. The chromophore is viewed (as for the Moscowitz Sector Rule) along the bisectrix of the O=C—N angle, and also from above, in projection on the lactam plane. The treatment considers the lactam group as a perturbed modification of the carboxylate anion which itself has C_{2v} symmetry (Fig. 6A). For small perturbation there is a curved sector boundary shown schematically in Fig. 6B; with greater perturbation the boundary would close round on itself (Fig. 6C), or even vanish, giving a quadrant rule (Fig. 6D) for some hitherto unexplored or unsuspected chromophores.

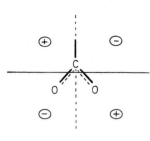

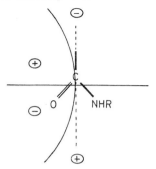

A. Carboxylate Ion

B. Small Perturbation

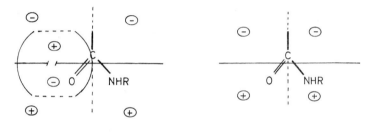

C. Moderate Perturbation

D. Infinite Perturbation

Fig. 6.

E. Planar and Quadrant Rules (*Schellman; Weigang*)

Planar and quadrant rules for the —CONH— chromophore particularly in peptides have been discussed by Schellman.[19] The peptide quadrant rule is shown schematically in Fig. 7.

Fig. 7. Peptide Quadrant Rule. Vertical surface not planar (Schellman[19]).

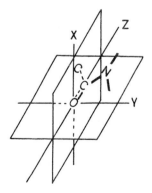

F. Coupling of Electric and Magnetic Moments in Two Chromophores: 'μ-m' mechanism (Tinoco; Schellman)

The μ-m treatment of Tinoco[20] and Schellman[11] is necessarily applicable only to compounds containing two identical or very similar chromophores, and is shown schematically in Fig. 8. It has been used chiefly for diketopiperazines but the large CD value for lactide studied by Toniolo *et al.*[21] ($\Delta\varepsilon - 5\cdot4$ at *c.* 220 nm) may perhaps be rationalized by this treatment. The application of bonding pattern ideas may also be of value here.

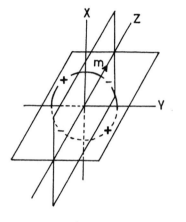

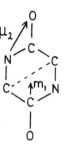

$n \rightarrow \pi^*$ transition.
Quadrupole and
magnetic moments

Diketopiperazine
μ_2 interacts with m_1

Fig. 8. *μ-m* Mechanism.

3.3.3   Factors for Consideration

The general factors mentioned in dealing with the carbonyl group (Chapter 3.1) are also of importance here, viz. rotational strengths, dissymmetry factors, bisignate curves, fine structure, solvent effects and temperature effects.

The suspicion that we may be dealing with two or more transitions in the short wavelength region for carboxyl and related groups makes the interpretation of any series of measurements all the more difficult.

Bisignate curves in carboxyl and related compounds may be due not only to a pair of conformations, or a combination of solvated and unsolvated forms, but also possibly to the existence of two different transitions in the same region of the spectrum. This must be considered an open question, at any rate for curves showing two features in the region below about 220 nm; for curves showing a small band at higher wavelengths (*c.* 240 nm) the explanation is probably to be sought in conformations or solvation (see below). Solvent effects are undoubtedly of much greater importance for carboxyl compounds than for ketones, especially for free carboxylic acids.

3.3.4 Survey of Data

The logical progression followed successfully in the ketone series was from *trans*-decalones to *cis*-decalones to (monocyclic) cyclohexanones and finally to open-chain ketones, with branches leading to cyclopentanones and cyclic ketones of other sizes; this represented a progression from almost rigid to very flexible structures.

Table 3

General Classification of Lactone Steric Types

Formula	Name	Conformational features
	1-Oxa-2-oxo-*trans*-decalin	Rigid
	2-Oxa-1-oxo-*trans*-decalin	Rigid
	2-Oxa-3-oxo-*trans*-decalin	Rigid
	1-Oxa-2-oxo-*cis*-decalin (a) Angular substituent X, axial with respect to C₉—O bond. (b) Angular substituent X-equatorial with respect to C₉—O bond.	Flexible if bicyclic; rigid if *trans*-fused to another six-membered ring
	2-Oxa-1-oxo-*cis*-decalin (a) Angular substituent X, axial with respect to C₉—C₁ bond. (b) Angular substituent X, equatorial with respect to C₉—C₁ bond.	Flexible if bicyclic; rigid if *trans*-fused to another six-membered ring
	2-Oxa-3-oxo-*cis*-decalin. (a) Angular substituent X, axial with respect to C₉—C₁ bond. (b) Angular substituent X, equatorial with respect to C₉—C₁ bond.	Flexible if bicyclic; rigid if *trans*-fused to another six-membered ring

Table 3—*continued*

Formula	Name	Conformational features
	1-Oxa-2-oxo-*trans*-hexahydroindane	Rigid
	2-Oxa-1-oxo-*trans*-hexahydroindane	Rigid
	1-Oxa-2-oxo-*cis*-hexahydroindane	Lactone ring essentially planar: flexible if bicyclic; rigid if *trans*-fused to another six-membered ring
	(a) Angular substituent X, axial with respect to O—C_8 bond. (b) Angular substituent X, equatorial with respect to O—C_8 bond.	
	2-Oxa-1-oxo-*cis*-hexahydroindane	Lactone ring essentially planar. flexible if bicyclic; rigid if *trans*-fused to another six-membered ring
	(a) Angular substituent X, axial with respect to O=C—C_8 bond. (b) Angular substituent X, equatorial with respect to O=C—C_8 bond.	
	1-Oxa-2-oxo-*trans*-[3,3,0]-bicyclooctane	Rigid (strained)
	2-Oxa-1-oxo-*trans*-[3,3,0]-bicyclooctane	Rigid (strained)
	1-Oxa-2-oxo-*cis*-[3,3,0]-bicyclooctane	Rigid
	2-Oxa-1-oxo-*cis*-[3,3,0]-bicyclooctane	Rigid

A similar progression will probably be followed in the carboxyl and related series; but with the difference that the initial basis is not so rigid and not of such well-defined geometry. Many of the compounds are conveniently considered as oxa- or aza-analogues of the corresponding ketones. An alternative logical, but in practice inconvenient, starting point is the carboxylate anion with its C_{2v} symmetry. This cannot however, be 'rigidified' and the preparation of salts on a milligram scale from rare compounds presents experimental difficulties.

A. Lactones

Table 3 shows the principle of such a classification of lactones. Only the most recent references are given here; for others see references 1 (pp. 75–77), 2, 3 and 22.

Only a few selected examples can be discussed here, but the classification shown in Table 3 is an attempt to provide an overall picture which will always be valid whatever mechanism and 'rules' are ultimately found appropriate for the CD of the lactone chromophore. A more detailed survey according to this classification will be published elsewhere.[23]

Table 4

CD Data for Some Steroid Ring-A Lactones
Solvent: methanol

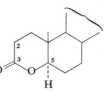

Substituents	$\Delta\varepsilon$	λ (nm)	Conformation	
			Ring	2-Substituents
None	+2·0	212	HB	—
2β-Me	+4·9	217	HB	eq.
2α-Me	$\begin{matrix} -0·3 \\ +0·7 \end{matrix}$	$\begin{matrix} 240 \\ 210 \end{matrix}$	$\begin{matrix} HC \\ HB \end{matrix}$	eq.
2β-Br	+4·1	214	HB[a]	eq.
2α-Br	+1·5	240	HC[a]	eq.

HB = half-boat; HC = half-chair. [a] Half-boat in solid; X-ray, Meier and Noack.[23a]

Table 4 summarizes results obtained in our laboratory for compounds kindly provided by Dr. W. Meier and Dr. K. Noack of F. Hoffmann-La Roche of Basel. CD results obtained in the Roche laboratories will be published elsewhere.[23a] These compounds which are oxa-*trans*-decalones provide us with reference values for structures some of which are known to be 'half-boats', at any rate in the crystalline state; they also give reference data for the CD contributions ($\Delta\Delta\varepsilon$ values) of methyl and bromine substituents 'α' to a lactone carbonyl.

Table 5 contains data for two series of oxa-hexahydroindanones which illustrate the dominance of the ring-chirality effect. Where the shape of the lactone-ring is reasonably certain, the ring-chirality rule is generally followed. Pairwise comparisons

Table 5

CD Data for Some *trans*-Fused Oxa-hexahydroindanones

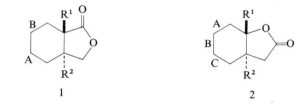

| 1 | 2 |

Type and general formula	Substituents	$\Delta\varepsilon$	λ (nm)
1. 16-Oxa-17-oxosteroid	R^1 = Me, R^2 = H; ring at A	+1·6	217–224
1. 16-Oxa-15-oxosteroid	R^1 = H, R^2 = Me; ring at B	+1·8	219–224
2. Enantiomer of eudesmane 12 → 6-lactones	R^1 = R^2 = H, ring at A	−1·0	217–220
2. Eudesmane 12 → 8-lactones	R^1 = R^2 = H; ring at B	−2·9	217
2. 17-Oxa-17-oxosteroid	R^1 = Me, R^2 = H; ring at C	−1·6	216

are most important in the present state of our knowledge of lactones. They suggest some preliminary thoughts regarding the contributions of substituents and of rings beyond the immediate environment of the chromophore.

A survey of λ_{max} values and the incidence of bisignate curves suggests that the use of the Curve Resolver in analysing curves which are (or might be) complex might help if we had some reference values for compounds of absolutely certain and fixed conformations.

B. Lactone–Lactam Comparisons

Spurred on by Professor Weigang's interest, we have been collecting CD data on pairs of corresponding lactones and lactams; unfortunately, few steroid or terpene lactams are available. What compounds we have (many of them from Dr. C. H. Robinson of Johns Hopkins University, Baltimore) suggest that for some rigid compounds a lactone and its corresponding lactam have CD maxima at about 220 nm of *opposite* signs. We understand from Professor Weigang that his latest theoretical treatment can easily rationalize this. Some results for rigid lactams are collected in Table 6. For a few flexible compounds however, the lactone and lactam have the same sign (see also comments on *O*-acetyl and *N*-acetyl compounds in Section D, below).

C. Carboxylic Acids and Their Esters

For carboxylic acids, conformational possibilities are much more numerous than for lactones. Even the relatively few papers which have extensive sets of data (many acids, or several acids in a range of solvents) have to make bold assumptions to interpret their results at all.

There has been much recent speculation on the preferred conformations of carboxylic acids and related compounds around the bonds joining the α-carbon atom

Table 6

Comparison of CD Data for Some Steroid Lactams and Lactones
Solvent: methanol. X = NH or O.

Position of chromophore in steroid nucleus	Lactam CO.NH		Lactone CO.O	
	$\Delta\varepsilon$	λ (nm)	$\Delta\varepsilon$	λ (nm)
(a) *Six-membered ring*				
2-CO, 3-X	+1·0	218	Not available	
3-CO, 2-X	+0·15	234	−0·4	232
	−0·64	218	+0·7	209
3-CO, 4-X (5α)	− (ORD)		+1·5	213
17-CO, 17a-X	+ (ORD)		+0·2	233
			−0·5	205
(b) *Five-membered ring*				
16-CO, 17-X	+10·7	216	−1·6	216[a]
17-CO, 16-X	−4·0	216	+1·5	224[a]
			+1·6	217
(c) *Five-membered ring in side-chain*				
24-CO, 20-X (R)	+5·0	213	− (ORD)	
24-CO, 20-X (S)	−3·2	214	+ (ORD)	

[a] Data, from Dr. M. Fétizon, are for dioxan solution.

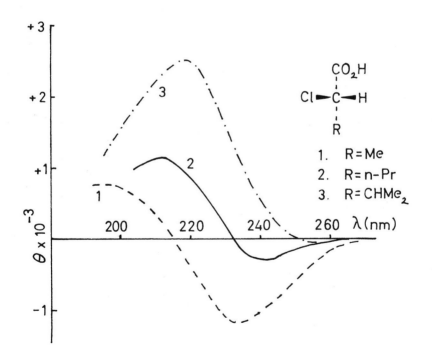

Fig. 9. (S)-α-chloro acids (Gaffield and Galetto[24]; MeOH).

to carboxyl and other substituents.[24–32] Studies of low-temperature CD will no doubt be useful here.

As for lactones, a large body of data is available and only some selected groups of acids are mentioned here.

α-Halogen acids. Gaffield[24] has made a careful study of a number of simple aliphatic α-chloro- and bromo-acids. All acids of the same stereochemical series give curves of the same antipodal type. Many curves are bisignate; the longer wavelength band decreases in magnitude with increasing substitution at the β-carbon atom; it increases in non-polar solvents. It usually disappears when the carboxylic acid group is transformed into the carboxylate anion; see Fig. 9.

Gaffield has rationalized these results in terms of two conformations II and III and an octant-type rule as shown in the perspective drawings. In II which is

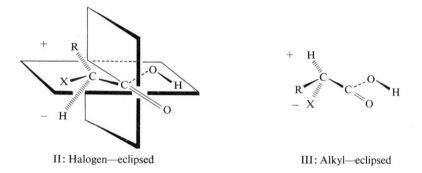

II: Halogen—eclipsed   III: Alkyl—eclipsed

responsible for the shorter wavelength band at 200–220 nm, the halogen is eclipsed with carbonyl and the alkyl group R makes a positive octant contribution; in the alternative conformation III, which gives rise to the longer wavelength band (usually the smaller band) at 240–260 nm, the alkyl group is eclipsed and the halogen X makes a negative octant contribution.

α-Hydroxy and α-amino acids. Listowsky[25] in a study of some α-hydroxy acids (and α-substituted succinic acids) presented a rather similar picture. The most preferred conformation (IV) has the α-hydroxyl group eclipsed with carbonyl, and the next preferred conformation (V) has alkyl eclipsed with carbonyl. The latter (V) is

IV   V

responsible for the longer wavelength band, which increases in intensity at higher temperature and in solvents of low dielectric constant.

Craig[26] has discussed both α-amino acids and α-hydroxy acids and has suggested that the longer wavelength band (usually weak and at about 240 nm) is due to interaction between the lone-pair on nitrogen or hydroxyl oxygen with the carbonyl in a less-preferred conformation (VI). The most preferred conformation responsible

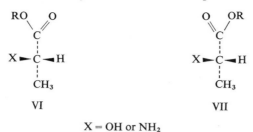

$$X = OH \text{ or } NH_2$$

for the main band at 210 nm is VII, in which the dipoles of C=O and αC—X (where X = OH or NH$_2$) are as far apart as possible. The less-favoured form disappears when the acid is converted into its anion, and, as expected, there is no indication of its presence in α-alkyl acids.

X-ray data indicate that in the solid state carbonyl and α-amino are eclipsed, and this may be taken to give some indication of the probable preferred conformation in solution. Other preferred conformations have been discussed by Listowsky.[25]

Our own empirical studies include an extensive survey of the CD of naturally occurring amino acids, both those from protein amino acids and those less commonly found.[27] For all these acids the same relationship holds between the absolute configuration at the α-carbon atom and the sign of the Cotton effect near 210 nm.

Studies on α-aryl acids by Craig[27a] may be considered in connection with work on α-hydroxy (or amino) α-aryl acids below.

α-Aryl-α-amino (and hydroxy) acids. Extensive work by Djerassi[28] (also by Korver[29]) on α-aryl α-hydroxy acids of the mandelic and atrolactic acid types may now be considered in parallel with our studies (with Professor H. Dahn, Lausanne)[30] on the corresponding α-amino acids (α-phenylglycine and α-phenylalanine).

All the compounds of the same absolute configuration show CD curves of the same pattern—and magnitudes are of the same order. This is true for α-hydroxy and α-amino acids, with and without an α-methyl group [Table 7(a)]; it is also true for the comparison acid, methyl ester, amide (at any rate in the amino series) see Table 7(b). All compounds of the S-configuration show a weak negative band at about 260 nm, which must be the aromatic ^1L_b band. There is a second, much stronger, band near 220 nm, which we suggest is due to interaction between the carboxyl n → π* transition and the aromatic ^1L_a band (Schellman in an important paper on tyrosines and related compounds[31] suggested that this band is essentially the ^1L_a aromatic band).

Results for α-cyclohexyl α-amino acids are similar to those for simple α-amino acids (cf. above) and show small positive Cotton effects near 210 nm [cf. Table 7(c) for a comparison of cyclohexyl amino acids with valine].

Steroid and terpene acids. Extensive studies on various steroid, diterpenoid and triterpenoid acids have been reported by one of us (P.M.S.[14]). There is probably less conformational mobility than for simple acids; this suggestion is supported by the smaller temperature indices (i.e. change in Δε with temperature); see below.

Comparison of acids, esters and amides. The work referred to above also includes a study of a useful homologous series of esters containing a steroid acid esterified with

Table 7

CD Data for Some α-Amino-α-aryl Acids and Related Compounds
Solvent: hydrochloric acid; values from Klyne *et al.*[30]

CO.X	CO$_2$H	CO$_2$H	CO$_2$H
R$^2{}_2$N►C◄R^1	HO►C◄R	NH$_2$►C◄R	NH$_2$►C◄H
Ph	Ph	C$_6$H$_{11}$	CHMe$_2$
(1)	(2)	(3)	(4)

---

a. Comparison between α-amino-α-aryl acids and α-hydroxy-α-aryl acids

Compound	Δε	λ (nm)
α-Amino-α-phenylglycine	−0·2	260
(1) R^1 = H, R^2 = H, X = OH	+9·9	217
α-Hydroxy-α-phenylglycine^a	−0·1	260
(2) R = H	+12·4	222
α-Amino-α-phenylalanine	−0·1	261
(1) R^1 = Me, R^2 = H, X = OH	+5·2	218
α-Hydroxy-α-phenylalanine^a	−0·3	260
(2) R = Me	+5·4	220

b. Comparison between various derivatives of α-amino-α-phenylglycine and α-dimethylamino-α-phenylalanine

Compound	R^2 = H		R^2 = Me	
	Δε	λ (nm)	Δε	λ (nm)
α-Amino-α-aryl acid	−0·2	260	−0·3	261
(1) R^1 = H, X = OH	+9·9	217	+7·6	217
α-Amino-α-aryl acid	−0·3	260	−0·2	261
Methyl ester	+11·8	217	+6·4	219
(1) R^1 = H, X = OMe				
α-Amino-α-aryl acid	−0·3	261	−0·3	262
Amide	+7·0	220	+5·4	221
(1) R^1 = H, X = NH$_2$				

c. Saturated-α-amino-α-cyclohexyl acids

Compound	Δε	λ (nm)
α-Amino-α-cyclohexylglycine	+1·6	209
(3) R = H		
α-Amino-α-cyclohexylalanine	+0·5	206
(3) R = Me		
Cf. L-valine (4)	+1·4	208

^{a} Values from Djerassi *et al.*[28] for aqueous solution.

Table 8

Low-temperature CD of Acids and Esters

$$I_{T_1}^{T_2} = \frac{\Delta\varepsilon_{max}(T_2) - \Delta\varepsilon_{max}(T_1)}{\Delta\varepsilon_{max}(T_1)} \cdot 100\%$$

where T_2 = higher temperature, T_1 = lower temperature.

Type	$I_{T_1}^{T_2}$
S-Methylmercaptopropionic acid	−75
Malic acid	−71
Chlorosuccinic acid	−64
Alkylsuccinic acids	−51
Triterpene-28-carboxylic acids (oleanane series)	−37
Steroid-17β-carboxylic acids	−29
Diterpene-4β-carboxylic acids	−25
Triterpene-28-carboxylic acids (lupene series)	−16
Diterpene-4α-carboxylic acids	Very small

a range of alcohols. The esters and the acid itself all show very similar $\Delta\varepsilon$ values. Other papers of this series include many comparisons of acids with methyl esters, which consistently show very similar values. Few examples are available for comparisons between amides and carboxylic acids, but most of them show the same sign for amide as for carboxylic acid.

Low-temperature studies on conformational flexibility. Low-temperature CD provides a valuable method for the study of conformational flexibility in acids and esters. Recent work includes studies of arylhydroxy acids[28] and of steroid and terpene acids.[32] Table 8 shows some values of the temperature index I for a variety of carboxylic acids. It is significant that this index has a larger value for those acids with greatest conformational freedom.

The carboxylate anion. The carboxylate anion has C_{2v} symmetry. Only a few comparisons of acid and anion are available, but there is one good recent set of CD figures by Listowsky.[25] This shows reversal of sign for many compounds on going from free carboxyl group to anion. This is confirmed by some of our own previous work; unfortunately, most of our own comparisons are from earlier work done on ORD, which gave incomplete curves.

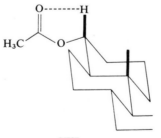

VIII

Table 9

CD Data for Some Acetamido-5α-steroids

Solvent: methanol. The Δε values quoted are for maxima at 212–216 nm for the position of substitution indicated. Signs agree with those for acetoxy-5α-steroids, except where marked with an asterisk. L. Bartlett and P. M. Scopes, 1971.

	Δε			Δε	
	α	β		α	β
1.	−3·9	—	6.	−0·6	−0·6*
2.	−1·1	−1·6	7.	+2·6	−3·6
3.	0	−0·6	11.	−3·6*	+2·2*
4.	+1·5	+0·9*	12.	−3·0	+4·6

D. Acetates of Chiral Alcohols

Acetates are similar in their general geometry to the methyl esters of chiral carboxylic acids, except that the chiral centre is on the opposite side of the chromophore. Early in our work on the carboxyl and related chromophores, we found to our surprise that many steroid acetates (excluding acetates at C-3) gave fairly strong Cotton effects at about 215 nm.[33] This can be useful empirically as one often makes acetates for other purposes. The signs can be rationalized—though *not* explained—in terms of the lactone sector rule, using a preferred conformation of the acetate group VIII which X-ray work shows is preferred in the crystal.[34]

E. Benzoates of Chiral Alcohols

These compounds including dibenzoates and the related *N*-benzoyl derivatives of amines, are more appropriately considered as having aryl chromophores (see Snatzke, Chapter 3.4).

F. N-Acyl Derivatives of Chiral Amines

These are nitrogen analogues of the acetates mentioned above. A series of acetamido steroids, recently made by Miss Lynne Bartlett in our laboratory gave CD results which are generally parallel with those for the steroid acetates, see Table 9. A few examples have also been published by Fétizon.[35] Some X-ray[36] and some NMR[37] work suggests a conformation for the acetamido group similar to that of acetate discussed above.

G. Miscellaneous Related Work

Sparteine alkaloids. A particularly valuable series of rigid *N*-alkyl-lactams is provided by the alkaloids of the sparteine group; we are engaged on the study of these compounds jointly with Professor M. Wiewiorowski of Poznan.

These compounds, e.g. IX, are complicated—but made the more interesting by reason of the fact that many of them include another type of chromophore, the

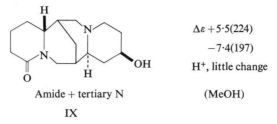

$\Delta\varepsilon +5\cdot5(224)$

$-7\cdot4(197)$

H⁺, little change

Amide + tertiary N

(MeOH)

IX

tertiary amine, e.g. X. This group is known to give a Cotton effect at about 200 nm which is presumably due to an n → σ* transition; this is completely obliterated by protonation, i.e. by the addition of acid to a methanol solution of the compound.

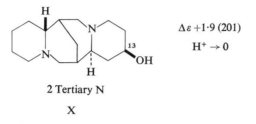

$\Delta\varepsilon +1\cdot9 (201)$

H⁺ → 0

2 Tertiary N

X

It is therefore possible, for compounds which contain both the *N*-alkyl-lactam and tertiary amine chromophores, to study the *N*-alkyl-lactam alone by protonation; an example is shown in formula IX; this compound after protonation shows two clear lactam Cotton effects at approximately 224 nm and 197 nm.

Anhydrides and imides. Two further groups related to carboxyl, where fortunately the symmetry of the group is not in question, are the anhydrides and imides. In these

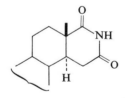

$\Delta\varepsilon +2\cdot18 (257 \text{ nm})$

XI

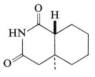

$\Delta\varepsilon -1\cdot42 (256 \text{ nm})$

XII

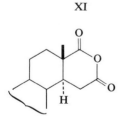

$\Delta\varepsilon +1\cdot86 (222 \text{ nm})$

XIII

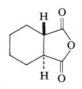

$a, +49$ (R. K. Hill[2])

XIV

compounds the chromophore is presumably all co-planar, and it must have local C_{2v} symmetry. In six-membered rings, anhydrides and imides of the same stereochemical type show similar curves; formulae XI to XIII illustrate examples of anhydrides and imides obtained from Dr. G. D. Meakins in Oxford (other examples, e.g. XIV, are illustrated in Crabbé's book,[2] French edition, as unpublished work by R. K. Hill of Princeton).

3.3.5 Conclusion

We come here to the end of a very incomplete story. We apologize for its incompleteness, but it is not for lack of hard work that relatively slow progress has been made since the Bonn meeting. From what we hear of our theoretical friends' discussions regarding the olefin chromophore, the picture may well remain confused for some time, because we certainly have at least two transitions close together in the far ultraviolet. We may console ourselves with the thought that perhaps the difficulties may in the end make it possible for us to learn a little more about the fundamental nature of chiroptical effects.

Our thanks are due to the research students and assistants who have done so much of the work, and to colleagues who have provided samples—as indicated in Chapter 3.1—regarding carbonyl.

We are greatly indebted to the Science Research Council for long-standing and continuing support.

References

1. P. Crabbé, *An Introduction to the Chiroptical Methods in Chemistry*. Mexico, 1971. This work gives principal references for all topics.
2. P. Crabbé, *Applications de la Dispersion Rotatoire Optique et du Dichroisme Circulaire Optique en Chimie Organique*. Gauthier Villars, Paris, 1968. This work gives full references for all topics.
3. P. M. Scopes, *Ann. Rep.* 34 (1969); 36 (1970); 102 (1971).
4. W. B. Gratzer, in G. D. Fasman, Ed., *Poly-α-amino Acids*. Dekker, New York, 1967.
5. W. B. Gratzer, *Proc. Roy. Soc. A* **297**, 163 (1967).
6. H. Basch, M. B. Robin and N. A. Kuehler, *J. Chem. Phys.* **49**, 5007 (1968).
7. K. K. Cheung, K. H. Overton and G. A. Sim, *Chem. Commun.* 634 (1965); R. C. Sheppard and S. Turner, *Chem. Commun.* 77 (1968).
8. A. McL. Mathieson, *Tetrahedron Lett.* 81 (1963).
9. J. S. McKechnie, I. Kubina and I. C. Paul, *J. Chem. Soc. B* 1476 (1970).
10. W. Meier, Paper at International Congress on Hormonal Steroids, Hamburg, 1970.
11. J. A. Schellman, *J. Chem. Phys.* **44**, 55 (1966).
12. W. Klyne and P. M. Scopes, in G. Snatzke, Ed., *Optical Rotatory Dispersion and Circular Dichroism in Organic Chemistry*. Heyden, London, 1967, p. 193.
13. J. P. Jennings, W. Klyne and P. M. Scopes, *J. Chem. Soc.* 7211, 7229 (1965); also collected references 1, 2 and 3.
14. G. Gottarelli, W. Klyne and P. M. Scopes, *J. Chem. Soc. C* 1366 (1967); G. Gottarelli and P. M. Scopes, *J. Chem. Soc. C* 1370 (1967); J. D. Renwick and P. M. Scopes, *J. Chem. Soc. C* 1949, 2574 (1968); J. D. Renwick, P. M. Scopes and S. Huneck, *J. Chem. Soc. C* 2544 (1969).
15. G. Snatzke, H. Ripperger, C. Horstmann and K. Schreiber, *Tetrahedron* **22**, 3103 (1966).
16. H. Wolf, *Tetrahedron Lett.* 1075 (1965) and 5151 (1966).
17. M. Legrand and H. Bucourt, *Bull. Soc. Chim. Fr.* 2241 (1967).
18. A. F. Beecham, *Tetrahedron Lett.* 2355, 3591 (1968); 4897 (1969).
19. J. A. Schellman, *Accounts Chem. Res.* **1**, 144 (1968).
20. I. Tinoco, *J. Chem. Phys.* **33**, 1332 (1960), **34**, 1067 (1961); I. Tinoco and R. W. Woody, *J. Chem. Phys.* **32**, 461 (1960); R. W. Woody and I. Tinoco, *J. Chem. Phys.* **49**, 2927 (1967).
21. C. Toniolo, V. Perciaccante, J. Falcetta, R. Rupp and M. Goodman, *J. Org. Chem.* **35**, 6 (1970).
22. F. I. Carroll, A. Sobti and R. Meck, *Tetrahedron Lett.* 405 (1971).

23. W. Klyne and P. M. Scopes. Forthcoming publication.
23(*a*). W. Meier and K. Noack, *Helv. Chim. Acta*. In press.
24. W. Gaffield and W. G. Galetto, *Tetrahedron* **27**, 915 (1971).
25. I. Listowsky, G. Avigad and S. Englard, *J. Org. Chem.* **35**, 1080 (1970).
26. J. C. Craig and W. E. Pereira, *Tetrahedron Lett.* 1563 (1970).
27. L. Fowden, P. M. Scopes and R. N. Thomas, *J. Chem. Soc. C* 833 (1971).
27(*a*). J. C. Craig, W. E. Pereira, B. Halpern and J. W. Westley, *Tetrahedron* **27**, 1173 (1971).
28. G. Barth, W. Voelter, H. S. Mosher, E. Bunnenberg and C. Djerassi *J. Amer. Chem. Soc.* **92**, 875 (1970).
29. O. Korver, *Tetrahedron* **26**, 3507 (1970).
30. W. Klyne, P. M. Scopes, R. N. Thomas and H. Dahn, *Helv. Chim. Acta* **54**, 2420 (1971).
31. T. M. Hooker and J. A. Schellman, *Biopolymers* **9**, 1319 (1970).
32. W. P. Mose and P. M. Scopes, *J. Chem. Soc. C* 2417 (1970); 1572 (1971).
33. J. P. Jennings, W. P. Mose and P. M. Scopes, *J. Chem. Soc. C* 1102 (1967).
34. A. McL. Mathieson, *Tetrahedron Lett.* 4137 (1965).
35. M. Fétizon and N. Moreau, *Bull. Soc. Chim. Fr.* 4387 (1969).
36. D. L. Peterson and W. T. Simpson, *J. Amer. Chem. Soc.* **79**, 2375 (1957).
37. C. R. Narayanan and B. M. Sawant, *Tetrahedron Lett.* 1321 (1971).

Aromatic Chromophores

G. SNATZKE

University of Bonn (F.R.G.)

M. KAJTÁR

University of Budapest (H)

and

F. SNATZKE (formerly WERNER-ZAMOJSKA)

Polish Academy of Sciences
Warsaw (PL)

3.4.1 Introduction

The early literature on the chiroptical properties of aromatic compounds has been thoroughly reviewed by Crabbé and Klyne.[1] Although a great bulk of material has been accumulated, only few general rules have been put forward. We shall discuss here the chiroptical data of the aromatic chromophores and especially those of the benzene derivatives from a general point of view. A detailed description of these general principles is given in Chapter 3.5 of this book.[2]

Any chiral aromatic molecule of general formula I (Fig. 1) is divided into different 'spheres', starting with the chromophore which by definition forms the first sphere. In compound I this would be ring A together with all other conjugated aromatic rings. That non-aromatic ring which is condensed with the first sphere comprises

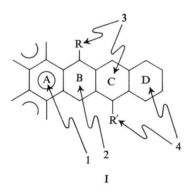

Fig. 1. Schematic representation of division of an aromatic polycyclic compound into spheres.

I

148

the second sphere (ring B of formula I); rings or substituents connected directly with the second sphere form the third one (ring C and group R of formula I), those rings and substituents which are bound to the third sphere (ring D and groups R' of formula I) build up the fourth, and so on. Our general rule[2, 3] states that the chiral sphere, which is nearest to the chromophore determines the sign and even a great deal of the magnitude of the Cotton effect within each absorption band. Examples of compounds with a chiral first sphere are, for example, those with a chiral σ-system, as hexahelicene (II),[4, 5] or the 3,4-benzophenanthrene III,[6] non-

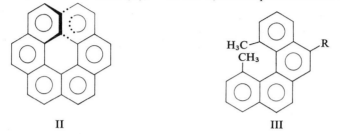

| II | III |

coplanar styrenes,[7] or compounds containing two achiral chromophores close to one another so that exciton splitting occurs.[8, 9] In a tetralin or tetrahydroisoquinoline the benzene ring is coplanar but the cyclohexene or piperidine ring is present in a half-chair conformation, containing only a C_2 axis of symmetry; thus for these compounds the second sphere is chiral. Mandelic acid or tyrosine are examples of compounds with achiral first and missing second but chiral third sphere.

3.4.2 The Chiral First Sphere

Compounds with a chiral first sphere belong to Moscowitz' class of 'inherently chiral chromophores'[10] (originally called 'inherently dissymmetric chromophores') and usually show very strong Cotton effects. In order to predict their signs from the geometry, highly sophisticated calculations are necessary, if the chirality of the π-system is caused by a chiral σ-skeleton, as in II and III. All but one calculation[11] predicted a positive rotation at the NaD line for the *P*-hexahelicene, and this has now been proved experimentally.[12]

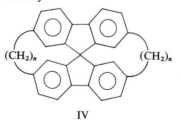

IV

Vespirenes of general formula IV contain two (achiral) fluorene chromophores connected by a spiro atom and within all absorption bands whose direction of polarization is (exactly or approximately) parallel to the 'pivot bond' of each 'biphenyl system', CD couplets[13] were found[8] if the two fluorene systems were not exactly perpendicular to each other. Deviation from this orthogonality is caused by ring strain (Baeyer and/or Pitzer type). Application of W. Kuhn's coupled oscillator theory[14, 15] is especially simple in this case because the two electric transition moment vectors are lying in two parallel planes (perpendicular to their connecting line).[8] The CD of some octahedral complexes between, for example, ruthenium and three bisdentate ligands, as α,α'-bipyridyl or phenanthroline within the strong 'aromatic' absorption bands can also be treated in this way.[9]

Biphenyl derivatives with an axis of chirality have been investigated by several groups of workers (e.g. Mislow et al.,[16], Mason,[17] Cymerman Craig and Roy,[18] etc.) and in this case those bands polarized perpendicular to the 'pivot bond' give rise to exciton couplets.[17] The sign of the CD bands at longer wavelengths depends strongly on the substitution pattern,[19] whereas the Cotton effect within the 'conjugation band' around 230 nm is determined only by the helicity of the biphenyl system.[16-18] Figure 2 shows the ORD curves[18] of bulbocapnine (V) and glaucine

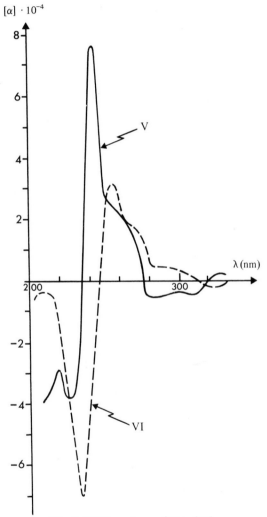

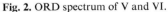

Fig. 2. ORD spectrum of V and VI.

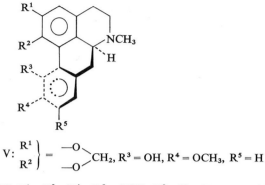

V: $\left.\begin{array}{c} R^1 \\ R^2 \end{array}\right\}$ = $\underset{-O}{\overset{-O}{\diagdown}}CH_2$, $R^3 = OH$, $R^4 = OCH_3$, $R^5 = H$

VI: $R^1 = R^2 = R^4 = R^5 = OCH_3$, $R^3 = H$ Hydrochloride

hydrochloride (VI): the Cotton effect of both homochiral aporphine alkaloids around 235–240 nm is positive, whereas within the bands at longer wavelengths the respective Cotton effects have opposite signs.

Dibenzoates show a very strong CD-couplet around 228 nm,[20] i.e. within the CT-absorption band, whereas monobenzoates give only a faint Cotton effect in this region. Application of the exciton theory explains this rule, according to which a positive torsion angle between the two OBz groups leads to a positive couplet—as, for example, in the case of VII (Fig. 3). This rule works also if the corresponding diol is not a vicinal glycol, as long as the two aromatic rings are close one to another.

This rule has recently[21] been extended to other compounds containing two non-conjugated substituted benzene rings with large transition moment vectors. For example, (−)-amurensine (VIII) shows negative couplets within each transition

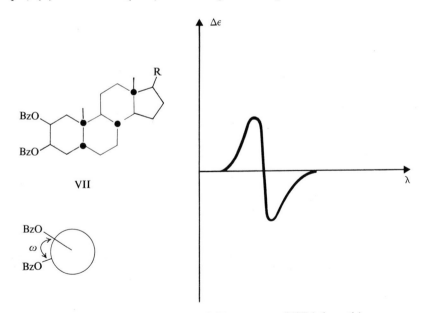

Fig. 3. Newman projection and CD spectrum of VII (schematic).

which indicates a negative torsion angle between the two moments.[22] For the
^1L_b band these bisect the two $(RO)_2$-groupings, for the ^1L_a band they are perpendicular to those of the ^1L_b band. The rhoeadine alkaloid (+)-oreodine (IX) shows such

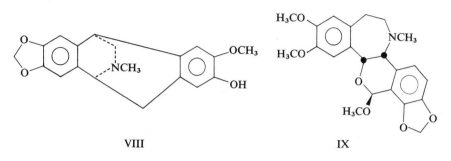

VIII   IX

a couplet just within the ^1B band[23] and it has been assumed that the transition
moments of the ^1L_b and ^1L_a bands are too small (and the two chromophores too
distant from each other) to give rise to exciton splitting; the couplet at short wavelengths was used to determine the absolute configuration. This band cannot be
utilized for this purpose, however, as the ^1B transition is degenerate in benzene,
and chiral compounds containing only one substituted benzene ring also show
such a couplet, which, of course, is not caused by such an exciton-splitting mechanism. The existence of a couplet within the ^1B band has been pointed out, for example,
by Miles et al.[24, 25] in discussing the CD spectra of pyrimidine nucleosides, and a very

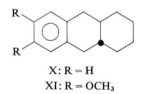

X: R = H
XI: R = OCH₃

simple example with a benzene chromophore is given by the octahydroanthracene
derivative XI[26] which shows (in iso-octane solution) a negative ^1L_b-band CD
[$\Delta\varepsilon_{max} = -0.71$ (295 nm), -1.02 (290 nm) and -1.07 (285 nm)], a negative ^1L_a-band
CD [$\Delta\varepsilon_{max} = -3.50$ (232 nm)] and a clear couplet for the ^1B transition [$\Delta\varepsilon_{max} = -13$
(205 nm), $+14$ (194 nm)].

Diphenylmethane derivatives obviously can give such a Davydov splitting, in
1,2-diphenylethane derivatives the distance between the aromatic rings seems to be
often too large to give rise to a pronounced exciton interaction.

Another interesting example for this treatment is the alkaloid cryptostyline II
(XII).[27] The hydrobromide of the synthetic enantiomer E-XII in the crystalline state
has the dimethoxyphenyl substituent pseudoequatorially arranged, and if the same
conformation holds in solution for the free alkaloid XII then for the ^1L_b transition
a negative couplet is expected and is indeed found [-5.88 (287 nm), $+3.33$ (273 nm)].
The transition moment vectors for the ^1L_a bands are, however, nearly parallel to
each other in this same conformation, thus we cannot expect a couplet within the
^1L_a transition and the CD is in fact only positive in this region [$+14.24$ (237 nm)].[27]

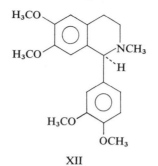

XII

For a simpler example without coupling see later (p. 155).

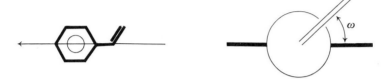

Fig. 4. Conformation of a styrene chromophore leading to a negative CD.

Non-coplanar styrenes have been investigated by Crabbé:[7] a positive torsion angle around the σ-bond between the double bond and the cisoid side of the benzene ring leads to a negative Cotton effect (Fig. 4). Oestra-1,3,5(10),6-tetraenes (XIII) of rigid conformation give a negative Cotton effect independent of the substitution at C-1 and C-3, whereas for example in the case of oestra-1,3,5(10),8-tetraenes (XIV) the preferred conformation of ring B can be deduced from its positive CD.[7]

XIII   XIV

There are reasons to believe, however, that for this rule also the substitution pattern of the aromatic ring cannot be always neglected.

3.4.3 The Chiral Second Sphere

Many of the more complex aromatic natural products contain a chiral second sphere and their CD can be explained by making use of the following rule, which is first applied to simpler compounds. If no pseudoaxial substituents are present at the benzylic carbon atoms, the *P*-helicity of the cyclohexene (piperideine, dihydropyrane, …) ring leads to positive Cotton effects within the ^1L_b and ^1L_a transition, and *M*-helicity to negative ones (Fig. 5). As is shown later the signs can be reversed by some patterns of substitution of the aromatic ring. If the chiral non-aromatic ring does not adopt a regular half-chair conformation but, for example, a sofa conforma-

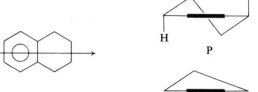

Fig. 5. *P*- and *M*-helicity of a tetralin (projection in direction of arrow, ▬▬ represents the benzene ring). Only the pseudoaxial hydrogen atoms are drawn.

tion (five atoms in one plane), we can still use the terms *P*- and *M*-helicity for describing the sense of its chirality.

Examples for this rule are the tetralins XV–XVII (Fig. 6); if the substituent preferentially adopts the equatorial conformation then *M*-helicity arises with the absolute configuration depicted, and negative Cotton effects were in fact found for

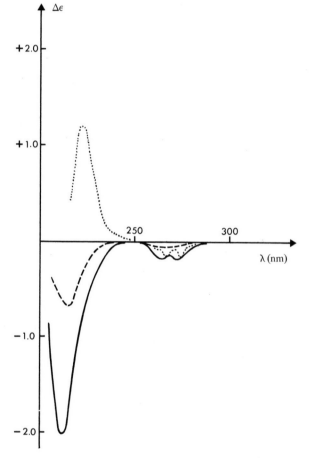

Fig. 6. CD curves of XV (— — —), XVI (———) and XX (·········).

the ^1L_b and ^1L_a transitions.[28, 29] The same CD signs were found[28] for compounds XVIII and XIX, and again it is reasonable to assume that the substituent at C-2 is equatorially, and that at C-1 pseudoaxially, disposed. For (1S)-methyl tetralin (XX) the ^1L_b-band CD is negative (Fig. 6) and that for the ^1L_a-band is positive (Fig. 6). We believe that the low-energy transition truly reflects the M-helicity of the

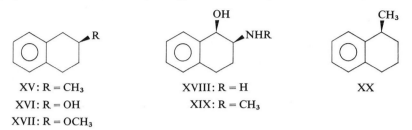

XV: R = CH₃

XVI: R = OH

XVII: R = OCH₃

XVIII: R = H

XIX: R = CH₃

XX

second sphere, and a sign inversion takes place within the ^1L_a band. For this higher-energy transition, interaction with σ^*-orbitals is more likely and a pseudoaxial bond at the benzylic atom is well positioned for σ–π-conjugation with the benzenoid π- and π^*-orbitals. The corresponding homochiral hydroxy and amino compounds also show a negative ^1L_b-band CD[30] and the pseudoaxial conformation of these substituents has been proved by NMR.[31]

Unlike an alkyl or OR group, a phenyl in the 1-position of a tetralin or tetrahydro-isoquinoline preferentially adopts the pseudoequatorial conformation, as already mentioned for XII. In the crystalline state this has been proved[32] also for the simple compound XXI, and according to the positive CD within the ^1L_b band[32] the same holds for solution. No exciton splitting is observed for this compound

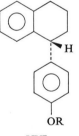

XXI

because the electric transition moment vector of a benzene ring without oxygen (nitrogen, . . .) substituents is too small to give rise to pronounced orbital inter-action.

In order to test this helicity rule, we[33] have synthesized the octahydro anthracenes X and XI and have found negative CD bands for both within the ^1L_b and ^1L_a transi-tion. The ^1B-couplet of XI has already been mentioned (p. 152). Many more complex alkaloids or other natural products contain the same substitution pattern in the aromatic ring and follow the same helicity rule. A particular case, argemonine (XXII) and some of its analogues must be treated, however, in more detail. Figure 7 shows the CD curve[34, 35] of this alkaloid which contains two identical chromo-phores (besides the N-methyl group). Mason *et al.*[35] have explained its CD by assuming exciton splitting between the two benzene rings, though only within the

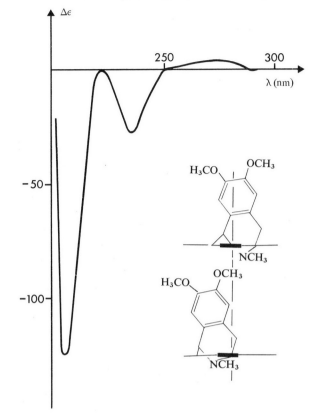

Fig. 7. CD curve and quadrant projections of argemonine (XXII) according to reference 39 (top) and reference 41 (bottom).

^1L_b band is bisignate CD found, and this is highly unsymmetric. For the reasons mentioned above, such an interaction does not seem to be very probable, furthermore other analogues, for example, norargemonine (XXIII) do not show this first small negative CD band at all.[34] We rather think that the CD of argemonine (XXII) and its analogues is merely the double of the Cotton effect of each half. In the usual projection two chiral second spheres can be seen, a six-membered half-chair, and an eight-membered chiral ring. As in the case of the corresponding ketones with a chiral second sphere (cf., for example, gibberellic acid derivatives,[36] kaurene derivatives,[36, 37] and camphor derivatives[38]) we can assume for these benzene derivatives also that the smaller ring builds up the 'determining' second sphere. Its *P*-helicity is in agreement with the positive sign of the ^1L_b-band CD (the small,

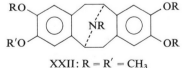

XXII: R = R′ = CH₃
XXIII: R = CH₃, R′ = H

negative 'Vorbande' appearing in some CD spectra around 290 nm may perhaps be attributed to a solvated species or to vibronic coupling, or may be due to a smaller negative contribution originating from the *M*-helicity of the second, eight-membered second sphere). The CD within the ^1L_a band is of opposite sign due to the presence of a pseudoaxial C—C bond at the allylic C-atom.

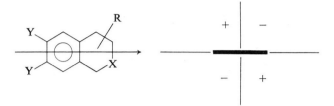

Fig. 8. Quadrant rule of Kuriyama *et al.*[39] for ^1L_b-band CD.

Kuriyama *et al.*[39] have published a quadrant rule for the ^1L_b-band CD which does not differentiate between second- and third-sphere contributions, and which is given in Fig. 8. It follows the general requirements for a C_{2v}-pseudoscalar[40] and the projection of Fig. 7 can also be used to apply this treatment.[39] According to it a positive CD is predicted. Furthermore it was often assumed that the sign of the CD within the ^1L_a band is opposite to that within the ^1L_b band, so the reverse sign pattern of Fig. 8 was assumed[39] to hold for the ^1L_a-band CD in general, and would be in agreement with the found values (Fig. 7). We have seen, however, that sign inversion may rather depend on the pseudoaxial substitution at the benzylic C-atom.

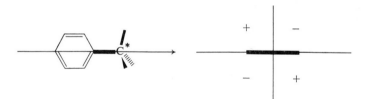

Fig. 9. Quadrant rule of DeAngelis and Wildman[41] for ^1L_a-band CD.

DeAngelis and Wildman[41] used another approach by stressing the influence of the nearest chiral centre to the aromatic ring. Their projection is given in Fig. 9, and the signs are this time valid for the ^1L_a-band CD. This rule has, however, several exceptions and Fig. 7 shows clearly that a positive CD is predicted for argemonine (XXII), whereas a strong negative one is found.

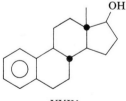

XXIV

Vibronic fine structure may sometimes obscure the easy correlation between CD and helicity of the second sphere, and in our experience this is especially the case with octahydrophenanthrene derivatives. For example, 1,3,5(10)-oestratrien-17β-ol (XXIV) within the ^1L_b band shows nearly equal positive and negative fine structure bands, whereas the ^1L_a-band CD (in the absence of a pseudoaxial C—C bond at the benzylic position) is regularly positive without fine structure.[33, 42] Nearly the same ^1L_b-band CD was observed for the homochiral trisnor-diterpenoid XXV.[43] In

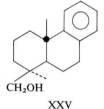

CH₂OH

XXV

such a case it is obviously the positive band at longer wavelengths which follows the helicity rule.

The influence of the substitution pattern on this helicity rule will be discussed later (p. 162).

3.4.4 The Chiral Third Sphere

As has already been mentioned, two rules have been formulated for third-sphere contributions by Kuriyama et al.[39] and by DeAngelis and Wildman[41] (Figs. 8 and 9). If one starts from the unsubstituted benzene chromophore with D_{6h}-symmetry, a rule with 24 sectors should hold, as this is the simplest corresponding pseudo-scalar.[40] On the other hand, the C_{2v}-symmetry of a mono-substituted benzene or the C_2 symmetry of a tetralin requires only a quadrant rule. In developing our original sector rule,[44, 45] we started from Platt's treatment[46] of the dipole strength of aromatic compounds and have recently[33, 47, 48] modified it to bring it into accord with the symmetry requirements of the skeleton.

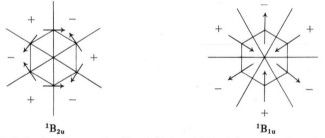

Fig. 10. Polarization diagram for $^1B_{2u}$ (=^1L_b) and $^1B_{1u}$ (=^1L_a) transition of benzene.

Platt[46] introduced the 'spectroscopic moment' of a substituent in order to explain quantitatively the change of the dipole strength by different substitution of the benzene ring. These moments are vectors perpendicular to the nodal planes of the respective transitions, and Fig. 10 shows them for the ^1L_b (=$^1B_{2u}$) and ^1L_a (=$^1B_{1u}$) bands.* The first sign in such a polarization diagram may be written arbitrarily, the

---

* It must always be kept in mind that '$^1B_{2u}$','$^1B_{1u}$', etc. refer to the unsubstituted benzene; any substitution changes symmetry and thus also group theory symbols. In this paper we have followed the usual practice (though very seldom explicitly stated) that, for example, '$^1B_{2u}$' should be understood as: the band of the compound in question which is analogous to the $^1B_{2u}$ band of benzene.

others then follow from this. By convention, the moment vectors are drawn from positive to negative sectors. It should be kept in mind that the plane of the benzene ring is not a nodal plane in these polarization diagrams of Platt!

In building up sector rules for third- (fourth-, ...) sphere contributions we start from these polarization diagrams and add all those planes which are required by the symmetry of the skeleton. For a (chirally) monosubstituted benzene we just have to add the plane of the ring in order to get a sector rule for the ^1L_b transition, whereas

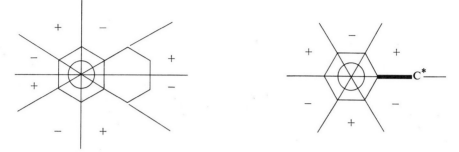

Fig. 11. Sector rules for third- (fourth-, ...) sphere contributions to the ^1L_b-band CD. The plane of the paper is also a nodal plane; signs are for upper sectors.

for tetralins (tetrahydroisoquinolines, etc.) one more plane (perpendicular to the benzene ring and containing the C_2 axis) has to be added. These rules are depicted in Fig. 11, the signs are introduced as found from experiment. In the case of the ^1L_a transition, the tetralin requires only one additional nodal plane (that of the benzene ring), the phenyl compounds two (Fig. 12).

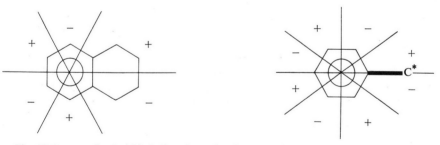

Fig. 12. Sector rules for third- (fourth-, ...) sphere contributions to the ^1L_a-band CD. The plane of the paper is also a nodal plane, signs are for upper sectors.

A certain similarity to the CD of ketones exists here. The two C atoms which are not lying in the plane of the carbonyl group of twist cyclohexanones or cyclopentanones are positioned in positive octants (according to the octant rule, valid only for third-sphere contributions) if the ring has P-helicity (second-sphere contribution), which leads to a positive Cotton effect. The two non-coplanar C atoms of a tetralin with P-helicity are, according to Figs. 11 and 12, also lying in positive sectors. Thus a simple relationship exists between second- and third-sphere contributions for benzene derivatives as for ketones. Within some sectors these four rules are identical with the other two quadrant rules mentioned,[39, 41] especially in the

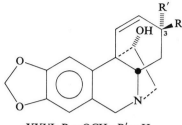

XXVI: R = OCH₃, R' = H
XXVII: R = H, R' = OCH₃

most important area around the C_2 axis at that side of the cyclohexene ring or chiral centre opposite the benzene ring.

A good example of the existence of additional nodal planes is the comparison of the CDs of the two epimeric alkaloids haemanthamine (XXVI) and crinamine (XXVII).[39] Within the ^1L_b band the CD values are +3·42 and +3·51, respectively; they are thus practically identical. Within the ^1L_a band on the other hand rotational strengths differ appreciably (−3·96 and −2·84, respectively). Indeed, one nodal plane of the ^1L_b sector rule just cuts C-3, and the OCH₃ group lies in it. Epimerization

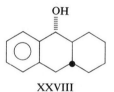

XXVIII

must therefore remain without influence. The same grouping lies, however, in the middle of a sector for the ^1L_a band Cotton effect, and the contributions of the methoxy group, which differ for the two epimers, are observed.

The CD of XXVIII within the ^1L_b band is negative as is required by the *M*-helicity of the second sphere, $\Delta\varepsilon_{max}$ is, however, smaller, as for the hydrocarbon X.[49] Thus the OH has a positive contribution to the CD, which contradicts Kuriyama's rule.[39] Indeed due to the nodal plane traversing C-9, this OH group falls into a positive (rear) sector according to the modified rules. Other examples in the series of tetra-hydroberberine alkaloids are cited in reference 45.

Some epimeric indanols XXIX–XXXII show the same sign of the CD independent of the configuration at C-1, the chiral centre next to the benzene ring.[28, 50] This

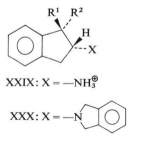

XXIX: X = —NH₃⊕

XXX: X = —N⟨image⟩

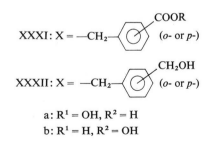

XXXI: X = —CH₂—⟨benzene⟩COOR   (*o*- or *p*-)

XXXII: X = —CH₂—⟨benzene⟩CH₂OH   (*o*- or *p*-)

a: R¹ = OH, R² = H
b: R¹ = H, R² = OH

strange result has been explained by us[28, 47, 50] by accepting the geometrical achirality of the second sphere (envelope form) but assuming that it is electronically chiral due to the different polarizabilities of the C-1/C-2 and C-2/C-3 bonds. Another explanation is, however, also possible. As mentioned, the plane of the benzene ring is no nodal plane for the $^1B_{2u}$ and $^1B_{1u}$ transitions. In a 2-substituted indane derivative, the cyclopentene ring has C_s and not C_2 symmetry (as in the case of the tetralins of Fig. 13) and thus we have only to add one nodal plane perpendicular to the

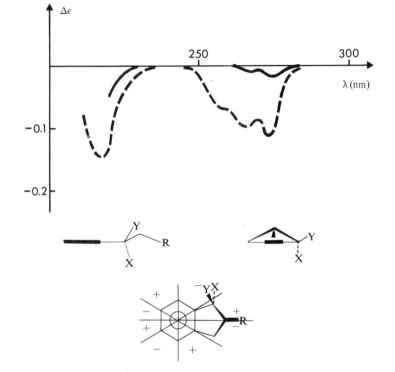

Fig. 13. CD curves and projections (perpendicular to and along the long axis of the benzene ring) of indanes XXIXa (----) and XXIXb (———); appropriate sector rule. The plane of the benzene ring is not a nodal plane.

benzene ring and hitting C-2. As the plane of the benzene ring itself is not a nodal plane, contributions have the same signs above and below this plane, epimerization

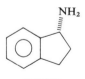

XXXIII

at C-1 thus does not in fact change the sign of the Cotton effect as long as the chirality of the envelope conformation is not changed, and the sector rule of Fig. 13 applies. From the positive sign of the ^1L_b-band CD of (1*R*)-amino indane

(XXXIII)[51] according to Fig. 14 we can deduce that in this compound the pseudo-equatorial conformation of the NH$_2$ group is more stable than the pseudoaxial

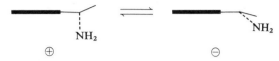

Fig. 14. Projections and predicted sign for two conformations of XXXIII.

form. From the examples XXIX–XXXII it follows that it is not always possible to use rigid compounds as models for assigning the signs of CD contributions in different sector rules for open-chain compounds, as is sometimes done (cf., for example, a recent example given in reference 52). The signs in the sector rules of Figs. 11 and 12 for the monosubstituted phenyl compounds have been derived from open-chain examples[33] and they are to be considered as only tentative, as long as conformational analysis of such phenyl compounds is not better developed. But they are, for example, also in agreement with CD data on phenyl cyclohexanes disclosed at this NATO Summer School by Verbit and Price.[53]

3.4.5 Influence of the Substitution Pattern of the Benzene Ring upon the Helicity and Sector Rules

In the literature, substitution of the benzene ring has only quite recently been taken into consideration (cf., for example, references 54 and 55) and a few determinations of absolute configuration from chiroptical methods have been proved to be wrong in the meantime [e.g. cularine (XXXIV)[56]]. In our first paper[44] we have already

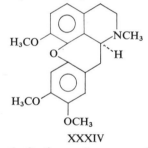

XXXIV

expressed the view that the substitution pattern may change the sign of a Cotton effect and the positive CD within the ^1L_b band of (−)-tetrahydropalmatine (XXXV)

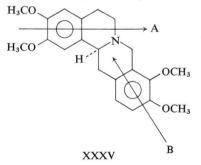

XXXV

led us[45] to assume that for the 'type B'-chromophore (formula XXXV) M-helicity of the second sphere corresponds to a positive CD. Recently,[47, 48] we have tried to explain this fact and to predict the influence of other substitution patterns and have obtained good agreement with experimental values.

Platt's theory,[46] which has been extended by Petruska,[57] has also shown that not only do the magnitudes of the spectroscopic moments of various substituents differ, but also the signs: alkyl, halogen, RO—, R_2N— and C=C, etc. have the same sign (deliberately chosen to be positive), CH_2OH, CHO, COOH, etc. have the opposite one (negative). For the polarization diagrams this means that the direction of the arrows has to be reversed for the appropriate substituents, and the CD data of the homochiral paracyclophane derivatives XXXVI and XXXVII could theoretically be explained only by taking into account such a change of sign.[58] The case of the secondary alcohol grouping >CHOH is difficult to treat as the data published[46, 57] are for (formally) freely rotating —CH_2OH groups, whereas

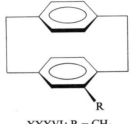

XXXVI: R = CH_3
XXXVII: R = CH_2OH

in compounds like XVIII or XXVIII their conformation is fixed. Furthermore, for groups giving rise to monoshifts of more than 1500 cm^{-1} (e.g. the important RO group), Petruska's calculations[57] do not apply quantitatively. Because of such difficulties in our simple approach we have assumed the moment vectors to be equally long.

At first this treatment will be applied to phenyl compounds (Fig. 15). R represents a chiral substituent, R' an achiral one having the same sign of the spectroscopic moment vector as R. On the left side of Fig. 15, polarization diagrams are depicted, and their sign patterns relative to R were chosen deliberately, but always the same. In the middle, the relative position of the sum vector with respect to R is drawn schematically. Figure 15 1c repeats this and gives the sector rule for third-sphere contributions to the ^1L_b-band CD as found experimentally.[33] From this we conclude that one can 'calibrate' the sector rule by putting a minus sign at the origin and a plus sign at the tip of the sum vector. As Fig. 15 2b shows, p-substitution does not change the orientation of the sum vector and thus the sector rule should have the same signs in all sectors, as for the non-substituted compound. For m- (3) and o-substitution (4) on the other hand the sum vector is rotated by 60° and this, by the same procedure as for 2, leads to inversion of the sign pattern in these sector rules.

An experimental verification can be found in amino-acid chemistry. L-Phenylalanine (XXXVIII) gives a very small positive Cotton effect within the ^1L_b band,[59, 60] and L-p-tyrosine (XXXIX) a bigger one of the same sign.[54, 59] The reason for this

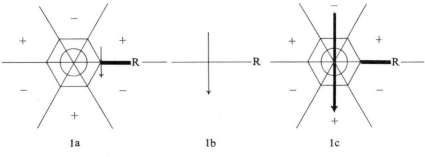

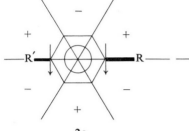

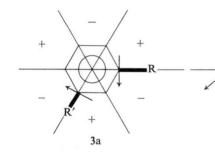

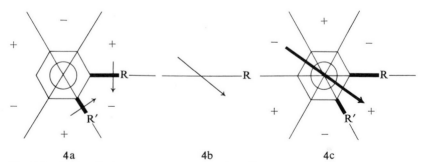

Fig. 15. Influence of substitution pattern upon sign of ^1L_b-band CD of phenyl derivatives:
    a: Platt polarization diagrams;
    b: schematic representation of direction of sum vector of spectroscopic moments;
    c: derived sector rules for third- (fourth-, . . .) sphere contributions.

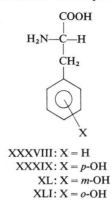

XXXVIII: X = H
XXXIX: X = *p*-OH
XL: X = *m*-OH
XLI: X = *o*-OH

difference in magnitudes is explained[61] by the fact that the electric and magnetic transition moment vectors are perpendicular in benzene, thus the rotational strength must be zero in a first approximation. Substitution by a group like OH can enhance the CD because interaction of the π- and π^*-orbitals of the benzene with the lone-pair orbitals on oxygen generates a component of the magnetic transition moment vector within the plane of the ring. For both acids similar conformations of the chiral side chains have been found in the crystalline state[62, 63] and may also be assumed in solution.

L-*m*- (XL) and L-*o*-Tyrosine (XLI), on the other hand, give negative ^1L_b-band Cotton effects[54] in full agreement with the predictions of Fig. 15, again when the same conformation of the side chain is present. Hooker and Schellman[54] have given a somewhat different explanation for the CD signs of XXXIX–XLI by assuming that only the OH group introduces an appreciable spectroscopic moment.

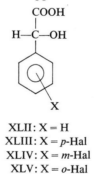

XLII: X = H
XLIII: X = *p*-Hal
XLIV: X = *m*-Hal
XLV: X = *o*-Hal

Korver[55] measured the CD of differently substituted mandelic acids (e.g. XLII–XLV) and also found the ^1L_b-band CD was dependent on substitution. Homochiral unsubstituted and *m*-substituted compounds gave analogous CD curves, *p*- and *o*- substituted ones those of enantiomorphous type.* The reason for this apparent discrepancy may be the following. For a compound Ph—CH₂—R with only one single substituent at the benzylic C atom, the conformational equilibrium will not depend very much on substitution, though calculations even in this case

* The absolute configuration of these compounds was not proved unambiguously at the time of publication.[55] This has, however, since been done independently by Dr. Guetté's group in Paris (private communication).

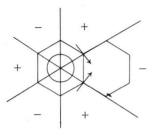
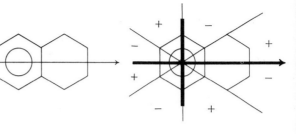

5a

5b

5c

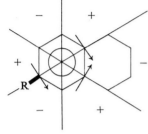
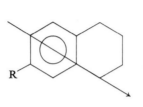
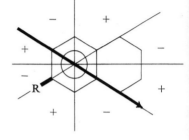

6a

6b

6c

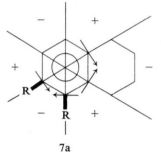
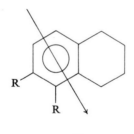
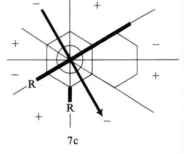

7a

7b

7c

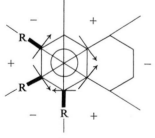
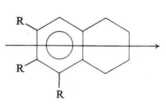
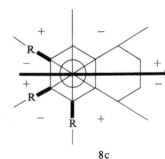

8a

8b

8c

Fig. 16. Influence of substitution pattern upon sign of ^1L_b-band CD of tetralins (tetrahydroisoquinolines, etc.):

a: Platt polarization diagrams;
b: schematic representation of direction of sum vector of spectroscopic moments;
c: derived sector rules for third- (fourth-, ...) sphere contributions.
   Extreme right column: sign of CD according to helicity rule (second-sphere
contributions) for *P*-helicity of nonaromatic ring.

have indicated some changes.[54] For compounds Ph—CHRR', two groups are available for hyperconjugation (σ–π conjugation) and it is reasonable to assume that different substitution of the aromatic ring will change the ability of the π-system to participate in such an interaction with the σ-bonds C—R and C—R'. Due to these phenomena (as well as for steric reasons in the case of the *o*-compounds, at least), the equilibrium between conformers can by altered which could reasonably explain the data observed by Korver.[55]

Much clearer results can be obtained for polycyclic compounds as usually no such difficulty with conformational equilibria exists. The already mentioned relationship between the helicity rule for second-sphere contributions and the sector rule for third-sphere contributions allows a similar treatment for the first. In Fig. 16, again at the left side, the polarization diagrams are drawn for one unsubstituted and three substituted tetralins (tetrahydroisoquinolines, etc.). In the second column is a schematic drawing of the direction of the sum vectors. In the third column sector rules for third-sphere contributions are depicted, and in the fourth the sign of the CD of the second-sphere contribution for *P*-helicity is given. The sector rules are found in the following way. In the polarization diagram, the sign patterns are chosen again deliberately, but alike for all compounds. Construction of the sum vector is straightforward, and Fig. 16 5c shows this sum vector once more, together with the experimentally found sector rule. This sum vector coincides in this case with the trace of one nodal plane and, in clockwise direction from the tip, a negative sector is situated above the plane of the paper. For Fig. 16 6c and 8c, the sum vector is first drawn into the 'empty' sector diagram, and the sector clockwise from the tip is made negative as for 5. This determines all signs, which are identical to those of 5c for 8c, but opposite for 6c. *P*-helicity of the non-aromatic ring thus gives a positive CD within the ^1L_b band for 8 as for 5, but a negative one for 6.

For Fig. 16 7c the sum vector does not coincide with a nodal plane. In this case we can refer to an auxiliary line perpendicular to it and also drawn in bold in diagram Vc. In a clockwise direction from the ends of this line, we again find negative sectors,

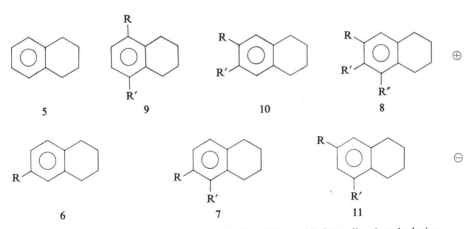

Fig. 17. Helicity rules for differently substituted homochiral tetralins (tetrahydroisoquinolines, etc.). The signs in the extreme right column refer to *P*-helicity of the non-aromatic ring.

and putting the same signs into the diagram 7c we also find the complete sign pattern, which is inverse to that of 5c. *P*-helicity thus leads to a negative CD for type 6.

This very simplified treatment has been applied to various substitution patterns and a summary of examples, which could be proved experimentally, is given in Fig. 17, which refers to *P*-helicity. Some unsubstituted compounds (type 5) and 6,7-disubstituted ones (type 10) have been discussed already and many more can be found in the literature.[1] Type 9 is realized in e.g. the steroid XLVI[64] or in chaparrol (XLVII)[65] which both give positive ${}^1L_b$-band CDs (*P*-helicity), type 8 in some

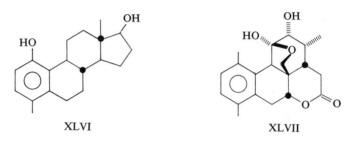

XLVI   XLVII

Amaryllidaceae alkaloids,[39, 41] phthalide isoquinoline alkaloids[44] and tetrahydroberberine alkaloids.[45]

Oestradiol (XLVIII),[64] which also has *P*-helicity of the ring (type 6) and its

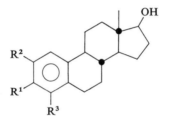

XLVIII : R¹ = OH, R² = R³ = H
XLIX: R¹ = OH, R² = CH₃, R³ = H
L: R¹ = OH, R² = H, R³ = CH₃

4-methyl derivative L[64] (type 7) give negative ${}^1L_b$-band CDs, whereas the 2-methyl isomer XLIX belongs to type 10 and shows, therefore, a positive CD.[64] Another example for type 6 is levorphanol (LIa)[66] (*P*-helicity, negative CD); many morphane alkaloids with or without an ether ring[67] [e.g. tetrahydrodeoxycodeine (LIb) or dihydrodeoxycodeine D (LII)] and rhoeadine alkaloids[68] belong to type 7 and give negative CDs for *P*-helicity.

Recently, Korver and Wilkins[69] described the CD curves for several flavanols (LIII) and found that chromane chromophores of type 6 or 11 give negative ${}^1L_b$-band CDs for *P*-helicity, in good agreement with our predictions.

Although this treatment of the Cotton effect of aromatic chromophores is very crude, it has given very good agreement with experiment. It must be emphasized, however, that it is more a guide to understanding why the CD can change with

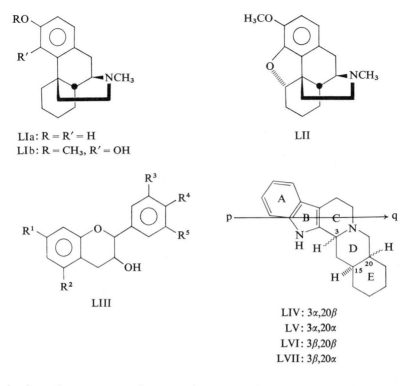

LIa: R = R′ = H
LIb: R = CH₃, R′ = OH

LII

LIII

LIV: 3α,20β
LV: 3α,20α
LVI: 3β,20β
LVII: 3β,20α

substitution, than a means for unequivocal prediction of signs. For this latter purpose at least the different lengths of the spectroscopic moment vectors have to be taken into account.

3.4.6 Heterocyclic Aromatic Chromophores

Some heterocyclic compounds like purines and pyrimidines give absorption bands which closely resemble those of the benzene chromophore (in addition to n → π* transitions),[24, 25] and interpretations of the CD spectra of their glycosides have been published (references 24 and 25 and newer ones by the same authors). Even if one does not know or is not sure about the transitions involved, this general treatment of the CD of aromatic chromophores can be useful in understanding the Cotton effects of heterocyclic compounds, as shown in Fig. 18 for some yohimbanes.[70] In these compounds, the indol system is the chromophore (=first sphere), ring C forms the (chiral) second sphere and rings D and E the third and fourth sphere, respectively. Yohimbane (LIV) and alloyohimbane (LV) have identical second and third spheres, and 3-epi-alloyohimbane (LVII) is heterochiral to them. Pseudoyohimbane (LVI), on the other hand, is the only one of these four stereoisomers which (being homochiral to LVII) differs in the conformation of the third (and fourth) sphere from the others. This result of the conformational analysis is nicely reflected in the CD spectra: those of LIV and LV are not only enantiomorphous to those of LVI and LVII, but the rotational strength and fine structure bands for

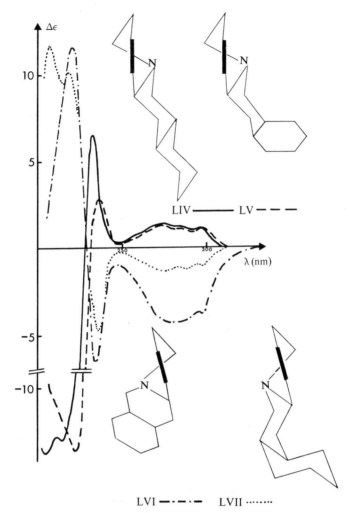

Fig. 18. CD-curves and projections along $p \rightarrow q$ for stereoisomeric yohimbanes LIV–LVII.

the three compounds with identical conformation of second and third spheres (besides absolute configuration), LIV, LV and LVII, are nearly identical or mirror images, whereas the CD of LVI, differing in conformation of the third sphere from the others, gives nearly three times as large a CD band at longest wavelengths, as LVII.

Many other interesting types of aromatic chromophores could not be dealt with in this short summary, but we believe that they all can be treated in a similar way to those described here.

Financial help from the Deutsche Forschungsgemeinschaft and the Fonds der Chemischen Industrie is highly appreciated. G.S. thanks also Miss L. Penzien and Mr. E. Kirmayr for skilful technical assistance, M.K. the A.-v-Humboldt-Stiftung and F.S. the German Academic Exchange Service for a grant.

Figs. 5, 7–11, 13, 15, 16 and 18 are completely or in part reproduced from *XXIIIrd International Congress of Pure and Applied Chemistry* 7, 117 (1971), and Fig. 3 is taken from E. Heftmann, Ed., *Modern Methods of Steroid Analysis*, J. Wiley, London. In press, with the permission of the editors.

References

1. P. Crabbé and W. Klyne, *Tetrahedron* **23**, 3449 (1967).
2. This book, p. 173.
3. G. Snatzke, *Tetrahedron* **21**, 413 (1965).
4. M. S. Newman, R. S. Darbek and L. Tsai, *J. Amer. Chem. Soc.* **89**, 6191 (1967).
5. This book, pp. 32 and 61.
6. C. M. Kemp and S. F. Mason, *Tetrahedron* **22**, 629 (1966).
7. P. Crabbé, *Chem. and Ind.* 917 (1969).
8. G. Haas, P. B. Hulbert, W. Klyne, V. Prelog and G. Snatzke, *Helv. Chim. Acta* **54**, 491 (1971).
9. This book, Chapters 2.4, 3.6, 3.7 and 4.3
10. A. Moscowitz, K. Mislow, M. A. W. Glass and C. Djerassi, *J. Amer. Chem. Soc.* **84**, 1945 (1962).
11. For a recent review and calculation cf. G. Wagnière, W. Hug and J. Kuhn. In press.
12. R. H. Martin. Private communication.
13. J. A. Schellman, *Accounts Chem. Res.* **1**, 144 (1968).
14. W. Kuhn, in K. Freudenberg, ed., *Stereochemie*. Deuticke, Leipzig, 1933, p. 317.
15. S. F. Mason, *Quart. Rev. Chem Soc.* **17**, 20 (1963).
16. K. Mislow, E. Bunnenberg, R. Records, K. Wellman and C. Djerassi, *J. Amer. Chem. Soc.* **85**, 1342 (1963).
17. S. F. Mason, in R. Bonnett and J. G. Davis, eds., *Some Newer Physical Methods in Structural Chemistry*. United Trade Press, London, 1967, p. 149.
18. J. Cymerman Craig and S. K. Roy, *Tetrahedron* **21**, 395 (1965).
19. C. Djerassi, K. Mislow and M. Shamma, *Experientia* **18**, 53 (1962).
20. N. Harada and K. Nakanishi, *J. Amer. Chem. Soc.* **91**, 3989 (1969).
21. N. Harada and K. Nakanishi, *Accounts Chem. Res.* **5**, 257 (1972).
22. M. Shamma, J. L. Moniot, W. K. Chan and K. Nakanishi, *Tetrahedron Lett.* 3425 (1971).
23. M. Shamma, J. L. Moniot, W. K. Chan and K. Nakanishi, *Tetrahedron Lett.* 4207 (1971).
24. D. W. Miles, R. K. Robins and H. Eyring, *Proc. Natl. Acad. Sci. U.S.A.* **57**, 1138 (1967).
25. D. W. Miles, M. J. Robins, R. K. Robins, M. W. Winkley and H. Eyring, *J. Amer. Chem. Soc.* **91**, 824 (1969).
26. P. C. Ho, Thesis, Bonn, 1971.
27. A. Brossi and S. Teitel, *Helv. Chim. Acta* **54**, 1564 (1971).
28. E. Dornhege and G. Snatzke, *Tetrahedron* **26**, 3059 (1970).
29. J. Barry, H.-B. Kagan and G. Snatzke, *Tetrahedron* **27**, 4737 (1971).
30. R. Weidmann and J.-P. Guetté, *C.R.H. Acad. Sci., Ser. C* **268**, 2225 (1969).
31. J.-P. Guetté. Private communication. In ref. 30 it was stated that these groups are pseudo-equatorially arranged. It has now been proved that this is not the case.
32. N. L. Bencze, B. Kisis, R. T. Puckett and N. Finch, *Tetrahedron* **26**, 5407 (1970).
33. G. Snatzke and P. C. Ho, *Tetrahedron* **27**, 3645 (1971).
34. R. P. K. Chan, J. Cymerman Craig, R. H. F. Manske and T. O. Soine, *Tetrahedron* **23**, 4209 (1967).
35. S. F. Mason, G. W. Vane and J. S. Whitehurst, *Tetrahedron* **23**, 4089 (1967).
36. A. I. Scott, F. McCapra, F. Comer, S. A. Sutherland, D. W. Young, G. A. Sim and G. Ferguson, *Tetrahedron* **20**, 1339 (1964).
37. A. I. Scott, G. A. Sim, G. Ferguson, D. W. Young and F. McCapra, *J. Amer. Chem. Soc.* **84**, 3197 (1962).
38. Cf. W. Kuhn and H. Kh. Gore, *Z. Phys. Chem.* **B 12**, 289 (1931).
39. K. Kuriyama, T. Iwata, K. Moriyama, K. Kotera, Y. Hamada, R. Mitsui and K. Takeda, *J. Chem. Soc.* **B** 46 (1967).
40. J. A. Schellman, *J. Chem. Phys.* **44**, 55 (1966).
41. H. H. DeAngelis and W. C. Wildman, *Tetrahedron* **25**, 5099 (1969).
42. We thank Dr. M. Legrand, Paris, for providing us with this CD-curve.

43. Unpublished results in collaboration with Professor R. C. Cambie, New Zealand.
44. G. Snatzke, G. Wollenberg, J. Hrbek, Jr., F. Šantavý, K. Bláha, W. Klyne and R. J. Swan, *Tetrahedron* **25**, 5059 (1969).
45. G. Snatzke, J. Hrbek Jr., L. Hruban, A. Horeau and F. Šantavý, *Tetrahedron* **26**, 5013 (1970).
46. J. R. Platt, *J. Chem. Phys.* **17**, 484 (1949); **19**, 263 (1951).
47. G. Snatzke, M. Kajtár and F. Werner-Zamojska, *Pure and Appl. Chemistry*, XXIIIrd International Congress of Pure and Applied Chemistry, **7**, 117 (1971).
48. G. Snatzke, M. Kajtár and F. Werner-Zamojska, *Tetrahedron* **28**, 281 (1972).
49. G. Poppe, *Diplomarbeit*, Bonn. 1971.
50. M. J. Luche, A. Marquet and G. Snatzke, *Tetrahedron* **28**, 1677 (1972).
51. J. H. Brewster and J. G. Buta, *J. Amer. Chem. Soc.* **88**, 2233 (1966).
52. H. E. Smith and T. C. Willis, *J. Amer. Chem. Soc.* **93**, 2287 (1971).
53. L. Verbit and H. C. Price. Lecture at this ASI, cf. *J. Amer. Chem. Soc.* **94**, 5143 (1972).
54. T. M. Hooker and J. A. Schellman, *Biopolymers* **9**, 1319 (1970).
55. O. Korver, *Tetrahedron* **26**, 5507 (1970).
56. J.-I. Kunimoto, K. Morimoto, K. Yamamoto, Y. Yoshikawa, K. Azuma and K. Fujitani, *Chem. Pharm. Bull* (*Japan*) **19**, 2197 (1971).
57. A. Petruska, *J. Chem. Phys.* **34**, 1120 (1961).
58. O. E. Weigang, Jr. and M. J. Nugent, *J. Amer. Chem. Soc.* **91**, 4555 (1969); M. J. Nugent and O. E. Weigang, Jr., *J. Amer. Chem. Soc.* **91**, 4556 (1969).
59. M. Legrand and R. Viennet, *Bull. Soc. Chim. France* 679 (1965).
60. J. Horwitz, E. H. Strickland and C. Billups, *J. Amer. Chem. Soc.* **91**, 184 (1969).
61. A. Moscowitz, A. Rosenberg and A. E. Hansen, *J. Amer. Chem. Soc.* **87**, 1813 (1965).
62. B. K. Vainshtain and G. V. Gurskaya, *Dokl. Akad. Nauk SSSR* **156**, 312 (1964).
63. A. Mostad, H. M. Nissen and C. Rømming, *Tetrahedron Lett.* 2131 (1971).
64. M. Legrand and R. Viennet, *Bull. Soc. Chim. France* 2798 (1966).
65. T. R. Hollands, P. de Mayo, M. Nisbet and P. Crabbé, *Can. J. Chem.* **43**, 3008 (1965).
66. A. F. Casy and A. P. Parulkar, *J. Med. Chem.* **12**, 178 (1969).
67. U. Weiss and Th. Rüll, *Bull. Soc. Chim. France* 3707 (1965).
68. J. Hrbek, Jr., L. Hruban, V. Šimánek, F. Šantavý and G. Snatzke, *Coll. Czechoslov. Chem. Commun.* In press.
69. O. Korver and C. K. Wilkins, *Tetrahedron* **27**, 5459 (1971).
70. L. Bartlett, N. F. J. Dastoor, J. Hrbek Jr., W. Klyne, H. Schmid and G. Snatzke, *Helv. Chim. Acta* **54**, 1238 (1971).

CHAPTER **3.5**

Other Chromophores

G. SNATZKE

University of Bonn (F.R.G.)

and

F. SNATZKE (formerly WERNER-ZAMOJSKA)

Polish Academy of Sciences
Warsaw (PL)

3.5.1 Introduction

In some of the preceding chapters the chiroptical properties of several special chromophores have been described. In this chapter we should first like to give a general procedure for finding the appropriate type of rule in each given case. Then we shall apply these rules to a greater variety of chromophores, whose chiroptical properties have been investigated in more detail.

3.5.2 General Treatment

When analysing the Cotton effects of many different chromophores we have found it useful to divide the whole molecule into spheres[1] which have been defined in the following way: the chromophore itself, by definition, is the first sphere, the ring into which it is incorporated forms the second one, the rings or groups directly connected to the second sphere build up the third sphere, and so on. In a modification of Tschugaeff's distance rule[2] (referring to rotations at the NaD line), which was revised by Klyne[3] for the Cotton effect of ketones, we proposed the generalization that the chiral sphere which is nearest to the chromophore determines the sign and, to a great extent, the magnitude of each Cotton effect. The contributions to the CD of different spheres are, however, not simply additive; the influence of the nth sphere seems to be smaller, if one of the other spheres $(n - i)$ $(i \geqslant 1)$ nearer to the chromophore is chiral. Formally this can be expressed in the following way.

If we call $R^{(i)}$ the contribution of the ith sphere to the rotational strength then the complete rotational strength R is not given by the sum

$$R = \sum_{(i)} R^{(i)}$$

but by the expression

$$R = \sum_{(i)} g^{(i)} \cdot R^{(i)}$$

in which the $g^{(i)}$ are weight factors with the following properties: $g^{(i)}$ is large if the *i*th sphere is the nearest chiral sphere to the chromophore, and it becomes smaller if this is not the case. Each $R^{(i)}$ may be described by a 'chirality function'[4-7] by which we may quantitatively characterize the chirality of each sphere. In that sense we can indeed speak of large and small chiralities and exceptions to the above-mentioned principle have their origin in the fact that the chiral sphere nearest to the chromophore may have a very small chirality whereas that of the next one may be much larger; in spite of its smaller $g^{(i)}$ weight factor it can then nevertheless over-compensate the contributions from the $(i-1)$th sphere, if both contributions have opposite signs.

Moscowitz[8] has already called those chromophores 'inherently dissymmetric' (this should now be replaced by 'inherently chiral'), which belong to that category having a chiral first sphere according to our definition. The rotational strength is one or two order(s) of magnitude stronger as in Moscowitz' second class[8] of compounds, to which belong those chromophores which are 'locally achiral, but chirally perturbed by their environment'. This second category is subdivided by us into a class of compounds containing a chiral second sphere, and another where also the second sphere is achiral.

Examples of compounds with a chiral first sphere are hexahelicene, for which the σ-skeleton is chiral and, therefore, also the π-system (cf. p. 149); some ketones whose n- and/or π^*-orbitals are chiral because of interaction with adjacent n- or π-orbitals (cf. p. 112), the disulphide chromophore (if the torsion angle around the S—S bond is not equal to $0°$, $90°$, or $180°$),[9] etc. A prediction of the correlation between the stereochemistry and the sign (and magnitude) of the Cotton effect by theoretical calculations is often very complicated. Only in the case of 'coupled oscillators' (cf. Chapter 2.3), i.e. in presence of two (or three) achiral chromophores which are not conjugated or only weakly conjugated with each other can the sign of the Cotton effect be obtained by applying simple geometric considerations.

If the second sphere is chiral this means that the ring containing the chromophore is chiral (or helical). In such a case [e.g. cycloalkanones in a twist-conformation (cf. p. 110), non-coplanar saturated lactones (cf. p. 130–37), tetralins (cf. p. 153), etc.] it is always the helicity (chirality) of this ring (named P or M according to Cahn *et al.*[10]) which determines the sign of the Cotton effect.

If the third sphere is the nearest chiral sphere to the chromophore, the latter and its local surroundings are achiral. For this case of an 'achiral skeleton substituted in a chiral manner by achiral ligands' Ruch's treatment[4-7] provides a general answer; the type of rule which can be applied depends on the symmetry of the skeleton. When this rule is of the sector type, Schellman's paper[11] on the simplest pseudoscalar function in each symmetry class can be consulted.

Ruch's approach was merely geometrical using group theory. He found the simplest 'chirality function' which 'qualitatively completely' describes any type of chirality observation, and thus also each Cotton effect. 'Qualitative complete' in this context means that chiral mixtures of chiral molecules (i.e. not racemates) are described correctly by such a chirality function. This chirality function can either be approximated by a polynomial or by a sum of functions, each of which depends on a single ligand $[\omega(i)]$, on the interaction between two ligands $[\omega(i,j)]$, or even on the interaction between three different ligands $[\omega(i,j,k)]$. The mathematical treat-ment makes use of 'Young Tableaux'[12] which correspond to the irreducible repre-

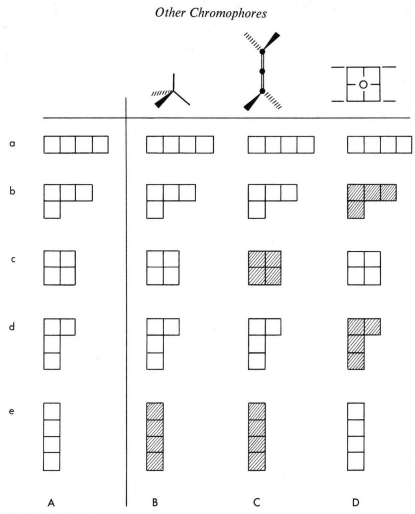

Fig. 1. Partition Tableaux for cases having four places on the (achiral) skeleton. A. The five possible partition diagrams; B. Partition Tableaux for an asymmetric C atom (T_d-symmetry); C. Partition Tableaux for allenes (D_{2d}-symmetry); D. Partition Tableaux for β-substituted adamantanones (C_{2v}-symmetry). The marked partition diagrams in Tableaux B, C and D correspond to 'active partitions'. For details see text.

sentations of the symmetric permutation group. A one-to-one correlation exists between these and the partition diagrams which give the different possibilities for arranging the (different or like) ligands on the n places of the skeleton. If there are, for example, four places ($n = 4$), we get the following five partitions (cf. Fig. 1): (a) represents the case of four like ligands, (b) the case of three like ligands and one different, (c) that of two pairs of identical ligands, (d) that of one pair of identical ligands and two others, and (e) that of four different ligands. Conventionally, the boxes are arranged in such a way that longer horizontal lines are positioned above shorter ones. All the different allowed permutations of the ligands present are represented in a single diagram.

The diagrams which belong to chiral mixtures ('active partitions' according to Ruch[6]) have been determined mathematically and these are marked. If the four places belong, for example, to an asymmetric C atom (centre of chirality, T_d-symmetry of the 'skeleton'), only the last diagram (Fig. 1B, e) is hatched, if the partition tableau represents the four substituents on an allene skeleton (D_{2d}-symmetry), the third and fifth diagrams are marked (Fig. 1C, c and e), and in the case of a ketone with (local) C_{2v}-symmetry, as a β-substituted adamantanone I it is the second and fourth (Fig. 1D, b and d). In the latter case only such places can be compared which

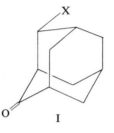

are correlated by the symmetry elements of the skeleton; they are said to belong to the same 'transitivity range'. For example, five different transitivity ranges are present for an adamantanone.

The number of boxes in the longest first line of marked diagrams is called 'chirality order o' and it can be shown that o can only be $(n - 1), (n - 2)$, or $(n - 3)$. In the first case the respective chirality function is of the type $\bar{\chi} = \sum \omega(i)$, thus each chirality observation is described by functions which depend solely on the individual ligands and not on interactions between them; the Cotton effect is governed by a sector type rule. If the chirality order $o = n - 2$, then the chirality function is of the form $\bar{\chi} = \sum \omega(i,j)$ and the Cotton effect depends on the interaction within pairs of ligands. Finally, in the case of $o = n - 3$, the chirality function is $\bar{\chi} = \sum \omega(i,j,k)$ and for such chromophores (molecules) the interaction between sets of three ligands has to be taken into account. If more than one partition diagram is marked within one tableaux, then the 'qualitative complete' chirality function contains ω-terms of different kinds corresponding to each marked diagram. In the latter case, however, that one coming from the topmost marked diagram alone describes the preponderant part of the Cotton effect: the other terms function only as corrections.

The chemist will not usually be able to ascertain these marked partitions but because of the aforementioned correlation can at least spot the topmost marked diagram. It corresponds to that molecule which has the maximum number of identical ligands and yet is chiral, because this is an identical definition of the chirality order o. Thus in the case of an asymmetric C atom all four ligands have to be different, in the case of an allene two pairs of ligands can lead to a chiral molecule, and the monosubstituted adamantanone I is an example of a chiral molecule where even three ligands (within one transitivity range, namely here that of the β-equatorial ligands*) can be identical. The corresponding partition diagrams are B, e; C, c; and D, b; respectively (of Fig. 1), i.e. they are indeed identical with the topmost marked diagrams in the respective Young tableaux. The allene example shows that

---

* Equatorial refers to that ring containing the carbonyl group.

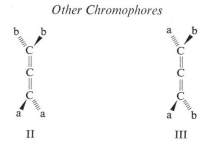

II   III

not every permutation of ligands leads to a chiral molecule. It is enough for this treatment that at least one permutation should do so. Both II and III contain two pairs of ligands, but only III lacks symmetry elements of the second order. The stereochemist thus very easily finds that, for example, for a compound with an asymmetric C atom as the only source of chirality, the chirality order $o = 1 = 4 - 3$, and therefore the Cotton effect is governed by a rule which has to take into account the interaction between three ligands. Thus Kauzmann's 'Principle of pairwise interaction',[13] which he used to build up the molecular rotation from increments, according to Ruch,[4, 6] is only an approximation.

The stereochemist, by simply investigating which *molecule* is chiral, finds only the first of the hatched partition diagrams related to the *chiral mixture*, but, as

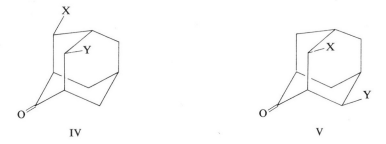

IV   V

explained above, this is usually the one of main interest. That such a description is, however, not complete can be seen from the following two examples. A 1:1 mixture of IV and V is a chiral ensemble, and the Cotton effect in principle must be unequal to zero, though in practice it may perhaps be very small. According

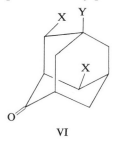

VI

to the simple octant rule (corresponding only to the topmost marked diagram with $o = 3$) for the mixture, a CD of zero will be predicted. Similarly, for VI according to the simple octant rule $\Delta\varepsilon \equiv 0$ is predicted, though this molecule is chiral. In these cases the second part of the chirality function containing the terms $\omega(i,j)$ becomes important. The latter example VI illustrates this nicely, although X and Y do not belong to the same transitivity range. In the language of the simple octant rule the contributions of the two substituents X are identical in magnitude but opposite in sign. The 'upper' X is, however, nearer to Y than the 'lower' one, and, when allowance is made for pairwise interactions, the two contributions are no longer of the same magnitude and a small CD should be found, although its sign cannot be predicted at the moment.

When, on the basis of Ruch's generalizations,[4-7] it has been found that a sector rule is applicable to the Cotton effect ($o = n - 1$), the precise form can be determined by Schellman's treatment.[11] Since the rotational strength R changes its sign if the coordinate system is inverted, R has the properties of a pseudoscalar. Schellman has calculated the simplest pseudoscalar functions for the symmetry groups of many important chromophores: e.g. for C_s-symmetry, a 'planar rule' is in agreement with pseudoscalar properties; for C_{2v}-symmetry, a 'quadrant rule' is appropriate; and for D_{2d}, an 'octant rule' should apply. Ketones belong to the symmetry class C_{2v} as long as the chromophore is regarded and Schellman[11] therefore predicted a quadrant rule, although, experimentally, an octant rule or an even more complex sector rule is favoured (cf. p. 89 and reference 14). These also have pseudoscalar properties in C_{2v}-symmetry, but they are not the simplest such functions. Schellman's paper[11] gives only the minimal requirement for each chromophore, the actual sector rule may, however, be more complicated. In general we may expect (a) Planar Rules, (b) Quadrant Rules, (c) Octant Rules, and (d) more complex Sector Rules for compounds with achiral first and second spheres; (e) Torsion Angle Rules, and (f) Helicity Rules for the latter type of compounds; (g) Rules taking into account Pairwise Interactions, and (h) Rules taking into account Interactions within Sets of Three Ligands for all compounds. Even if no sector rule is allowed, within a given group of related compounds one can build up approximate rules of type (a)–(f), provided that it is realized that they are restricted in their applicability. Some examples are given in the following. A recent monograph by Crabbé[15] contains a good compilation of papers on the chiroptical properties of many different chromophores. Instead of attempting the impossible task of covering all or even most chromophores in such a short review, we should like to give a few typical examples for the general treatment outlined above.

3.5.3   The Chiral First Sphere

CT-Complexes between tetracyanoethylene (TCE) and ketones. The CT-complexes of TCE and ketones have been found to give Cotton effects within the CT bands[16] and they are good examples for demonstrating the basic principles of generating rotational strength. In these complexes charge from the lone pair orbital of the carbonyl group is transferred into the free π^*-orbital of the TCE molecule, producing an electric transition moment vector $\vec{\mu}$. For best overlap the plane of the carbonyl

VII

VIII

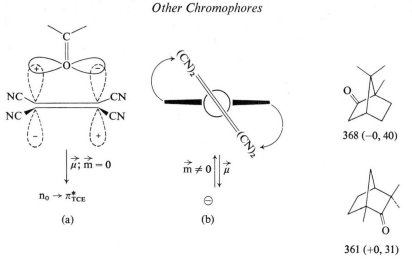

368 (−0, 40)

361 (+0, 31)

Fig. 2. Charge-transfer complexes between ketones and tetracyano-ethylene: (a) optimal geometry for orbital overlap does not cause a magnetic transition moment;(b) twisted complex, due to steric interaction with chiral ketone—the example shown gives a negative Cotton effect.

group must coincide with the symmetry plane of the π^*-orbital (Fig. 2) and thus no magnetic moment is introduced (in first approximation) by this CT. In complexes with chiral hindered ketones like (+)-camphor (VII) or (+)-fenchone (VIII) steric interaction will tend to twist the TCE molecule with respect to the ketone, and by this chirality of the first sphere (cf. Fig. 2) a rotation of charge, i.e. a magnetic transition moment vector $\vec{m}$ is also generated. According to the general formula

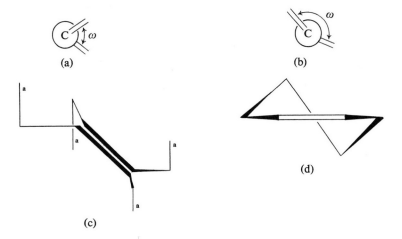

Fig. 3. Rules for conjugated dienes: (a) Helicity rule for cisoid dienes leading to a positive CD; (b) Helicity rule for transoid dienes leading to a positive CD; (c) 'Allylic axial chirality contribution'—the four groups (including hydrogen) marked with 'a' give positive contributions to the CD; (d) Ring helicity rule—a double bond (as part of a diene) incorporated into a ring of P-helicity as shown gives a positive contribution to the CD.

$R = |\vec{\mu}| . |\vec{m}| \cdot \cos(\vec{\mu}, \vec{m})$, a positive CD arises if $\vec{\mu}$ and $\vec{m}$ are parallel, and a negative one if they are antiparallel. Thus the sense of twist may be deduced from the sign of the CD within the CT-band. The CD is relatively small, but for other reasons, e.g. dissociation.

Conjugated dienes. Conjugated dienes form a chiral chromophore and the empirical helicity rules proposed for cisoid*[17] and transoid*[18] dienes (Fig. 3, a and b) have been interpreted theoretically.[19-21] The rule of Fig. 3b shows exceptions as does that of Fig. 3a with dienes which are not homoannular.[22] Burgstahler and Barkhurst[22] gave another interpretation for the long wavelength $\pi \rightarrow \pi^*$ transition of conjugated dienes by incorporating the σ-bonds to the allylic axial substituents (including hydrogen) into the chromophore and assuming that this 'allylic axial chirality contribution' (i.e. $\sigma - \pi$ homoconjugation) is more powerful in determining the sign of the Cotton effect, than the helicity of the diene system (i.e. $\pi - \pi$ conjugation) (Fig. 3c). For homoannular dienes both rules (Fig. 3a and c) lead to identical predictions. We should like to propose another approach, which also can explain the published data: the contribution of each olefinic bond of a diene to the Cotton effect is determined by the helicity of the ring into which it is incorporated (Fig. 3d). Actually there is no fundamental difference between rules c and d of Fig. 3.

The CD of α-phellandrene (IX) illustrates the application of this rule. At room temperature a negative Cotton effect is observed[17] which points to a pseudoaxial conformation of the isopropyl group. As this was assumed to be the less preferred conformer, the temperature was raised and the ORD-amplitude increased. As expected, on lowering the temperature the Cotton effect becomes first zero and then positive,[23] proving that the conformer with the pseudoequatorial isopropyl group is the energetically preferred one. By referring to a conformationally rigid diene, the differences in free enthalpy and entropy between the two conformers have been

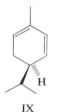

IX

found to be $\Delta H = 0.28$ kcal/mole and $\Delta S = 2.2$ cal/degree.mole. A comparison for the application of the different rules for two steroidal dienes[22] is given in Fig. 4.

Disulphides. Disulphides give two CD bands at 250–300 nm and at 230–250 nm[24-26] and for torsion angles between ~30–60° the first band depends mainly on the helicity of the system; the second depends also on contributions from more distant spheres. For torsion angles approaching 90° the sign of the first CD band (at 250–260 nm) is, however, solely governed by the environment of the chromophore.[27] This discrepancy has been solved by a theoretical treatment of the

---

*The helicity of a and b (Fig. 3) is often referred to as 'right-handed' helix, and by this it is implied that one considers the two double bonds as steps of a spiral staircase. Looking along the C_2-axis of the diene system however, the two C=C double bonds form an M-helix (left-handed screw) as does the helix built from the three bonds of the C=C—C=C system (axis parallel to C—C). The torsion angle along the single bond is positive for a and b. In mentioning the helicity of such a system, the mode of projection must always be defined in order to avoid ambiguity.

—S—S— chromophore by Lindenberg and Michl[9] who showed that at 90° degeneracy occurs (Fig. 5) and the helicity of the system therefore has no influence upon the CD. The prediction[9] of sign inversion at torsion angles larger than 90°, which is also in agreement with a more general treatment of systems belonging to C_2-symmetry[28] has recently been proved[29] to be correct by investigating the CD

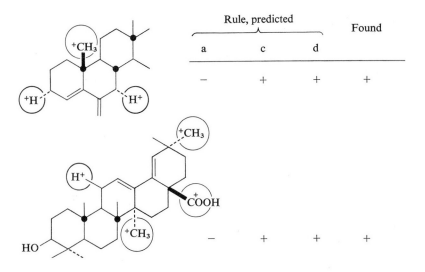

Fig. 4. Application of the rules of Fig. 3 to a 6-methylene-Δ^4-ene-steroid (top) and another heteroannular diene of the triterpene series (bottom). Letters a, c and d refer to the rules in Fig. 3.

of (2,7-cystine)-gramicidine S containing the disulphide bridge in a P-helical conformation with a torsion angle of about +120° (negative CD at 271·5 nm).

Azochromophore, perturbed by a C(=O) *group.* The N=N chromophore in chiral environments gives rise to optical activity within both n → π* transitions.[30-32] In the special case of a pyrazoline ring these bands appear at about 330 and 230 nm and have a small rotational strength. If however a C(=O) group (carbonyl or carboxyl) is present in the α-position to one of the nitrogens very large ellipticities can be observed,[31, 32] whereas the corresponding carbonyl Cotton effects retain their original magnitudes. In such an arrangement (Fig. 6) the orbital system of the azo chromophore is thus perturbed by the CO group, but the orbitals of the latter are not significantly influenced by the N=N moiety. As spiropyrazolines are easily prepared from naturally occurring methylene lactones (e.g. in sesquiterpene

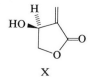

X

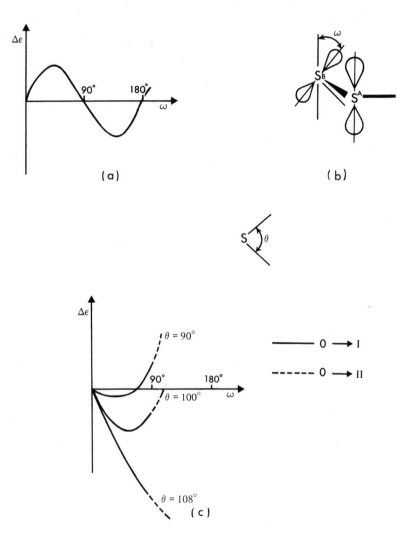

Fig. 5. CD of disulphides. The excited state is split, a Hückel treatment leads to a dependence of the CD on the torsion angle ω of the disulphide [shown in (b) as the angle between
the lone-pair p-orbitals on the S atoms] as shown in (a). A more sophisticated CNDO
treatment also shows a dependence upon the bond angle θ at the S atom, degeneracy again
occurs at $\omega = 90°$, but the crossover point (i.e. change of sign) appears within a wider
range (c).

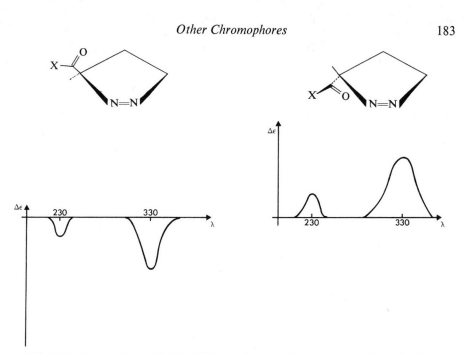

Fig. 6. CD of pyrazolines with C(=O)X group in α-position (schematic), X may be OR or alkyl.

series), this rule (Fig. 6) can be used to determine the stereochemistry of such compounds. For example, the aglycone X of tuliposide A[33] gave on CH_2N_2 addition two spiropyrazolines XI and XII of which only XI showed internal hydrogen bonding from OH to N (by IR spectroscopy). The CD bands [XI: 324 (+8·8), 236 (+3·3); XII: 323 (−7·7), 232 (−5·1)] characterize the absolute configuration of

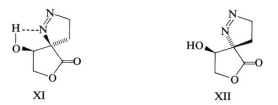

| XI | XII |

the newly introduced auxiliary centre of chirality to be (R) and (S) for XI and XII respectively, and together with the IR results this determines the absolute configuration of X to be (S).

3.5.4 The Chiral Second Sphere

Azomethines. The C=N chromophore gives rise to a CD band at about 250 nm;[34−36] for those containing this grouping in a six-membered ring the helicity of this ring determines the sign of the Cotton effect[35] according to Fig. 7. Thus the 18-homo-conanine derivative XIII with M-helicity of ring E gives a negative Cotton effect.[36]

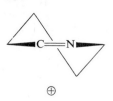

Fig. 7. Cyclic azomethines. The half-chair conformation drawn leads to a positive CD.

Oxathiolanes. Oxathiolanes give a Cotton effect around 250 nm, for which two
rules have been published. One correlates the helicity (or chirality) of the five-
membered ring with the sign of the CD[37] according to Fig. 8a (P-helicity leading to

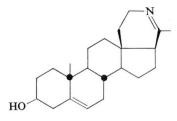

XIII

positive CD; second-sphere contribution), the other[38] is a sector rule (Fig. 8b) for
third-sphere contributions. The former rule is, of course, more powerful than the
latter.[37]

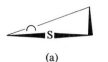

(a)

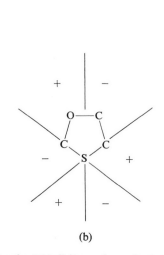

(b)

Fig. 8. Oxathiolanes. (a) Ring-chirality (helicity) rule: M-helicity as drawn leads to
negative Cotton effect. (b) Sector rule for third-sphere contributions. Signs refer to
upper sectors (the plane of the paper is another nodal plane of this sector rule).

Trithiocarbonates. An $n \rightarrow \pi^*$ band is found in the CD spectra of trithiocarbonates at about 450 nm, and a $\pi \rightarrow \pi^*$ band around 315 nm. Both are optically active

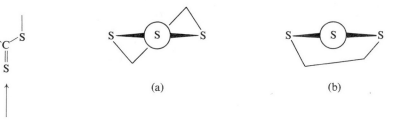

Fig. 9. Trithiocarbonates. The arrow shows direction of projection. M-Helicity [(a) C_2-symmetry; (b) C_1-symmetry] leads to positive CD at 450 and negative CD at 315 nm.

and their signs are determined by the helicity (or chirality) of the ring if this grouping is incorporated into a 1,3-dithiane according to Fig. 9.[38, 39]

Axial nitrocompounds. In Chapter 3.2 (p. 111) we have shown that the helicity (chirality) of the second sphere can also be interpreted by referring to the torsion angle around the nearest bonds to the chromophore. Axial nitro compounds, for which the chromophore never can be part of a ring, have thus also been treated in a similar way[40] with reference to the torsion angle around the C—N bond; if this is positive (defined as the angle between the bond to the geminal hydrogen and the nearest N—O bond), a positive CD is found around 280 nm. No simple correlation could be found for the other band at around 330 nm.[40, 41]

Axial thiolacetates. Thiolacetates give a CD band at about 270 nm which most probably is of n → π* origin.[38, 42] An octant rule (see Fig. 10a) has been proposed for this chromophore,[38] the CD data of axial acetylmercapto compounds can, however, equally well be explained by referring to the chirality of the second sphere: a positive torsion angle around the C—S(Ac) bond (with respect to the geminal hydrogen) correlates with a positive CD (Fig. 10b).

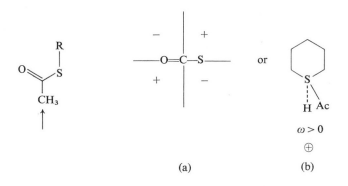

Fig. 10. Axial thiolacetates. (a) Octant rule for third-sphere contributions (the plane of the paper is also a nodal plane, the signs refer to back octants). The arrow in the left formula indicates the direction of projection. (b) Chirality rule (projection along the S—C bond). A positive torsion angle ω as drawn leads to a positive CD contribution of the second sphere.

3.5.5 The Chiral Third (Fourth, ...) Sphere

A. Planar rule

N-Chloro compounds. *N*-Chloro compounds of secondary amines give a CD band around 270 nm,[43, 44] whose sign could be correlated in the case of *N*-chloropiperidines with the absolute configuration according to the planar rule depicted in Fig. 11a.[44]

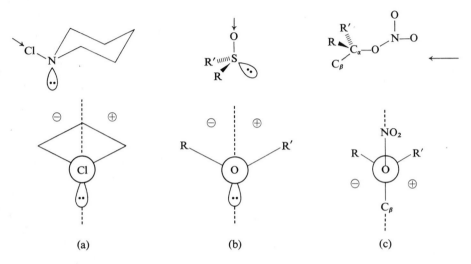

Fig. 11. Planar Rules. (a) *N*-Chloro-amines, projection along Cl—N bond (arrow). (b) 210 nm band CD of dialkyl sulphoxides, projection along O—S bond (arrow). (c) *o*-Nitrates (230 nm CD band only), projection along O—C$_\alpha$ bond (arrow).

Sulphoxides. Saturated sulphoxides give a Cotton effect at 210 nm, which follows the planar rule of Mislow[45] shown in Fig. 11b. In the original paper this rule is called a chirality rule (positive CD belongs to *S*-configuration at the sulphur atom). Some sulphoxides like XIV give an additional CD band at 230 nm[46] with opposite sign to that at 210 nm; this was explained by the presence of a second rotamer.[46] Double bonds in the vicinity of the sulphur atom may influence the sign of the CD.

O-Nitrates. Nitrates of chiral alcohols, as e.g. sugar derivatives[47, 48] or steroids[49] give up to three CD bands around 270, 230 and 210 nm. Recently, a planar rule (Fig. 11c) has been proposed for the correlation of the 230 nm band CD with the

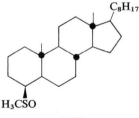

XIV

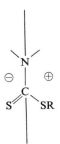

Fig. 12. Quadrant rule for dithiocarbamates. The plane of the paper is also a nodal plane, signs refer to the upper quadrants.

stereochemistry of the nitrate ester,[50] we believe, however, that additional nodal surfaces must also be taken into account.

B. Quadrant Rule

N-Dithiocarbamates of secondary amines. N-Dithiocarbamates give an n → π* band CD at around 340 nm and a π → π* band CD at about 280 nm. For the first a quadrant rule has been proposed,[51, 52] which is depicted in Fig. 12. Such a rule which gave good results for various aliphatic and ring compounds implies that the two sulphur atoms are equivalent, which is, however, only approximately true (resonance).

Olefin–Pt complexes [PtCl₄]²⁻ salts form square planar complexes with olefins in which one corner is occupied by the C=C grouping and which show several Cotton effects. That at 430 nm was correlated[53] with the stereochemistry of the olefin and the quadrant rule of Fig. 13 was proposed. It suffers, however, from the fact that the complexes formed are transient, and after decomposition not always the original olefins, but isomeric ones, have been recovered. Furthermore, in order to explain some of the exceptions, it has been assumed that from some distance on another quadrant rule holds in which the signs are inverted ('double quadrant rule'). We believe that another reason for the frequent failures is the fact that, for complexes in which the C=C double bond is not exactly perpendicular to the 'plane' of the complex, chirality of the second sphere is introduced.

C. Octant Rule

Ketones with achiral first and second spheres follow at least an octant rule,[14] though local symmetry of the C=O chromophore requires only quadrant behaviour.[11] This rule is discussed extensively in Chapter 3.1 of this book.

Azides and thiocyanates show n → π* CD bands at 280 and 250 nm, respectively. Theory predicts for both an octant rule with the same signs as for ketones[54, 55] (Fig. 14). In the steroid series[54] results were not unambiguous, better correlations were possible for azido sugars.[56, 57] The problem in the application of these rules lies in the uncertainty of the preferred conformation of the rod-like chromophore around the C—N and C—S bonds, respectively.

Olefins. The CD of the longest wavelength band of chiral olefins has been accessible for direct measurements only during the last few years.[58] Yogev *et al.*,[59] from ORD measurements, were the first to propose a rule by assuming that the position of the axial allylic groups (including hydrogen) determines the sign of the

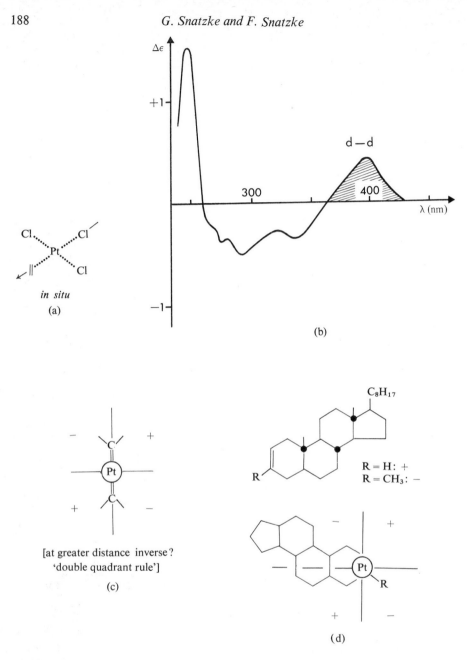

Fig. 13. Olefin–Pt complexes. (a) Structure of the complexes formed *in situ*; arrow gives the direction of projection for the quadrant rule. (b) Typical CD-spectrum; rule refers only to one of the d—d bands (hatched). (c) Quadrant rule for olefin–Pt complexes in the vicinity of the central atom, viewed from the Pt atom towards the olefin. (d) Illustration of the rule by application to a Δ^2-ene-steroid and its 3-methyl substitution product. The signs given next to the formulae are the experimental ones.

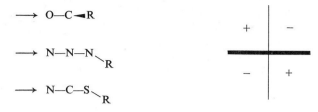

Fig. 14. Schematic representation of the octant rule for ketones, azides and thiocyanates. Arrow indicates direction of projection. The plane of the paper is also a nodal plane, the signs refer to the back octants.

Cotton effect. As mentioned already, this approach has been taken up by Burg-stahler and Barkhurst[22] in their treatment of the Cotton effect of conjugated dienes. Assuming that the band in question is of $\pi_x \to \pi_x^*$ origin, Scott and Wrixon[60] proposed an octant rule (Fig. 15),* the application of which to (R)-*trans*-cyclo-octene[61] $[\Delta\varepsilon_{max}(196) = -31\cdot7]$ is also shown in Fig. 15†. Some of the exceptions[62] to this rule are believed[63] to be only apparent ones, because the $\pi_x \to \pi_y^*$ (or $\sigma \to \pi^*$) transitions, usually assumed to lie at higher energies and following an inverse rule to that just described, occasionally may appear at longer wavelengths. Gawroński and Kiełczewski[64] explained the same data,[62] however, by also taking into account 'homoallylic axial bond contributions'. The presence of two CD bands of opposite signs whose relative positions cannot be predicted unequivocally is a severe drawback for this rule. Furthermore, a small distortion of the double bond (deviation from coplanarity = chirality of the first sphere) should have a much greater influence[65] upon the sign of the Cotton effect than third-sphere

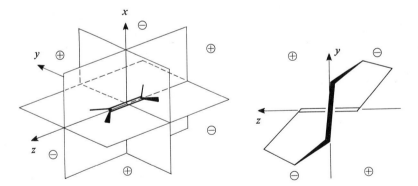

Fig. 15. Octant rule for olefins, and application to (R)-*trans*-cyclo-octene (right). The signs in the right figure refer to upper octants ($x > 0$).

† Sometimes this rule for olefins is called an octant rule, and that for ketones an inverse octant rule, because in a right-handed coordinate system with the z-axis along the C=X double bond and the y-axis perpendicular to it and in the plane of the ethylene grouping, the sign of the Cotton effect is the same as that of the product of the coordinates, i.e. of $x.y.z$ in the case of olefins, but opposite to it in the case of ketones. For the latter substances a left-handed coordinate system is, therefore, often used.

contributions. We believe also, that the helicity of the ring into which the double bond is incorporated (chirality of the second sphere) must not be neglected. During a round-table discussion at this Summer School, it was also suggested by theoreticians that the longest-wavelength absorption (sometimes called 'mystery band[66]') is most probably of $\pi \rightarrow \sigma^*$ rather than $\pi \rightarrow \pi^*$ origin.

D. More Complex Sector Rules

Benzoates show a strong absorption around 225 nm assigned to an intramolecular charge transfer[67] ($\pi \rightarrow \pi^*$). A sector rule has been proposed[68] on theoretical grounds[67] (Fig. 16) and for its application to cycloalkanol benzoates it is assumed

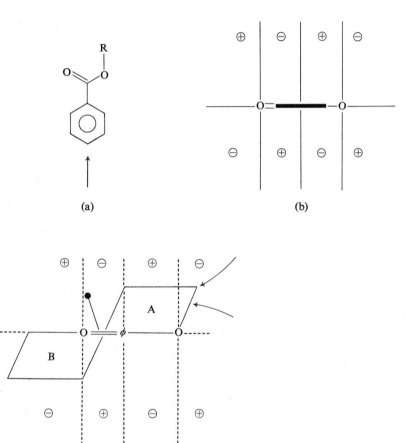

(a)   (b)

(c)

Fig. 16. Sector rule for benzoates. (a) Arrow indicates direction of projection and assumed preferred conformation of the benzoate. (b) The horizontal and the three vertical nodal planes. The benzene ring is indicated by the thick bar. (c) Application to steroid benzoate XV; only rings A and B are drawn, the benzene ring is indicated this time by ϕ, the arrows point to the two most important bonds [C(1)—C(2), C(2)—C(3)].

that the phenyl ring of the (coplanar, transoid) benzoate grouping is positioned between the smaller side of the cycloalkane and the geminal hydrogen, the C(=O) bond thus eclipsing the larger side of the ring. Only the nearest two bonds are con-

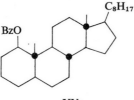

XV

sidered, double bonds seem to have a stronger influence than single bonds. In a projection of, for example, 1β-benzoyloxy-5α-cholestane, XV (Fig. 16) the bonds in question are C(1)—C(2), C(2)—C(3), C(1)—C(10), C(5)—C(10), and C(10)—C(19).

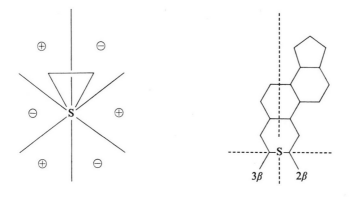

(a)   (b)

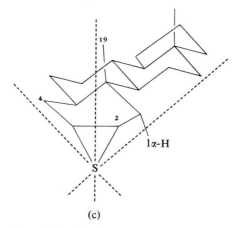

(c)

Fig. 17. Sector rule for episulphides. (a) General rule; signs refer to the upper sectors. (b) and (c) Two projections of the episulphide XVI.

The first two lie in a negative sector, the third in a nodal plane, and the latter two compensate each other, The prediction (negative sign) is thus correct (found: amplitude in ORD $a = -100$).

Our *Lactone rule*[69] is discussed in Chapter 3.3 (p. 126). It was based on the assumption that atoms act as perturbers,[70] not bonds, and the nodal surfaces of the n- and π_3^*-orbital were taken to construct the boundary between the sectors. As all atoms in a γ- or δ-lactone ring lie in nodal surfaces, second-sphere contributions have been thought to be negligible.[69] It has now been shown[71] that the dynamic coupling theory can also correctly predict the octant behaviour of analogous ketones and thus bond positions and not atom positions have to be taken into account; second-sphere chirality is, therefore, governing the Cotton effect, as expressed by the rules of Legrand and Bucourt[72] and Wolf.[73] We believe, however, that our rule is applicable to aliphatic esters.

Episulphides can readily be prepared from olefins, and their chiroptical properties were discussed by Kuriyama and Komeno[74] during the Summer School at Bonn (see also references 38, 75). Figure 17 shows the sector rule proposed by them for the CD of the 270-nm band, and its application to a steroidal $2\alpha,3\alpha$-episulphide (XVI).

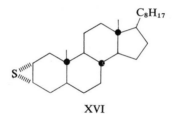

XVI

For *N-nitroso derivatives* the sector rule given in Fig. 18 has been proposed;[69] the surfaces separating the sectors have been constructed in a similar way to that discussed above for lactones. Later on from NMR work it became evident that the conformation assumed at that time to be the preferred one (NO directed away

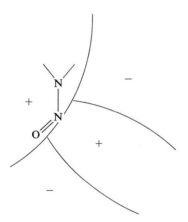

Fig. 18. Sector rule for *N*-nitroso compounds. The plane of the paper is also a nodal plane, signs refer to the upper sectors.[69] Recently,[76] sign inversion was suggested.

from the α-substituent at a piperidine ring, equatorial conformation of such a substituent) is, in fact, not always preponderant, and thus recently[76] sign inversion was suggested. More examples have still to be investigated both by chiroptical and NMR measurements in order to decide unequivocally between these two sign patterns.

E. Chirality Rules

Several 'cottonogenic derivatives' of alcohols have been used to determine their absolute configuration. The *O-nitrites* give a band around 350–400 nm, which shows a pronounced fine structure;[77-79] but since remote groups can change the sign of this Cotton effect, any simple chirality rule must be regarded as tentative. *Xanthates* have also frequently been used for the determination of the stereochemistry of an OH group.[80, 81] For the 350-nm CD band of these derivatives of secondary alcohols the chirality rule of Fig. 19 was put forward.[81]

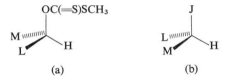

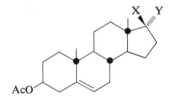

Fig. 19. Chirality rules. (a) Xanthates of secondary alcohols, (b) secondary iodo-alkanes. Both give rise to positive Cotton effects. L refers to a large, M to a medium-size alkyl group.

(a)　　　　(b)

Iodo-alkanes show a Cotton effect around 250–270 nm, and for secondary ones the chirality rule of Fig. 19 applies.[82, 83] Heteroatoms or double bonds in the vicinity to the iodine may, however, in this case invert the sign of the Cotton effect. According to this rule the 17β-iodo steroid XVII, for example, gives a positive and its 17α-epimer XVIII a negative CD.[84]

XVII: X = J, Y = H
XVIII: X = H, Y = J

Financial help from the Deutsche Forschungsgemeinschaft and the Fonds der Chemischen Industrie is highly appreciated (G.S.). Figs. 8, 10, 14 and 18 are reproduced completely or in part from E. Heftmann, Ed. *Modern Methods of Steroid Analysis*, J. Wiley, London. In press, and Fig. 17 from reference 1, p. 374, with the permission of the editors.

References

1. G. Snatzke, *Optical Rotatory Dispersion and Circular Dichroism in Organic Chemistry*. Heyden, London 1967, p. 208.
2. L. Tschugaeff and A. Ogorodnikoff, *Z. phys. Chem.* **85**, 481 (1913).
3. W. Klyne, *Tetrahedron* **13**, 29 (1961).
4. E. Ruch and A. Schönhofer, *Theor. Chim. Acta* **10**, 91 (1968).
5. E. Ruch, *Theor. Chim. Acta* **11**, 183 (1968).
6. E. Ruch and A. Schönhofer, *Theor. Chim. Acta* **19**, 225 (1970).

7. E. Ruch, *Accounts Chem. Res.* **5**, 49 (1972).
8. A. Moscowitz, K. Mislow, M. A. W. Glass and C. Djerassi, *J. Amer. Chem. Soc.* **84**, 1945 (1962).
9. J. Lindenberg and G. Michl, *J. Amer. Chem. Soc.* **92**, 2619 (1970).
10. R. S. Cahn, C. K. Ingold and V. Prelog, *Angew. Chem.* **78**, 413 (1966).
11. J. A. Schellman, *J. Chem. Phys.* **44**, 55 (1966).
12. Cf., for example, M. Hamermesh; *Group Theory and its Application to Physical Problems.* Addison-Wesley, Reading, 1964, p. 198.
13. W. Kauzmann, F. B. Clough and I. Tobias, *Tetrahedron* **13**, 57 (1961).
14. D. N. Kirk, W. Klyne and W. P. Mose, *Tetrahedron Lett.* 1315 (1972).
15. P. Crabbé, *ORD and CD in Chemistry and Biochemistry.* Academic Press, New York, 1972.
16. G. Briegleb, H.-G. Kuball and K. Henschel, *Z. phys. Chem., N.F.* **46**, 229 (1965); G. Briegleb, H.-G. Kuball, K. Henschel and W. Euing, *Ber. Bunsen-Ges. phys. Chem.* **76**, 101 (1972).
17. A. Moscowitz, E. Charney, U. Weiss and H. Ziffer, *J. Amer. Chem. Soc.* **83**, 4661 (1961).
18. E. Charney, H. Ziffer and U. Weiss, *Tetrahedron* **21**, 3121 (1965).
19. E. Charney, *Tetrahedron* **21**, 3127 (1965).
20. R. R. Gould and R. Hoffmann, *J. Amer. Chem. Soc.* **92**, 1813 (1970).
21. G. Wagnière and W. Hug, *Helv. Chim. Acta* **54**, 633 (1971).
22. A. W. Burgstahler and R. C. Barkhurst, *J. Amer. Chem. Soc.* **92**, 7601 (1970).
23. G. Snatzke, E. sz. Kováts and G. Ohloff, *Tetrahedron Lett.* 4551 (1966).
24. M. Carmack and L. A. Neubert, *J. Amer. Chem. Soc.* **89**, 7134 (1967).
25. R. M. Dodson and V. C. Nelson, *J. Org. Chem* **33**, 3966 (1968).
26. G. Claeson, *Acta Chem. Scand.* **22**, 2429 (1968).
27. D. L. Coleman and R. E. Blout, *J. Amer. Chem. Soc.* **90**, 2405 (1968).
28. G. Wagnière and W. Hug, *Tetrahedron Lett.* 4765 (1970).
29. V. Ludescher and R. Schwyzer, *Helv. Chim. Acta* **54**, 1637 (1971).
30. D. J. Severn and E. M. Kosower, *J. Amer. Chem. Soc.* **91**, 1710 (1969).
31. G. Snatzke and J. Himmelreich, *Tetrahedron* **23**, 4337 (1967).
32. G. Snatzke, H. Langen and J. Himmelreich, *Liebigs Ann. Chem.* **744**, 142 (1971).
33. R. Tschesche, F.-J. Kämmerer and G. Wulff, *Chem. Ber.* **102**, 2057 (1969).
34. R. Bonnett and T. R. Emerson, *J. Chem. Soc.* 4508 (1965).
35. H. Ripperger, K. Schreiber and G. Snatzke, *Tetrahedron* **21**, 1027 (1965).
36. J. Kalvoda and G. Anner, *Helv. Chim. Acta* **52**, 2106 (1969).
37. D. A. Lightner, C. Djerassi, K. Takeda, K. Kuriyama and T. Komeno, *Tetrahedron* **21**, 1581 (1965).
38. K. Kuriyama, T. Komeno and K. Takeda, *Ann. Rep. Shionogi Res. Lab.* **17**, 66 (1967).
39. C. Djerassi, H. Wolf, D. A. Lightner, E. Bunnenberg, K. Takeda, T. Komeno and K. Kuriyama, *Tetrahedron* **19**, 1547 (1963).
40. G. Snatzke, *J. Chem. Soc.* 5002 (1965).
41. C. Djerassi, H. Wolf and E. Bunnenberg, *J. Amer. Chem. Soc.* **85**, 2835 (1963).
42. K. Takeda, K. Kuriyama, T. Komeno, D. A. Lightner, R. Records and C. Djerassi, *Tetrahedron* **21**, 1203 (1965).
43. H. Ripperger, K. Schreiber and G. Snatzke, *Tetrahedron* **21**, 727 (1965).
44. H. Ripperger and H. Pracejus, *Tetrahedron* **24**, 99 (1968). Recently, R. G. Kostyanovsky, V. I. Markov and I. M. Gella, *Tetrahedron Lett.* 1301 (1972) have applied the octant rule for ketones without any proof to the n → σ* CD- band of *N*-chloro and *N*-bromo aziridines and azetidines. Their few results could also be explained by using a planar rule, the signs should then, however, be opposite to those given by Ripperger and Pracejus.
45. K. Mislow, M. M. Green, P. Laur, J. T. Melillo, T. Simmons and A. L. Ternay, Jr., *J. Amer. Chem. Soc.* **87**, 1958 (1965).
46. D. N. Jones and M. J. Green, *J. Chem. Soc. C* 532 (1967); D. N. Jones, M. J. Green, M. A. Saeed and R. D. Whitehouse, *J. Chem. Soc.* 1362 (1968).
47. Y. Tsuzuki, K. Tanabe and K. Okamoto, *Bull. Chem. Soc. Japan* **38**, 274 (1965); **39**, 761 (1966); Y. Tsuzuki, K. Tanabe, K. Okamoto and N. Yamada, *Bull. Chem. Soc. Japan* **39**, 1391, 2269 (1966).
48. L. D. Hayward and S. Claesson, *Chem. Commun.* 302 (1967).
49. G. Snatzke, H. Laurent and R. Wiechert, *Tetrahedron* **25**, 761 (1969).
50. R. E. Barton, Thesis, Vancouver, 1971; R. E. Barton and L. D. Hayward, *Can. J. Chem.* **50**, 1719 (1972).

51. H. Ripperger, *Angew. Chem., Intern. Ed.* 6, 704 (1967).
52. H. Ripperger, *Tetrahedron* 25, 725 (1969).
53. A. I. Scott and A. D. Wrixon, *Tetrahedron* 27, 2339 (1971).
54. C. Djerassi, A. Moscowitz, K. Ponsold and G. Steiner, *J. Amer. Chem. Soc.* 89, 347 (1967).
55. C. Djerassi, D. A. Lightner, D. A. Schooley, K. Takeda, T. Komeno and K. Kuriyama, *Tetrahedron* 24, 6913 (1968).
56. H. Paulsen, *Chem. Ber.* 101, 1571 (1968).
57. T. Sticzay, P. Šipoš and Š. Bauer, *Carbohyd. Res.* 10, 469 (1969).
58. M. Legrand and R. Viennet, *C.R.H. Acad. Sci.* 262 C, 1290 (1966).
59. A. Yogev, D. Amar and Y. Mazur, *Chem. Commun.* 339 (1967).
60. A. I. Scott and A. D. Wrixon, *Tetrahedron* 26, 3695 (1970).
61. A. C. Cope and A. S. Mehta, *J. Amer. Chem. Soc.* 86, 5626 (1964). cf. also R. D. Bach, *J. Chem. Phys.* 52, 6423 (1970), and O. Schnepp, E. F. Pearson and E. Sharman, *J. Chem. Phys.* 52, 6424 (1970).
62. M. Fétizon and I. Hanna, *Chem. Commun.* 462 (1970).
63. M. Fétizon, I. Hanna, A. I. Scott, A. D. Wrixon and T. K. Devon, *Chem. Commun.* 545 (1971).
64. J. K. Gawroński and M. A. Kiełczewski, *Tetrahedron Lett.* 2493 (1971).
65. M. Yaris, A. Moscowitz and R. S. Berry, *J. Chem. Phys.* 49, 3150 (1968).
66. M. B. Robin, R. R. Hart and N. A. Kuebler, *J. Chem. Phys.* 44, 1803 (1966).
67. N. Harada and K. Nakanishi, *J. Amer. Chem. Soc.* 90, 7351 (1968).
68. N. Harada, M. Ohashi and K. Nakanishi, *J. Amer. Chem. Soc.* 90, 7349 (1968).
69. G. Snatzke, H. Ripperger, Ch. Horstmann and K. Schreiber, *Tetrahedron* 22, 3103 (1966).
70. A. Moscowitz, *Advan. Chem. Phys.* 4, 67 (1962).
71. E. G. Höhn und O. E. Weigang, Jr., *J. Chem. Phys.* 48, 1127 (1968).
72. M. Legrand and R. Bucourt, *Bull. Soc. Chim. France* 2241 (1967).
73. H. Wolf, *Tetrahedron Lett.* 1075 (1965); 5151 (1966).
74. K. Kuriyama and T. Komeno, in G. Snatzke, Ed., *Optical Rotatory Dispersion and Circular Dichroism in Organic Chemistry*. Heyden, London, 1967, p. 366.
75. K. Kuriyama, T. Komeno and K. Takeda, *Tetrahedron* 22, 1039 (1966).
76. W. Gaffield, L. Keefer and W. Lijinsky, in press.
77. L. Velluz, M. Legrand and M. Grosjean, *Optical Circular Dichroism*. Verlag Chemie, Weinheim, 1965, p. 149.
78. C. Djerassi, H. Wolf and E. Bunnenberg, *J. Amer. Chem. Soc.* 85, 2835 (1963).
79. C. Djerassi, I. T. Harrison, O. Zagneetko and A. L. Nussbaum, *J. Org. Chem.* 27, 1173 (1962).
80. L. Velluz, M. Legrand and M. Grosjean, *Optical Circular Dichroism*. Verlag Chemie, Weinheim, 1965, p. 145.
81. B. Sjöberg, D. J. Cram, L. Wolf and C. Djerassi, *Acta Chem. Scand.* 16, 1079 (1962).
82. H. A. Chaudri, D. G. Goodwin, H. R. Hudson, L. Bartlett and P. M. Scopes, *J. Chem. Soc. C* 1329 (1970).
83. R. C. Cookson and J. M. Coxon, *J. Chem. Soc. C* 1466 (1971).
84. M. Biollaz and J. Kalvoda, *Helv. Chim. Acta* 55, 366 (1972).

Optical Activity and Molecular Dissymmetry in Coordination Compounds

S. F. MASON

Chemistry Department
King's College, Strand
London WC2R 2LS, U.K.

3.6.1 Introduction

Although molecular circular dichroism was first observed in the visible absorption bands of transition metal complexes by Cotton[1] (1895) the optical activity of chiral coordination compounds is understood in less detail than that of dissymmetric organic molecules as yet. The problem derives from the greater number and variety of excitation processes in transition metal complexes where, to the electronic transitions of the organic ligand, are added those of the metal ion and the metal-ligand charge-transfer excitations. In favourable cases the three types of electronic excitation in a coordination complex are discrete in good approximation, having large frequency separations and small mixing energies. An individual consideration is then feasible of the Cotton effects associated with each type, namely, (a) the d-electron transitions of the coordinated metal ion, (b) metal-ligand charge-transfer excitations, and (c) internal ligand transitions.

3.6.2 Classical Studies of d-Electron Optical Activity

Over the period 1911–19 Werner[2] resolved into optical isomers a range of bis- and tris-chelated complexes containing achiral ligands and transition metal ions from each of the three long periods. The work established the octahedral structure of hexacoordinated complexes and posed the problems of the absolute configuration of these complexes and of the origin of their optical activity. Classical studies of the optical properties of the Werner complexes were carried out, notably, by Jaeger[3] (ORD) and Mathieu[4] (CD), while Kuhn and Bein[5] in 1934 developed a coupled-oscillator model to relate the absolute configuration to the sign and the form of the visible Cotton effects in chiral complexes.

During the 1930s the ligand field theory and the quantum theory of optical activity were not yet developed in detail nor generally appreciated, and only the empirical correlations of this period between relative configuration and optical activity remain at all substantial. The theory of Kuhn and Bein[5] envisaged that charge-displacements

196

along the three octahedral edges spanned by chelate rings in a tris-chelated complex were correlated coulombically one with the other and with a linear charge displacement at the metal ion to generate optical activity in the visible region. The ligand field theory subsequently indicated that the charge displacements at the metal ion were circular (magnetic dipole) rather than linear (electric dipole), and the first definitive absolute configuration of a metal complex, determined by Saito and co-workers[6] (1955), using the anomalous X-ray scattering method, showed that the configurational assignment[7] of the Kuhn and Bein model was incorrect.

Saito and co-workers[6] found that the tris(ethylenediamine)cobalt(III) isomer which is dextrorotatory at the sodium D-line, $(+)$-$[Co(en)_3]^{3+}$, has the Λ-configuration[8] (I). An absolute basis was thus provided for the empirical relation of Mathieu[9] who had proposed (1936) that tris-chelated complexes with the same configuration as $(+)$-$[Co(en)_3]^{3+}$ give a predominantly positive circular dichroism in the region of the lowest-energy absorption band. Subsequent X-ray diffraction studies support Mathieu's generalization in the cases of the (R)-$(-)$- and (S)-$(+)$-propylenediamine complexes,[10] Λ-$(-)$-$[Co(R$-$pn)_3]^{3+}$ and Λ-$(-)$-$[Co(S$-$pn)_3]^{3+}$, the (S,S)-$(+)$-*trans*-1,2-cyclohexanediamine complex,[10] Λ-$(-)$-$[Co(S,S$-$chxn)_3]^{3+}$, the oxalato and malonato complexes,[11, 12] Λ-$(-)$-$[Co(ox)_3]^{3-}$, Λ-$(+)$-$[Cr(ox)_3]^{3-}$, and Λ-$(+)$-$[Cr(mal)_3]^{3-}$, the $(+)$-3-acetylcamphor complex,[13] Λ-$(+)$-*trans*-$[Cr(+atc)_3]$, the acetylacetone complex,[14] Λ-$(-)$-$[Co(acac)_3]$, the (R,R)-$(-)$-1,3-pentanediamine complex,[15] Λ-$(+)$-$[Co(R,R$-$ptn)_3]^{3+}$ and the biguanide complex,[16] Λ-$(-)$-$[Cr(bgd)_3]^{3+}$; but the trimethylenediamine complex,[17] Λ-$(-)$-$[Co(tn)_3]^{3+}$, the (S,S)-$(+)$-*trans*-1,2-cyclopentanediamine complex,[18] Λ-$(-)$-$[Co(S,S$-$cptn)_3]^{3+}$, and the 1,10-phenanthroline complex,[11] Λ-$(+)$-$[Ni(phen)_3]^{2+}$, are exceptional.

3.6.3 Ligand Field and Spectroscopic Studies

The early quantum theories of d-electron optical activity were directed towards dihedral trigonal complexes of D_3 symmetry, notably the tris-chelated complexes of cobalt(III) and chromium(III). In the first of these theories Moffitt[19] showed that the lowest-energy spin-allowed d-electron transition of cobalt(III), $^1A_{1g} \rightarrow {}^1T_{1g}$ in O_h, and the analogous $^4A_{2g} \rightarrow {}^4T_{2g}$ transition of chromium(III), are magnetic dipole-allowed, and that their D_3 components in a tris-chelated complex acquire a first-order rotational strength by mixing with the 3d $\rightarrow$ 4p transitions of the metal ion under the perturbation of an ungerade ligand field potential due to the atoms of the chelate rings. In a trigonal coordinate frame (Fig. 1) the potential has the polar (R, θ, ϕ) or cartesian (X, Y, Z) form

$$(Y_3^3 + Y_3^{-3}) \approx \sin^3 \theta \sin^3 \phi \approx Y(3X^2 - Y^2) \tag{1}$$

where Y_L^M is the spherical harmonic of degree L and order M. In a cartesian octahedral frame (Fig. 1) the ungerade potential [1] assumes the form,

$$(X - Y)(Y - Z)(Z - X) \tag{2}$$

Equation [1] or the equivalent form [2] represents the first ungerade term which is totally symmetric for the group D_3 in the expansion over the spherical harmonics of the crystal-field potential in the ionic model for metal complexes. The potential

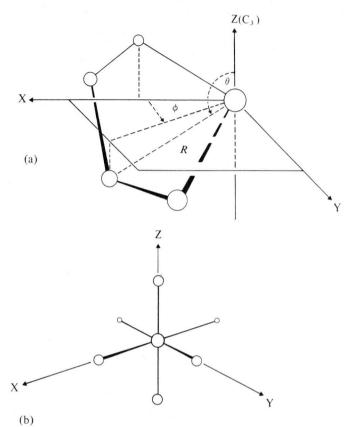

Fig. 1. Coordinate frames, (a) the spherical polar (R, θ, ϕ) and cartesian (X, Y, Z) trigonal frame, and (b) the corresponding octahedral or tetragonal frame.

[1] or [2] connects the 3d with 4p or 4f orbitals of the metal ion but does not mix the 3d orbitals amongst themselves, so that the D_3 components, $A_1 \to A_2$ and $A_1 \to E$ of the octahedral $A_{1g} \to T_{1g}$ cobalt(III) d-electron transition remain degenerate.

Subsequently, Sugano[20] found that a potential of the form [1] or [2], which has T_{2u} octahedral parentage, gives first-order rotational strengths of equal magnitude but opposite sign to the D_3 components of the d-electron transition from the A_1 ground state to the A_2 and E excited states

$$R'(A_2) + R'(E) = 0 \qquad\qquad [3]$$

whereas Moffitt[19] had deduced, owing to an error in sign, that the two rotational strengths have a like sign. Since the A_2 and E excited states remain degenerate under the potential [1] or [2], a D_3 complex ion randomly oriented in solution would give no net optical activity in the region of the octahedral $A_{1g} \to T_{1g}$ absorption.

However, for an assembly of D_3 complex ions oriented with their C_3 axis parallel to the optic axis in a single crystal only the doubly-degenerate D_3 component,

$A_1 \rightarrow E$, polarized in the plane perpendicular to the C_3 axis of the complex ion, is excited by radiation propagated along the optic axis of the crystal. The axial circular dichroism spectrum of a D_3 complex ion in a uniaxial crystal thus measures $R'(E)$ of [3] directly, the d-electron transition $A_1 \rightarrow A_2$ remaining inactive. It has been found generally[21-25] that the lowest-energy single-crystal CD band of a D_3 complex ion is an order of magnitude larger than the corresponding CD band or bands observed in solution (Fig. 2, Table 1). Accordingly, equation [3] is correct to within 10%, $R(A_2)$ and $R(E)$ largely cancelling one another when the complex ion is randomly orientated in solution.

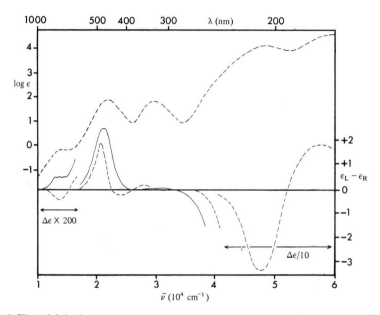

Fig. 2. The axial single-crystal circular dichroism spectrum ($\Delta\varepsilon/10$) of [Λ-(+)-Co(en)$_3$Cl$_3$]$_2$. NaCl. 6H$_2$O (full line) and the absorption and CD spectrum of the salt in water. (The CD spectrum 40–60 kK is kindly provided by Dr. W. C. Johnson, Jr.)

For a randomly-orientated D_3 metal complex, Sugano demonstrated[20] that only a pseudoscalar ligand field, with A_{1u} symmetry in O_h, induces a net first-order rotational strength in the d-electron transitions. The simplest octahedral pseudoscalar potential has the form[26] in a cartesian octahedral frame (Fig. 1)

$$[XYZ(X^2 - Y^2)(Y^2 - Z^2)(Z^2 - X^2)] \tag{4}$$

and, being of the ninth order with respect to the electronic coordinates, it can mix the 3d orbitals ($l = 2$) only with orbitals of large angular momentum and high energy at the central metal ion ($l = 7, 9, 11$).

A solution to the problem, proposed by Sugano and Shinada[27] and worked out in detail by Shinada,[28] is the assumption that the electrons of a metal ion in a D_3 complex are subject not only to the ungerade field [1] or [2] but also to a gerade

Table 1

The circular dichroism in the region of the lowest-energy spin-allowed d-electron absorption of trigonal dihedral complex ions in a uniaxial single crystal for radiation propagated along the optic axis and the corresponding CD for the randomly orientated complex ion in microcrystalline form in a potassium bromide matrix or in aqueous solution. The assignment refers to the D_3 component of the corresponding octahedral excited state.

	Single crystal		Random orientation				
Complex salt	λ (nm)	$\Delta\varepsilon$	λ (nm)	$\Delta\varepsilon$	Medium	Assignment	Ref.
$2[\Lambda\text{-}(+)\text{-Co(en)}_3]\text{Cl}_3].\text{NaCl}.6\text{H}_2\text{O}$	475	+23	490	+1·1 ⎫	KBr	^1E	22–24
			430	−0·2 ⎭		$^1\text{A}_2$	
$\Delta\text{-}(+)\text{-[Co(tn)}_3]\text{Cl}_3.4\text{H}_2\text{O}$	483	+3·0	490	+0·36	KBr	^1E	25, 50
$2[(+)\text{-Cr(en)}_3]\text{Cl}_3].\text{NaCl}.6\text{H}_2\text{O}^a$	458	+15	456	+1·36	H_2O	^4E	c
$(-)\text{-[Rh(en)}_3]\text{Cl}_3.\text{H}_2\text{O}$	<325	>+15	320	+2·0 ⎫	H_2O	^1E	23
			287	−0·1 ⎭		$^1\text{A}_2$	
$\Lambda\text{-}(-)\text{-NaMg[Co(ox)}_3].9\text{H}_2\text{O}^b$	620	+39	617	+3·0	KBr	^1E	23, c
$\Lambda\text{-}(+)\text{-NaMg[Cr(ox)}_3].9\text{H}_2\text{O}^b$	561	+20	546	+2·9	KBr	^4E	23, c
$(+)_{546}\text{-NaMg[Rh(ox)}_3].9\text{H}_2\text{O}^b$	395	+49	388	+4·1	KBr	^1E	23, c

[a] In $2[\text{Rh(en)}_3]\text{Cl}_3].\text{NaCl}.6\text{H}_2\text{O}$. [b] In $\text{NaMg[Al(ox)}_3].9\text{H}_2\text{O}$. [c] S. F. Mason, B. J. Peart and J. W. Wood. Unpublished measurements.

potential of the form

$$Y_2^0 \approx (3\cos^2\theta - 1) \approx (3Z^2 - R^2) \qquad [5]$$

in a trigonal frame or the equivalent form

$$(XY + YZ + ZX) \qquad [6]$$

in an octahedral frame (Fig. 1). The gerade potential [5] or [6] is of T_{2g} parentage in O_h and gives with the T_{2u} field [1] or [2] a direct product containing the octahedral pseudoscalar representation, A_{1u}.

The gerade field [5] or [6] mixes the 3d-orbitals amongst themselves, breaking the degeneracy of the D_3 components of the d-electron transition from the A_1 ground state to the A_2 and E excited states. The frequency separation between the component transitions measures the trigonal-splitting parameter, K

$$\Delta v = [v(\text{E}) - v(\text{A}_2)] = (3/2)\,\text{K} \qquad [7]$$

The combined ungerade [1] or [2] and gerade fields [5] or [6] give the D_3 component transitions second-order rotational strengths of unequal magnitude. Neglecting smaller terms, the rotational strengths of the A_2 and E components in D_3 are:[34, 35]

$$R(\text{E}) = R'(\text{E})\,[1 + (9/2)\,(\text{K}/\Delta)] \qquad [8]$$

and

$$R(\text{A}_2) = -R'(\text{E}) \qquad [9]$$

where $R'(E)$ is the first-order rotational strength of [3] and Δ is the frequency interval between the octahedral $^1T_{1g}$ and $^1T_{2g}$ d-electron states of cobalt(III) or the equivalent separation for other d-configurations. Hence for a randomly-orientated D_3 complex a net circular dichroism should be observed in the region of the lowest-energy spin-allowed band, firstly, because the first-order rotational strengths [3] do not cancel completely due to the splitting of the A_2 and E dihedral states and, secondly, because of the second-order contributions, principally to $R(E)$ in [8].

The plane-polarized single-crystal spectrum[29] of $2[Coen_3Cl_3]. NaCl.6H_2O$ shows, however, that the O—O band origins of the transitions to the A_2 and E states of $[Co(en)_3]^{3+}$ are virtually coincident, although the band maxima are split, lying at 21,285 and 21,425 cm^{-1}, respectively. The CD data for $(+)-[Co(en)_3]^{3+}$ (Fig. 2) indicate a contrary energy-order, as the major positive CD band at 20,300 cm^{-1} in solution is due to the E component, having the same sign as the axial crystal CD band, and the minor negative CD band at 23,400 cm^{-1} arises from the A_2 component.[22] The axial crystal CD spectrum and a gaussian analysis of the solution CD bands[30] indicate that $R(E)$ and $R(A_2)$ have maxima at 21,050 and 21,170 cm^{-1}, respectively.

In the case of $(+)-[Co(en)_3]^{3+}$ therefore the trigonal splitting parameter K of [7] due to the gerade potential [5] is virtually zero at the band origin, but at the band maximum is +93 cm^{-1} for the isotropic absorption and −80 cm^{-1} for the circular dichroism. Vibrational modes additional to those active in the circular dichroism evidently contribute to the isotropic absorption, although there is a close correspondence between the vibrational structure observed in the absorption and in the CD near to the band origin,[24] and the potential energy surfaces for these additional modes are shallower for the A_2 than the E excited state.[31] However, if any of the three possible values of K are inserted into the rotational strength expressions [8] and [9], the expected CD spectrum of $(+)-[Co(en)_3]^{3+}$ in solution has a form different from that observed (Fig. 2), i.e. either zero, or a minor and a major CD band at lower and higher frequency, respectively.

In the particular physical model adopted by Sugano and Shinada[27, 28] two sets of point-dipoles are located on the ligand atoms coordinated to the metal ion, one set producing the ungerade potential [1] and the other set the gerade field [5]. In a number of other theories it was similarly assumed that the main dissymmetric perturbation of a ML_6 chromophore in a chiral complex is a coulombic field, or the molecular-orbital equivalent, due to the distortion of the ligand atoms directly coordinated to the metal ion, or their orbitals, or their charge distributions, from the octahedral disposition. The chelate ring atoms not directly bonded to the central metal ion are assumed to be essentially passive in relation to the electrons of the ML_6 chromophore, and their primary role is to produce mechanically, or electrically by polarization effects, the necessary distortions of the ligand atoms or their charges.

Piper and Karipides extended Moffitt's treatment[19] to include 3d − 4f orbital mixing in a crystal field model,[32] and subsequently developed a molecular orbital model in which the d-electron transitions of the metal ion mixed with metal–ligand charge-transfer excitations due to the displacement of the coordinated ligands from the octahedral position.[33] In the theory of Liehr[34] the optical activity of a chiral metal complex is ascribed to a basic 'mis-match' between the directions of maximum charge density of the metal-ion and the coordinated ligand-atom orbitals. The 'mis-match', or deviations from the octahedral disposition, arise from constraints imposed by the non-coordinated groups of the chelate rings, and they produce metal-ligand molecular orbitals which are inherently dissymmetric.

The angle of 'mis-match' is not a readily accessible quantity and, as yet, no specific predictions arise from the model of Liehr.[34] However, Piper and Karipides[32, 33] underlined an important consequence of the ungerade potential [1]. The form of the potential [1] indicates that for a particular absolute stereochemical configuration of a D_3 complex the rotational strength of a given transition changes sign as the L–M–L bond angle within a chelate ring passes from higher to lower values through $\pi/2$ if the displacement of the coordinated atoms L from the octahedral orientation is the principal source of the optical activity. The inference is supported by the data for $\varLambda$-(+)-[Co(en)$_3$]$^{3+}$ (I) and the trimethylenediamine analogue $\varLambda$-(−)-[Co(tn)$_3$]$^{3+}$ (II)

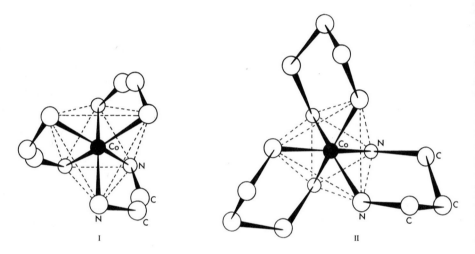

for which the N–Co–N angle within a ring is 85·3° and 94·5°, respectively,[35] and the rotational strength $R(E)$, from the axial crystal circular dichroism,[22, 25] is positive and negative, respectively (Table 1).

In these two complexes, however, the angular distortions from $\pi/2$ are comparable in magnitude yet $R(E)$ is substantially larger for $\varLambda$-(+)-[Co(en)$_3$]$^{3+}$ than for $\varLambda$-(−)-[Co(tn)$_3$]$^{3+}$ (Table 1), suggesting that perturbations from the non-coordinated atoms of the chelate rings are significant. Moreover, $R(E)$ is positive for a number of tris-oxychelate complexes with the $\varLambda$-configuration whether the O–M–O ring angle is greater or less than $\pi/2$ (Tables 1 and 2). For $\varLambda$-(−)-[Co(ox)$_3$]$^{3-}$ the O–Co–O ring angle[11] is 84·3° compared with 97·3° for[36] [Co(acac)$_3$] and the O–Cr–O ring angle in [Cr(ox)$_3$]$^{3-}$ is[37] 85°, compared with 91° for[36] [Cr(acac)$_3$], or with 92·4° for[12] $\varLambda$-(+)-[Cr(mal)$_3$]$^{3-}$.

The sign of the rotational strength of a given transition, e.g. $R(E)$, is provided by the single-crystal CD spectrum (Table 1) or, with less certainty, by the frequency separation $(v_\sigma - v_\pi)$, i.e. equation [7], or the intensity ratio, (I_π/I_σ), from the plane-polarized single-crystal spectrum taken in conjunction with the solution CD spectrum (Table 2). Of the latter two procedures, the intensity-ratio method appears to be the more reliable. The frequency sequence of two CD bands due to the D_3 components of an octahedral transition is expected to follow the frequency order of the

Table 2

The intensity ratio (I_π/I_σ) and the frequency separation ($v_\sigma - v_\pi$) at the band maxima of the D_3 components of the lowest-energy spin-allowed octahedral d-electron transition obtained from the plane-polarized single crystal spectra of trigonal metal complexes and the derived assignments of the corresponding solution circular dichroism spectra. The doubly-degenerate E-component is polarized perpendicular (σ) and the non-degenerate A_2-component parallel (π) to the C_3 axis of the complex. Each component is denoted by the direct product of the D_3 states connected by the transition considered.

	Single crystal absorption			Solution circular dichroism[h]		
Complex	(I_π/I_σ)	($v_\sigma - v_\pi$) (cm^{-1})	Ref.	λ (nm)	$\Delta\varepsilon$	Assignment
Λ-(+)-[Co(en)$_3$]$^{3+}$	1·34	+140	a	493	+1·89	E (intensity; converse
				428	−0·17	A_2 for frequency)
(+)-[Cr(en)$_3$]$^{3+}$	1·47	Small	b	456	+1·36	E (intensity)
Λ-(−)-[Co(ox)$_3$]$^{3-}$	1·33	−150	c	617	+3·30	E (intensity)
Λ-(+)-[Cr(ox)$_3$]$^{3-}$	1·46	+300	c	630	−0·58	A_2 (intensity and
				552	+2·83	E frequency)
(+)$_{546}$-[Rh(ox)$_3$]$^{3-}$	1·45	−100	d	395	+2·98	E (intensity)
Λ-(+)-[Cr(mal)$_3$]$^{3-}$	1·4	−180	e	620	−0·07	A_2 (intensity; converse
				555	+0·20	E for frequency)
Λ-(−)-[Co(acac)$_3$]	1·02	+800	f	645	−2·0	A_2 (intensity and
				571	+5·6	E frequency)
Λ-(+)-[Cr(acac)$_3$]	1·50	+800	g	606	−0·5	A_2 (intensity and
				538	+1·6	E frequency)

[a] R. Dingle and C. J. Ballhausen, *Mat. Fys. Medd. Dan. Vid. Selsk.* **35**, No. 12 (1967). [b] A. G. Karipides and T. S. Piper, *J. Chem. Phys.* **40**, 674 (1964). [c] T. S. Piper and R. L. Carlin, *J. Chem. Phys.* **35**, 1809 (1961). [d] J. W. Wood, Thesis, University of East Anglia, 1968. [e] W. E. Hatfield, *Inorg. Chem.* **3**, 605 (1964). [f] T. S. Piper, *J. Chem. Phys.* **35**, 1240 (1961). [g] T. S. Piper and R. L. Carlin, *J. Chem. Phys.* **36**, 3330 (1962). [h] Reference 23, except for the [M(acac)$_3$] data (R. C. Fay and S. F. Mason. Forthcoming publication).

isotropic absorption due to those components, but the well explored case of Λ-(+)-[Co(en)$_3$]$^{3+}$ shows that this expectation is not necessarily realized when the trigonal-splitting is small (Tables 1 and 2).

The intensity-ratio method depends upon the inference that, if the sum-rule [3] were valid, the isotropic absorption intensity of the non-degenerate dihedral component, with π-polarization, should be twice as large as that due to the doubly-degenerate component (σ-polarized), since the latter has a zero-order magnetic-dipole transition moment $\sqrt{2}$ times as large as that of the former component. After allowing for a zero-order octahedral contribution to the absorption intensity, e.g. by sub-tracting from the tris-diamine absorption the absorption of the corresponding [M(NH$_3$)$_6$]$^{3+}$ complex, it is found in all cases as yet studied that the ratio (I_π/I_σ) is less than 2 (Table 2). Thus the doubly-degenerate D_3 component has a larger dipole strength than expected if the sum-rule [3] held, implying that the sign of the major and of the minor CD band associated with the lowest-energy absorption band give the sign of R(E) and R(A_2), respectively, or, where a single CD band is observed, that band reflects the sign of R(E). The intensity-ratio method affords generally the same assignment as the axial crystal CD procedure (Tables 1 and 2), but assignments based upon a small trigonal frequency-splitting[23] are not reliable. The empirical correlation[23] of the Λ-configuration with a positive R(E) is not general, Λ-(−)-[Co(tn)$_3$]$^{3+}$ (II) being the important exception.

The displacement of the coordinated ligand atoms from the octahedral position provides an important contribution to the optical activity of dihedral and other chiral metal complexes, but the limitations of the simple relation between the L–M–L ring-angle, or the derived polar (θ) and azimuthal (ϕ) angle of [1], and the sign of that activity suggest that the contributions of the non-coordinated atoms of the chelate rings are also significant. Moreover, the CD spectra of two chiral complexes distinguished solely by the conformation of the chelate rings generally differ appreciably, as do the positions of the non-coordinated atoms of the chelate rings in the coordination sphere, whereas the L–M–L ring angle and the displacements of the ligand atoms from the octahedral disposition in general are not necessarily dissimilar.

3.6.4   Configurational and Conformational Optical Activity

The principles of conformational analysis were first applied to chelated metal complexes by Corey and Bailar[38] who showed in 1959 that five-membered chelate rings formed by 1,2-diamines exist preferentially in one of two enantiomeric puckered conformations. In the IUPAC nomenclature[8] these conformations are δ when the C—C bond of the chelate ring forms a segment of a right-handed helix with respect to the N$\cdots$N direction or λ for the antipodal left-handed conformation. The two conformations are energetically non-equivalent for a chiral C-substituted 1,2-diamine, owing to the equatorial preference of the substituent: (S)-(+)-1,2-propylenediamine and, more particularly, (S,S)-(+)-1,2-cyclohexanediamine, give predominantly a δ-chelate ring whereas the (R)-(−)-isomers preferentially form a λ-ring.

In a bis- or tris-chelate complex the two conformations are energetically non-equivalent even for achiral 1,2-diamines on account of steric interactions between each pair of chelate rings. For a tris-ethylenediamine complex the C—C bond of each chelate ring is approximately parallel to the C_3 axis of the complex in the most-favoured *lel*-conformation, $\Lambda(\delta\delta\delta)$ or $\Delta(\lambda\lambda\lambda)$, whereas each C—C bond is obliquely inclined with respect to the C_3 axis in the least-favoured *ob*-conformation, $\Lambda(\lambda\lambda\lambda)$ or $\Delta(\delta\delta\delta)$. For the Λ-configuration the order of decreasing stability is

$$\Lambda(\delta\delta\delta) > \Lambda(\lambda\delta\delta) > \Lambda(\lambda\lambda\delta) > \Lambda(\lambda\lambda\lambda)$$

with an enthalpy increment of approximately 0·6 kcal mole^{-1} for each δ to λ ring inversion.[38] Piper and Karipides[39] subsequently pointed out that the intermediate forms ($\lambda\delta\delta$) and ($\lambda\lambda\delta$) are statistically favoured by the factor $R\ln 3$ (0·7 kcal mole^{-1}) over the extreme *lel* and *ob* forms.

For chiral C-substituted 1,2-diamines the steric interactions favouring an equatorial rather than an axial disposition of the substituent are generally greater than those giving a preferred ring conformation, so that chiral 1,2-diamines form diastereoisomeric *lel* and *ob* tris-complexes. The X-ray diffraction studies of Saito and co-workers[10] show that (S)-(+)-propylenediamine gives the *lel*-complex, $\Lambda(\delta\delta\delta)$-(+)-[Co($S$-pn)$_3$]$^{3+}$ (III) and the *ob*-isomer, $\Delta(\delta\delta\delta)$-(−)-[Co($S$-pn)$_3$]$^{3+}$ (IV) and that, in a number of crystals, [Co(en)$_3$]$^{3+}$ adopts the *lel*-conformation (I). Dwyer and co-workers[40, 41] found that III and IV are formed in the ratio of 14·6/1 under thermodynamically controlled preparative conditions, so that the free-energy difference between the *lel* (III) and *ob* (IV) forms is 1·6 kcal mole^{-1}, compared with the enthalpy difference of 1·8 kcal mole^{-1} estimated by Corey and Bailar.[38]

Larger cations are less selective, however, and (+)- and (−)-[Pt(R-pn)$_3$]$^{4+}$ are formed only in the ratio 3/2 in dimethylformamide or 5·7/1 in ethanol solution.[42]

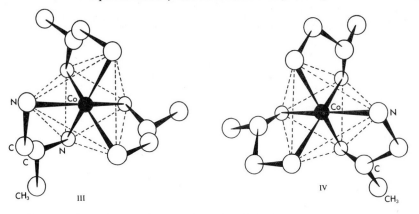

Recent X-ray studies of crystals containing $[Cr(en)_3]^{3+}$ and large anions show the presence of intermediate $\Lambda(\delta\delta\lambda)$ and $\Lambda(\delta\lambda\lambda)$ forms and the *ob*-conformation $\Lambda(\lambda\lambda\lambda)$ of the complex cation, due to hydrogen bonding with the anion.[43] Moreover, NMR studies of $[M(en)_3]^{n+}$ complexes in solution indicate that generally only 60–70% of the ligands have a *lel*-orientation, the most abundant conformation being $(\delta\delta\lambda)$ for the Λ-configuration.[44]

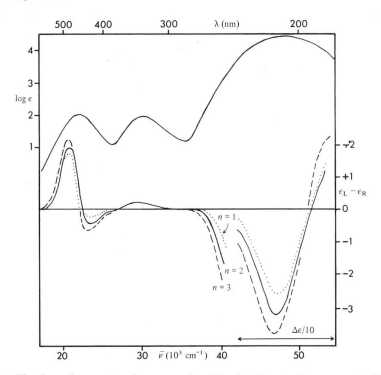

Fig. 3. The absorption spectrum (upper curve) and circular dichroism (lower curves) of the (*S*)-(+)-1,2-propylenediamine complexes, Λ-(+)-$[Co(S\text{-pn})_n(en)_{3-n}]^{3+}$ in water for $n = 1\ (\cdots\cdots)$, $n = 2\ (\text{————})$, and the *lel*-conformation, $n = 3\ (\text{— — — —})$.

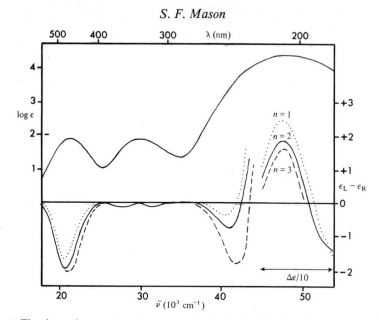

Fig. 4. The absorption spectrum (upper curve) and circular dichroism (lower curves) of the (*S*)-(+)-propylenediamine complexes, Λ-(−)-[Co(S-pn)$_n$(en)$_{3-n}$]$^{3+}$ in water for $n = 1$ (··········), $n = 2$ (————), and the *ob*-conformation, $n = 3$ (— — — —).

The CD spectra of the complexes, Λ-(+)-[Co(S-pn)$_n$(en)$_{3-n}$]$^{3+}$, with one or more ring fixed in the *lel*-orientation (Fig. 3), and Δ-(−)-[Co(S-pn)$_n$(en)$_{3-n}$]$^{3+}$, with at least one ring in the *ob*-orientation (Fig. 4), recently remeasured and extended,[45] indicate that the lowest-energy d-electron and the metal-ligand charge-transfer Cotton effects are sensitive to chelate ring conformation as well as to the configuration of the rings about the metal ion. The minor A_2 component of the CD associated with the lowest-energy d-electron transition appears only in the Λ-(+) series and increases in area with the number of rings with a fixed *lel*-orientation (Fig. 3), suggesting that a majority of the rings of Λ-(+)-[Co(en)$_3$]$^{3+}$ in aqueous solution (Fig. 2) have that orientation.

The area of the main accessible charge-transfer CD band near 210 nm is less sensitive to ring-conformation than earlier measurements with a now-obsolescent CD instrument suggest.[46] The recent measurements[45] indicate contributions in $\Delta\varepsilon$ units (1.mole^{-1} cm^{-1}) to the CD band near 210 nm of +25 for the Δ or −25 for the Λ configuration of the rings around the metal ion, and of +3 for the λ-conformation or −3 for the δ-conformation of each diamine chelate ring. The charge-transfer CD bands of the diastereoisomeric complexes (+)- and (−)-[Pt(R-pn)$_n$(en)$_{3-n}$]$^{4+}$, where $n = 1, 2, 3$, are instrumentally inaccessible, but Drude plots of the ORD indicate these CD bands dominate the sodium D-line rotation.[47] An analysis of the rotation data for the six complexes of these series, together with (+)-[Pt(en)$_3$]$^{4+}$ and (+)- and (−)-[Pt(S-pn)$_2$(R-pn)]$^{4+}$, indicates[47] that the contributions to the molecular rotation, $[M]_D$, are +618° for the Δ or −618° for the Λ configuration of the three rings about the platinum(IV) ion and −204° for the δ or +204° for the λ conformation of each chelate ring. The analysis suggests[47] little or no preference of conformation in the chelate rings of [Pt(en)$_3$]$^{4+}$ whereas the NMR evidence indicates a preference of some 65% for the *lel*-orientation.[44]

Like cyclohexane, the six-membered chelate ring of a trimethylenediamine complex has two main low-energy conformations, the chair and the twist form, which are favoured in a complex by the ligands *meso* and *active* 2,4-pentanediamine, respectively, on account of the equatorial preference of the methyl groups with respect to the chelate ring. The principal conformations of the tris-chelated complex $[Co(tn)_3]^{3+}$ are the tris-chair (II), the *lel*-twist (V), and the *ob*-twist (VI), where *lel* and *ob* now

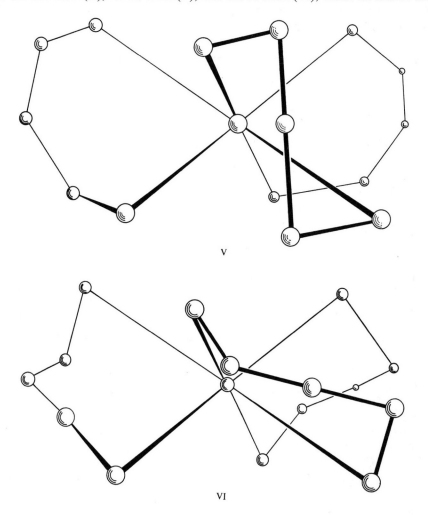

V

VI

refer, respectively, to the parallel or oblique orientation of the C—C—C ligand chain with respect to the C_3 axis of the complex. The ligand, (S,S)-(+)-2,4-pentanediamine forms preferentially a tris-chelate complex with the *lel*-twist conformation for the Λ-configuration (V), whereas (R,R)-(−)-2,4-pentanediamine gives the *ob*-twist conformation for the Λ-configuration (VI), and *meso*-(R,S)-2,4-pentanediamine assumes the tris-chair conformation for either configuration.

The CD spectra of $(+)_{546}$- and $(-)_{546}$-$[Co(R,R\text{-ptn})_3]^{3+}$ and $(-)_{546}$-$[Co(R,S\text{-ptn})_3]^{3+}$, isolated and characterized by K. Saito and co-workers,[48] show (Fig. 5) that changes of ring conformation have a more profound effect upon both the d-electron and charge-transfer Cotton effects in the six-membered than the five-membered chelate ring series. The X-ray diffraction analysis of Y. Saito and colleagues[15] shows that $(+)_{546}$-$[Co(R,R\text{-ptn})_3]^{3+}$ has the Λ-ob-twist structure (VI) with a N–Co–N ring angle of 87·9°, compared with 94·5° for the tris-chair structure of Λ-$(-)$-$[Co(tn)_3]^{3+}$ (II) in the crystal[10, 35] $(-)$-$[Co(tn)_3]Br_3 . H_2O$.

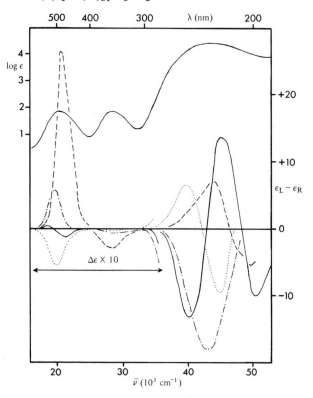

Fig. 5. The absorption spectrum (upper curve) and circular dichroism (lower curves) of Λ-$(-)$-$[Co(tn)_3]^{3+}$ (———), Λ-$(+)_{546}$-$[Co(R,R\text{-ptn})_3]^{3+}$ (ob-twist) (— — —), Λ-$(+)_{546}$-$[Co(S,S\text{-ptn})_3]^{3+}$ (lel-twist) (—·—·—·—), and $(-)_{546}[Co(R,S\text{-ptn})_3]^{3+}$ (tris-chair) (· · · · · ·) in water. The spectra of the tris-2,4-pentanediamine isomers are adapted from originals kindly provided by Professor K. Saito and co-workers.[48]

A conformational analysis of $[Co(tn)_3]^{3+}$ by Butler and Snow[49] indicates that the steric interactions are at a minimum for a N–Co–N ring angle of 93·7° in the tris-chair form or of 88·4° in the lel-twist form. The strain energy is 0·9 kcal mole^{-1} less for the lel-twist than the tris-chair form, whereas the ob-twist conformation lies at a substantially higher energy.[49] The CD spectrum of microcrystalline Λ-$(-)$-$[Co(tn)_3]Br_3 . H_2O$ in a potassium bromide matrix, where the complex has the tris-chair conformation, as in the single crystal, differs in form from the corresponding solution CD spectrum which is found to be temperature-sensitive[50] (Fig. 6). On cooling, the solution CD spectrum changes towards the form of the KBr matrix CD spectrum, suggesting that the tris-chair conformation is the more stable, and an analysis, on the assumption that the tris-chair and *lel*-twist conformation are the sole species in equilibrium, places the latter 0·5 kcal mole^{-1} higher in energy.[50]

Changes in the solution CD spectrum of Λ-(−)-[Co(tn)$_3$]$^{3+}$ similar to those produced by lowering the temperature are observed on adding polarizable oxy-anions, notably, phosphate or selenite.[51, 52] The effect arises, in part, from the formation of an orientated ion-pair favouring the tris-chair conformation, probably by hydrogen bonding between the N—H groups of the complex cation and the oxygen atoms of the anion. In part, however, the effect is due to interionic charge-transfer interactions as new absorption and CD bands appear in the spectrum of the complex ion when an excess of the oxy-ion is added to the solution.

Moreover the gegenion effect upon the CD spectrum is observed when the conformation of the chelate rings is fixed by alkyl substitution,[53, 54] notably, the *lel* complex, Λ-(+)-[Co(*S*-pn)$_3$]$^{3+}$ (III) but less so for the *ob*-isomer, Δ-(−)-[Co(*S*-pn)$_3$]$^{3+}$

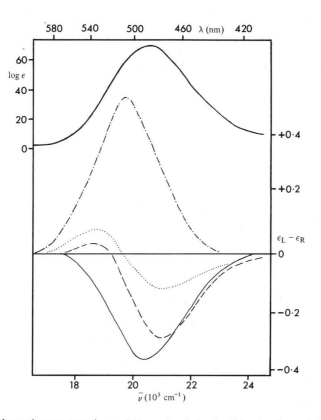

Fig. 6. The absorption spectrum (upper full curve) and circular dichroism (lower full curve) of tris-chair Λ-(−)-[Co(tn)$_3$]Br$_3$.H$_2$O in a potassium bromide matrix, and the CD of Λ-(−)-[Co(tn)$_3$]$^{3+}$ in water at 330°K (· · · · · · ·), and in ethylene glycol-water (7/3) at 198°K (— — — —), and of *lel*-twist Λ-(+)-[Co(*S*,*S*-ptn)$_3$]$^{3+}$ in water (—·—·—·—).

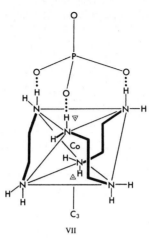

VII

(IV). In the case of Λ-(+)-[Co(en)$_3$]$^{3+}$ the formation of the orientated ion-pair (VII) with an oxy-anion[53] favours the *lel*-conformation of the complex, since the A$_2$ component of the CD due to the lowest-energy d-electron transition is enhanced (Fig. 7), as in the series Λ-(+)-[Co(S-pn)$_n$(en)$_{3-n}$]$^{3+}$ with progressive *lel*-orientation of the ligands from $n = 1$ to $n = 3$ (Fig. 3). However, the additional source of the gegenion effect, an interionic charge-transfer CD and absorption, is prominent near 250 nm (Fig. 7).

The structure proposed[53] for the stereospecific outer-sphere complex of Λ (+)-[Co(en)$_3$]$^{3+}$ with [PO$_4$]$^{3-}$, VII, is supported by the X-ray diffraction analysis[55] of the crystal [Co(en)$_3$]$_2$[HPO$_4$]$_3 \cdot 9$H$_2$O, where the monohydrogen phosphate ion is disposed with the phosphorus atom on the C$_3$ axis of the complex cation and the oxygen atoms are hydrogen bonded to the N—H groups of the cation. The proposed structure VII is simulated[56] in the cobalt(III) complex of 1,1,1-tris(2'-amino-ethylamino)ethane (sen), and the CD spectrum of (+)-[Co(sen)]$^{3+}$, VIII, resembles

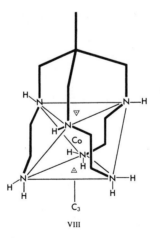

VIII

that of the ion-pair VII (Fig. 7). The complex VIII exhibits a marked gegenion effect (Fig. 7) which is attributed[56] to the introduction of new chiral centres at the hydrogen-bonded nitrogen atoms on the formation of an orientated ion-pair analogous to VII.

The gegenion effect has been used[57] to assign CD bands to particular components of the lowest-energy d-electron transition since the effect consists, in cases where the components have been identified by other criteria, of a decrease and an increase in the respective CD band areas due to the E and A_2 components. Caution is required in this application, as is illustrated by the case[51, 52] of Λ-(−)-[Co(tn)$_3$]$^{3+}$ where a major part of the ion-pairing effect appears to consist of a ring-conformation change. In five-membered ring complexes conformation changes may be appreciable as the addition of phosphate sharpens up[54] the otherwise broad NMR spectrum of

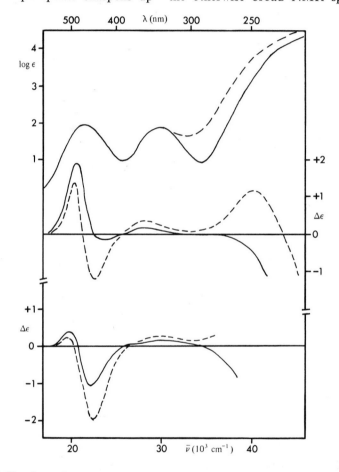

Fig. 7. The absorption spectra (top curves) and circular dichroism (middle curves) of Λ-(+)-[Co(en)$_3$](ClO$_4$)$_3$ in water (———) and in 0·1 M-aqueous phosphate (————), and (bottom curves) the circular dichroism of the corresponding 1,1,1-tris(2′-amino-ethylamino methyl)ethane complex (+)-[Co(sen)]$^{3+}$ (VIII) in water (———), and in 0·1 M-aqueous phosphate (————). The bottom curves are adapted from Sarneski and Urbach.[56]

[Co(en)₃]³⁺ and an analysis of the NMR spectrum of [Rh(en)₃]³⁺ indicates[44] a substantial increase in the fraction of the ligands with a *lel* orientation on the addition of phosphate.

A pseudoracemate of *lel* and *ob* diastereoisomers is not optically inactive, and the CD spectrum of an equimolecular mixture of $\Lambda(\delta\delta\delta)$-(+)-[Co($S$-pn)₃]³⁺ (III) and $\Delta(\delta\delta\delta)$-(−)-[Co($S$-pn)₃]³⁺ (IV) records the Cotton effects due to three puckered 1,2-propylenediamine rings with the δ-conformation, the optical activity due to the Λ and Δ configuration of the rings around the metal ion being internally compensated in the mixture.[46, 58, 59] On the other hand, the CD spectrum of an equimolecular mixture of $\Lambda(\delta\delta\delta)$-(+)-[Co($S$-pn)₃]³⁺ and $\Lambda(\lambda\lambda\lambda)$-(+)-[Co($R$-pn)₃]³⁺ gives the Cotton effects due to the Λ-configuration of three hypothetically-planar 1,2-propylenediamine rings about the metal ion, the conformational effect now being internally compensated.[46, 58, 59]

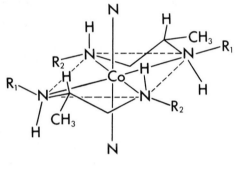

IX R₁ = R₂ = H
X R₁ = Me, R₂ = H
XI R₁ = H, R₂ = Me

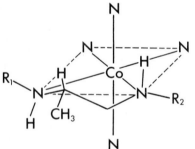

XII R₁ = R₂ = H
XIII R₁ = Me, R₂ = H
XIV R₁ = H, R₂ = Me

The *trans*-bis-diamine complexes, IX–XI, and the corresponding monochelate complexes, XII–XIV, where the diamine is (S)-(+)-propylenediamine or a N-methyl derivative,[60] are devoid of configurational optical activity and their CD spectra afford the Cotton effects due respectively to two *trans*-rings and to one 1,2-propylenediamine ring with the δ-conformation (Fig. 8). An approximate measure of the conformational effect of two *cis*-rings is provided by the CD spectra of (+)- and (−)-[Co(R-pn)₂(ox)]⁺, the oxalato ring being planar, and of the configurational effect of two *cis*-rings by the CD spectrum of *cis*-(+)-[Co(en)₂-(NH₃)₂]³⁺ compared with that of (+)-[Co(en)₃]³⁺ (Table 3).

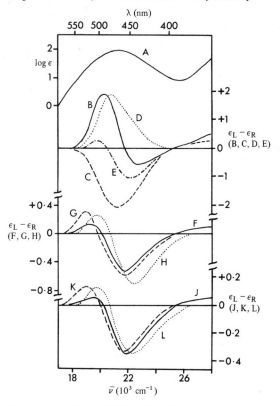

Fig. 8. The absorption spectrum (A) of [Co(pn)₃]³⁺ and the circular dichroism of: (B) the *lel*-isomer Λ-(+)-[Co(S-pn)₃]³⁺ (III), (C) the *ob*-form Δ-(−)-[Co(S-pn)₃]³⁺ (IV), (D) the equimolar mixture of (+)-[Co(R-pn)₃]³⁺ and (+)-[Co(S-pn)₃]³⁺ giving the Λ-configurational effect of three, hypothetically-planar, diamine rings, (E) the equimolar mixture of (+)- and (−)-[Co(S-pn)₃]³⁺, giving the δ-conformational effect of three puckered diamine rings, (F) *trans*-[Co(S-pn)₂(NH₃)₂]³⁺ (IX), (G) *trans*-[Co(N₁Me-S-pn)₂(NH₃)₂]³⁺ (X), (H) the δ-conformational effect of two puckered diamine rings (curve E reduced by 2Δε/3), (J) [Co(S-pn)(NH₃)₄]³⁺ (XII), (K) [Co(N₂Me-S-pn)(NH₃)₄]³⁺ (XIV), and (L) the δ-conformational effect of one (S)-(+)propylenediamine ring (curve E reduced by Δε/3).

The data indicate (Fig. 8, Table 3) that the conformational Cotton effect of propylenediamine chelate rings is additive, the magnitude being proportional to the number, but not the mutual disposition in the complex, of the rings. The result suggests that the conformational effect arises from a first-order perturbation of the d-electrons of the metal ion by the atoms of the chelate ring, or a sum of one-centre second-order perturbations. The configurational Cotton effect is some three times larger for (+)-[Co(en)₃]³⁺ than *cis*-(+)-[Co(en)₂(NH₃)₂]³⁺ (Table 3), suggesting that the effect is second-order, arising from pair-wise interactions between the chelate rings involving the d-electrons of the metal ion.

The conformational or vicinal effect is found to be approximately additive for a range of ligands in cobalt(III) complexes, notably, (R,R)-(−)-stilbenediamine (Table

3), (R,R)-(−)-cyclohexanediamine,[39, 61] and the L-amino acids.[62–66] A ligand for which the effect is not additive is (R,R)-(−)-2,4-pentanediamine,[67] as the conformational Cotton effect derived from the CD spectra[48] of $(+)_{546}$- and $(−)_{546}$-[Co$(R,R$-ptn)$_3$]$^{3+}$ is larger and has a form different from the Cotton effect near 500 nm given by [Co(NH$_3$)$_4(R,R$-ptn)]$^{3+}$. The steric restraints on the flexible (R,R)-ptn ligand are more severe in the tris- than the mono-chelate complex, and it is likely that the twist ring conformation is the less preferred in the latter complex.

Table 3

The frequency, ν (10^3 cm^{-1}), and the rotational strength, R (10^{-40} c.g.s.), of the circular dichroism given by cobalt(III) complexes in the region of the octahedral $^1A_{1g} \rightarrow {}^1T_{1g}$ absorption, and the derived rotational strength for the Λ-configurational effect and the λ-ring conformational effect

	(+)-isomer		(−)-isomer		R (10^{-40} c.g.s.)	
Complex	ν	R	ν	R	Λ-configuration	λ-conformation
[Co(R-pn)$_3$]$^{3+}$	21·2	+8·05	20·2	−5·35	+6·1	+1·9
			22·7	+1·15		
[Co(R-pn)$_2$(ox)]$^+$	19·4	+10·5	19·1	−7·9	+9·2	+1·3
[Co(R-pn)$_2$(en)]$^{3+}$	20·8	+7·05	20·5	−5·4	+5·7	+1·3
			22·9	+0·9		
[Co(R,R-stien)$_3$]$^{3+}$	20·3	+5·5	21·2	−19·5	+12·0	−7·5
	22·4	−1·0				
trans-[Co(R,R-stien)$_2$(NH$_3$)$_2$]$^{3+}$			21·3	−5·0		−5·0
trans-[Co(R-pn)$_2$(NH$_3$)$_2$]$^{3+}$	19·3	−0·2				+1·2
	21·6	+1·4				
[Co(R-pn)(NH$_3$)$_4$]$^{3+}$	19·2	−0·07				+0·65
	21·7	+0·72				
[Co(en)$_3$]$^{3+}$	20·3	+4·8			+4·4	
	23·5	−0·4				
cis-[Co(en)$_2$(NH$_3$)$_2$]$^{3+}$	20·3	+1·5			+1·4	
	23·3	−0·1				

A similar relaxation of steric constraints is probably responsible for the small conformational Cotton effect of (R)-(−)-propylenediamine in a four-coordinate tetragonal complex, compared to that of the corresponding (R,R)-(−)-cyclohexanediamine complex (Table 4). In the six-coordinate tetragonal complexes the Cotton effects of corresponding R-pn and R,R-chxn complexes are more nearly comparable, the magnitudes in the latter cases being some 20 % larger (Table 5) as opposed to a factor of 2 or more in the four-coordinate complexes, except for copper(II) which is likely to be hexacoordinate by apical solvation (Table 4). The steric restrictions to the axial conformation of the methyl group in a 1,2-propylenediamine ring are substantially reduced in a square planar complex whereas the assumption of an analogous conformation is precluded in a 1,2-cyclohexanediamine chelate owing to the fused ring.

The tetragonal bis-diamine complexes of a range of transition metal ions show overall conformational Cotton effects of the same sign for a given ligand (Tables 3, 4 and 5). In the hexacoordinated (d)^6 complexes containing the trans-[MN$_4$Cl$_2$]$^{n+}$ chromophore (Table 5), and other trans-[MA$_4$B$_2$] complexes where the ligands A

Table 4

The circular dichroism spectra of tetragonal $[MN_4]^{2+}$ complexes in the region of the d-electron absorption bands

Complex[a]	v_1 (10^3 cm^{-1})	$\Delta\varepsilon_1$	v_2 (10^3 cm^{-1})	$\Delta\varepsilon_2$	Ref.
$[Cu(R\text{-pn})_2]^{2+}$	15·2	+0·04	19·6	+0·27	b
$[Cu(R,R\text{-chxn})_2]^{2+}$	16·0	+0·05	19·2	+0·40	c
$[Cu(R,R\text{-stien})_2]^{2+}$	18·0	−0·50			d
$[Cu(N_1Me\text{-}S\text{-pn})_2]^{2+}$	16·5	−0·098	19·6	+0·050	e
$[Cu(N_2Me\text{-}S\text{-pn})_2]^{2+}$	15·5	−0·049	19·0	+0·044	e
$[Ni(R\text{-pn})_2]^{2+}$	21·7	+0·15			f
$[Ni(R,R\text{-chxn})_2]^{2+}$	22·0	+0·45			c
$[Ni(R,R\text{-stien})_2]^{2+}$	22·5	−1·0			d
$[Pd(R\text{-pn})_2]^{2+}$	29·0	+0·06	35·5	+1·22	g
$[Pd(R,R\text{-chxn})_2]^{2+}$	29·1	+0·13	35·3	+2·94	g
$[Pt(R\text{-pn})(NH_3)_2]^{2+}$	35·2	+0·22	44·8	+0·51	g
$[Pt(R\text{-pn})(en)]^{2+}$	35·7	+0·29	45·1	+0·54	g
$[Pt(R\text{-pn})_2]^{2+}$	35·7	+0·54	45·2	+1·03	g
$[Pt(R,R\text{-chxn})(NH_3)_2]^{2+}$	35·0	+0·40	45·0	+0·86	g
$[Pt(R,R\text{-chxn})_2]^{2+}$	35·5	+0·94	45·3	+2·02	g

[a] The ligands are (R)-$(-)$-propylenediamine $(R\text{-pn})$; (R,R)-$(-)$-1,2-cyclohexanediamine $(R,R\text{-chxn})$; (R,R)-$(-)$-1,2-stilbenediamine $(R,R\text{-stien})$; (S)-3-methyl-4-amino-2-azabutane $(N_1Me\text{-}S\text{-pn})$; and (S)-4-amino-4-methyl-2-azabutane $(N_2Me\text{-}S\text{-pn})$. [b] J. P. Mathieu, *Ann. Phys. Paris* **19**, 335 (1944). [c] R. S. Treptow, Thesis, University of Illinois, 1966. [d] P. L. Fereday and S. F. Mason. Forthcoming publication. [e] M. Morita and S. Yoshikawa, *Chem. Commun.* 578 (1972). [f] B. Bosnich, J. H. Dunlop and R. D. Gillard, *Chem. Commun.* 274 (1965). [g] H. Ito, J. Fujita and K. Saito, *Bull. Chem. Soc. Japan* **40**, 2584 (1967).

and B occupy different positions in the spectrochemical series, an additional source of optical activity is apparent in the resolved D_4 components of the octahedral $^1A_{1g} \rightarrow {}^1T_{1g}$ transition.

The tetragonal effect is the more apparent where the conformation effect is weak, as in the case of *trans*-$[Co(R,R\text{-ptn})_2Cl_2]^+$ where the chelate rings are more labile

Table 5

The circular dichroism spectra of *trans*-dichloro-bis-diamine (d)^6 transition metal complexes in the region of the octahedral $^1A_{1g} \rightarrow {}^1T_{1g}$ absorption

Complex	$^1A_1 \rightarrow {}^1E$ component		$^1A_1 \rightarrow {}^1A_2$ component		Ref.
	v (10^3 cm^{-1})	$\Delta\varepsilon$	v (10^3 cm^{-1})	$\Delta\varepsilon$	
trans-$[Co(R\text{-pn})_2Cl_2]^+$	16·6	+0·76	21·6	−0·10	a
trans-$[Co(R,R\text{-chxn})_2Cl_2]^+$	16·4	+0·93	21·4	−0·10	b
trans-$[Co(R,R\text{-stien})_2Cl_2]^+$	16·9	−1·0	21·8	−1·4	c
trans-$[Co(R,R\text{-ptn})_2Cl_2]^+$	16	+0·5	21	−0·6	d
trans-$[Rh(R\text{-pn})_2Cl_2]^+$	24·6	+0·59	31·0	−0·03	a
trans-$[Pd(R\text{-pn})_2Cl_2]^{2+}$	24·5	+0·4			a
trans-$[Pt(R\text{-pn})_2Cl_2]^{2+}$	30·5	+0·27			a
trans-$[Pt(R,R\text{-chxn})_2Cl_2]^{2+}$	30·1	+0·35			a, b

[a] H. Ito, J. Fujita and K. Saito, *Bull. Chem. Soc. Japan* **42**, 1286 (1969). [b] R. S. Treptow, Thesis, University of Illinois, 1966; *Inorg. Chem.* **5**, 1593 (1966). [c] P. L. Fereday and S. F. Mason, *Chem. Commun.* 1314 (1971). [d] F. Mizukami, H. Ito, J. Fujita and K. Saito, *Bull. Chem. Soc. Japan* **45**, 2129 (1972). B. Bosnich and J. MacB. Harrowfield gives the values, $\Delta\varepsilon_{16} + 0\cdot78$ and $\Delta\varepsilon_{21} - 0\cdot80$ [*J. Amer. Chem. Soc.* **94**, 3425 (1972)].

conformationally than those of the 1,2-diamines, and it consists of CD bands nearly equal in magnitude and opposed in sign associated with the two D_4 components of the d-electron transition to the octahedral T_{1g} state (Fig. 9). When the conformational effect is strong, as in the case of the (R,R)-$(-)$-stilbenediamine ligand (Table 3) the tetragonal effect is not seen and CD bands of the same sign, reflecting that of conformational effect, are observed (Table 5, Fig. 10). The ligands, R-pn and R,R-chxn

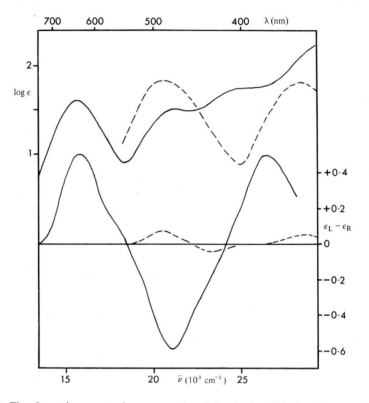

Fig. 9. The absorption spectra (upper curves) and the circular dichroism (lower curves) of *trans*-[Co(R,R-ptn)$_2$Cl$_2$]$^+$ (———) and [Co(R,R-ptn)(NH$_3$)$_4$]$^{3+}$ (— — — —). Adapted from original spectra kindly provided by Professor K. Saito.[67]

are intermediate cases where the tetragonal and conformational effects are more nearly comparable, CD bands of opposite sign but unequal magnitude being associated with the D_4 components (Table 5, Fig. 11).

The magnitude of both the tetragonal and the conformational Cotton effects decreases in the *trans*-[MN$_4$Cl$_2$]$^{n+}$ series as the atomic number and the oxidation number of the metal ion increase. However, the decreases are not parallel, the tetragonal effect vanishing between rhodium(III) and palladium(IV), whereas the platinum(IV) complexes retain some 40% of the conformational optical activity of the corresponding cobalt(III) complexes (Table 5). The different trends suggest that the tetragonal and the conformational optical activity may have different physical origins.

Although the electronic excitations of the *trans*-$[MN_4Cl_2]^{n+}$ complexes listed (Table 5) may be classified in the group D_4 these complexes structurally have D_2 symmetry or, in the case of the *R*-pn complexes, an approximate D_2 symmetry. If that symmetry is lowered to C_2, e.g. by *N*-alkylation, the CD due to the doubly-degenerate D_4 component is resolved (Fig. 11). The splitting identifies the E parentage of the CD bands in D_4 symmetry, and the corresponding A_2 component of the

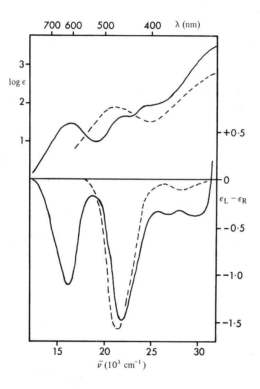

Fig. 10. The absorption spectra (upper curves) and circular dichroism (lower curves) of *trans*-$[Co(R,R\text{-stien})_2Cl_2]^+$ (———) and *trans*-$[Co(R,R\text{-stien})_2(NH_3)_2]^{3+}$ (– – – –).

trans-$[MN_4Cl_2]^{n+}$ Cotton effects is located by the expectation that it lies at the same frequency as the $A_{1g} \rightarrow T_{1g}$ absorption of the corresponding $[MN_6]$ chromophore.[68] Similarly, the reduction in symmetry of a tris-chelated complex to C_2 may resolve the CD due to the doubly-degenerate D_3 component, giving three CD bands in the region of the octahedral $A_{1g} \rightarrow T_{1g}$ absorption, as in the case[69] of Δ-(+)-$[Co(mal)_2(en)]^-$, and the parent triple-degeneracy is also lifted in mono-chelate amino-acid complexes,[63] e.g. $[Co(NH_3)_4(L\text{-alanine})]^{2+}$.

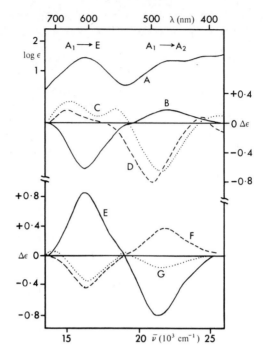

Fig. 11. The absorption spectrum (A) and the circular dichroism (B) of *trans*-[Co(*S*-pn)$_2$Cl$_2$]$^+$ (XVI), and the circular dichroism of (C) (−)-*trans,trans*-[Co(NMeen)$_2$Cl$_2$]$^+$ (XV), and (D) *trans*-[Co(N$_1$Me-*S*-pn)Cl$_2$]$^+$ (XVII) in water. Curve E represents the specific tetragonal effect of the two *N*-methyl groups of XV or of XVII, curve F the specific tetragonal effect of the chelate-ring groups in XV, XVI or XVII, and curve G the specific octahedral (conformational) effect of two 1,2-diamine rings with the δ-conformation. Curve G is obtained by partitioning the observed conformational effect of two δ-rings on the [CoN$_6$] chromophore (Fig. 8) in the ratio (1/3) and (2/3), respectively, over the wavelength regions of the A$_1$ → A$_2$ and A$_1$ → E tetragonal components given by the [CoN$_4$Cl$_2$] chromophore in XV–XVII. Curves B, C and D are given approximately by the sums appropriate for XVI, XV, and XVII, respectively, of the curves E, F and G.

3.6.5   Regional Rules for d-Electron Optical Activity

Hamer,[70] developing Sugano's discussion[20] of Moffitt's theory,[19] showed that a first-order rotational strength is generated in a centrosymmetric metal complex only by a ligand field which transforms under the pseudoscalar Γ_{1u} representation of the point group of the complex. The result was developed further by Schellman[26] for the general case of a symmetric chromophore disposed in a dissymmetric molecular environment where the electronic states of the chromophore are mixed by the encompassing static coulombic field of the substituents. The effective component of the perturbing potential from the substituent groups has pseudoscalar symmetry in the point group of the symmetric chromophore, and pseudoscalar functions expressing the form of that component, e.g. [4] for the octahedron, provide the basis for a theoretical perturbation treatment. Equally the pseudoscalar functions provide working sector rules for the empirical correlation of the position of a substituent in the chromophoric coordinate frame with the sign and the magnitude of the rotational strength induced by the substituent in a particular electronic transition of the symmetric chromophore.[26]

In an alternative or complementary general treatment, due to Höhn and Weigang[71] and based on Kirkwood's dynamic coupling model,[72] it is assumed that a charge displacement in the substituent, i.e. a transient dipole induced by the chromophore field, correlates coulombically with the charge displacements involved in the particular electronic transition of the symmetric chromophore. According to this model the optical activity of a symmetric chromophore in a dissymmetric molecular environment arises from the coupling of the moment of the chromophoric transition, electric or magnetic, with the transient electric dipole induced in the substituent. Sector rules relating the substituent disposition in the chromophoric frame to the form of the induced rotational strength are provided in the dynamic-coupling model by the geometric or orientational factors governing the potential between the electric multipole charge distribution of the chromophoric transition and the transient electric dipole induced in the substituent.[71]

The static-field and the dynamic-coupling mechanism emerge as discrete terms in the perturbational treatment of the optical activity of a symmetric chromophore in a dissymmetric molecular environment carried to first order, although cross-terms between the two mechanisms appear in the second and higher orders.[73] For a symmetric chromophore with zero-order electronic states A_i and a perturbing substituent with an analogous set of electronic states B_j the rotational strength of the chromophoric transition, $A_0 \rightarrow A_n$, has the form

$$R_{0n} = -i\langle A_0\,B_0|\,\hat{\mu}\,|A_n\,B_0\rangle \cdot \langle A_n\,B_0|\,\hat{m}\,|A_0\,B_0\rangle \qquad [10]$$

where $\hat{\mu}$ and $\hat{m}$ are the electric- and the magnetic-dipole operators, respectively. The expansion of the correct wave functions $|A_n B_0\rangle$ to first order in terms of the zero-order basis set $|A_i B_j)$, on the assumption that there is no electron-exchange between the chromophore and the substituent, gives

$$|A_n\,B_0\rangle = |A_n\,B_0) + \sum_i \sum_j \frac{(A_i\,B_j|\,V\,|A_n\,B_0)}{(E_n - E_i - E_j)}\,|A_i\,B_j) \qquad [11]$$

with $n = 0$ for the ground-state function $|A_0 B_0\rangle$. The perturbation V is the coulombic potential between the transition charge distributions $(A_i|A_n)$ of the chromophore and $(B_j|B_0)$ of the perturbing substituent.

For a magnetically-allowed excitation of the chromophore the magnetic moment of the transition $A_0 \rightarrow A_n$ is taken as the zero-order value

$$m_{n0} = \langle A_n\,B_0|\,\hat{m}\,|A_0\,B_0\rangle = (A_n\,B_0|\,\hat{m}\,|A_0\,B_0) \qquad [12]$$

but the electric dipole moment of the transition is wholly borrowed, with the following components[71]

$$\langle A_0 B_0| \, \mu |A_n B_0\rangle = \sum_{i\neq 0} (-E_i)^{-1}(A_i B_0| \, V |A_0 B_0) \, \mu_{ni} \qquad [13a]$$

$$+ \sum_{k\neq n} (E_n - E_k)^{-1}(A_k B_0| \, V |A_n B_0) \, \mu_{0k} \qquad [13b]$$

$$+ \sum_{j} (-E_n - E_j)^{-1}(A_n B_j| \, V |A_0 B_0) \, \mu_{0j} \qquad [13c]$$

$$+ \sum_{l} (E_n - E_l)^{-1}(A_0 B_l| \, V |A_n B_0) \, \mu_{0l} \qquad [13d]$$

The first two terms [13a, b] refer to the mixing of the transition $A_0 \rightarrow A_n$ with other transitions of the chromophore, e.g. $A_0 \rightarrow A_k$, which are electric-dipole allowed and have a component of the moment μ_{0k} collinear with m_{n0} [12] to give a non-zero R_{0n} [10]. These two terms [13a, b] arise from the static field due to the ground-state charge distribution of the perturbing substituent $(B_0|B_0)$, and the perturbation element $(A_k B_0|V|A_n B_0)$ is non-zero only if V has the direct-product symmetry of the polar and axial vectorial representations under which A_k and A_n respectively transform. The particular pseudoscalar function describing the potential V of [13a] or [13b] depends upon the form of the electric-dipole states A_i or A_k chosen to mix with the magnetic-dipole state A_n, and there is some latitude in the design of sector rules by the static field procedure, e.g. a quadrant or an octant rule for the $n \rightarrow \pi^*$ Cotton effect of chiral ketones depending upon the selection of the $\pi \rightarrow \pi^*$ or the $n \rightarrow 3d$ perturbing excitation.

The dynamic-coupling mechanism, embodied in the latter two terms [13c, d], is more restrictive, for explicit summation of these terms gives the rotational strength [10] as a function of the zero-order magnetic moment m_{n0} [12] and electric multipole moment P_{0n}^{lm} of the chromophoric transition and the polarizability of the substituent at the transition frequency, $\alpha(\nu_{0n})$. For an isotropic polarizability and a z-polarized magnetic transition moment the dynamic-coupling rotational strength becomes

$$R_{0n} = -i m_{n0}^z \, P_{0n}^{lm} \, G_{1m,z} \, \bar{\alpha}(\nu_{0n}) \qquad [14]$$

where $G_{1m,z}$ is the geometric factor governing the radial and angular dependence of the coulombic potential between the mth component of the 2^l electric multipole P^{lm} and the z-component of an electric dipole. A residual latitude of the dynamic coupling mechanism derives from the relative importance of the mean polarizability of the substituent, $\bar{\alpha}$, and of the anisotropy of that polarizability $(\alpha_\| - \alpha_\perp)$ when the chromophoric transition is magnetically allowed. For the anisotropic contribution to the rotational strength an expression analogous to [14] obtains, but the geometric factor and the consequent sector rule has a different form.[71] In the case of an electric-dipole chromophore transition only the anisotropy of the substituent's polarizability is significant, and the expression for the rotational strength corresponding to [14] is then definitive.[71]

A number of sector rules correlating the substituent disposition in a chiral metal complex with the d-electron Cotton effects have been proposed in recent years,[74–81] particularly after the formulation of the static-field[26] and dynamic-coupling[71] procedures. The earliest of these, the octant-sign rule,[74] was of a general nature, relating the sign of the Cotton effect due to a particular component descended from the $(d)^6$ octahedral $A_{1g} \rightarrow T_{1g}$ transition in a tetragonal, trigonal, orthorhombic, or lower-symmetry ligand environment to the sum of the signs of the coordinate function $[Z(X^2 - Y^2)]$ for each substituent (Fig. 12a). As the principal types of d-electron optical activity became the more fully distinguished, the octant-sign rule was found to lack adequate discrimination, and it is now apparent that the different types, often superposed, follow different sector rules.

The main types of d-electron optical activity requiring distinct sector rules are: (A) the conformational or octahedral effect, (B) the configurational or trigonal effect, (C) tetragonal optical activity, and (D) orthorhombic and lower-symmetry optical activity manifest in resolved CD bands with $E(D_3)$ or $E(D_4)$ parentage.

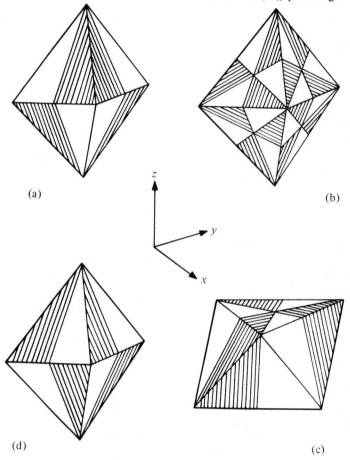

Fig. 12. Regional rules relating the position of substitution to optical activity: (a) the octant-sign rule; substitution in a hatched sector gives a positive Cotton effect for the $A_1 \rightarrow E$ trigonal component or the $A_1 \rightarrow A_2$ tetragonal component; (b) the octahedral rule for the conformational effect; substitution in a hatched sector gives a net positive circular dichroism in the region of the $A_{1g} \rightarrow T_{1g}$ octahedral cobalt(III) absorption; (c) the sextant rule for the configurational optical activity of trigonal complexes; substitution in a hatched region gives the $A_1 \rightarrow A_2$ trigonal component a positive rotational strength; and (d) the rule for the specific tetragonal optical activity; substitution in a hatched sector gives the tetragonal components $A_1 \rightarrow A_2$ and $A_1 \rightarrow E$ a positive and a negative rotational strength, respectively.

(A). The Conformational Effect

The form of an appropriate sector rule for the conformational effect is determined by the symmetry properties of the effect. The primary octahedral symmetry elements of the conformational effect are C_3, $(C_4)^2$, and C_2', from the CD data for the CoN_6 complexes devoid of configurational activity, i.e. the mono-chelate, *trans*-bis-diamine, and diastereoisomeric pseudoracemic tris-diamines (Table 3, Fig. 8). The conformational effect is nodal for the secondary elements, σ_h, since the effect vanishes for planar rings, and σ_d, since the *N*-methyl group of N_1- or N_2-methyl-(+)-1,2-propylenediamine makes little contribution to the Cotton effects of the CoN_6 chromophore in the complexes IX–XIV (Fig. 8) compared with the notable sign-reversals produced in the case of the tetragonal *trans*-CoN_4Cl_2 chromophore in the complexes XV–XVII (Fig. 11). An X-ray diffraction analysis[82] of the *N*-methyl-

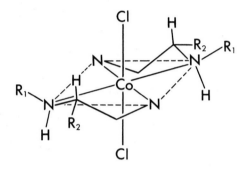

XV R_1 = Me, R_2 = H
XVI R_1 = H, R_2 = Me
XVII R_1 = R_2 = Me

ethylenediamine complex, (–)-*trans, trans*-[Co(Meen)$_2$Cl$_2$]$^+$ (XV) and an analysis[83] of the chelate ring conformation in [Co(NH$_3$)$_4$(Meen)]$^{3+}$ show that the *N*-methyl group of a *N*-methyl-1,2-diamine chelate ring has a preferred orientation in, or close to, a σ_d plane of the octahedron (Fig. 13).

The antisymmetry of the conformational effect with respect to the σ_h and σ_d planes and the implied other secondary operations of the octahedron, and the totally symmetric behaviour of the effect under the primary operations, indicate that the conformational rotational strengths are spanned by the A_{1u} representation of O_h and, more specifically, that the appropriate sector rule is described by the lowest pseudoscalar function in O_h (equation [4]). The hatched sectors of the octahedral regional rule depicted (Fig. 12b) correspond to positive values of the O_h pseudoscalar function [4] as illustrated (Fig. 13) and correlate with the net positive conformational rotational strength observed generally for the λ-ring conformation of alkyl-substituted (R)-(–)-diamines (Table 3). Conversely, unhatched sectors (Fig. 12b) correspond to negative values (Fig. 13) and correlate with the net positive conformational CD of alkyl-substituted (S)-(+)-1,2-diamines (Fig. 8). The aryl-substituted (R,R)-(–)-stilbenediamine complexes with a λ-ring conformation but a large negative conformational Cotton effect (Table 3, Fig. 10) are only apparently exceptional, since the benzene rings are disposed in sectors with a negative sign and exercise an opposed and stronger perturbation than the chelate ring atoms in positive sectors[84] (Fig. 14).

The CD spectra of the stilbenediamine complexes, compared with those of analogous alkyl-substituted 1,2-diamines, suggest that the conformational optical activity originates more probably through the dynamic-coupling than the static-field

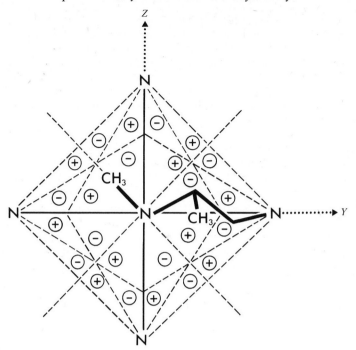

Fig. 13. The projection of the chelate ring and the ligand atoms of $[Co(N_1Me\text{-}S\text{-}pn)(NH_3)_4]^{3+}$ (XIII) on the YZ planar section of the octahedral pseudoscalar function (4), i.e. Fig. 12(b).

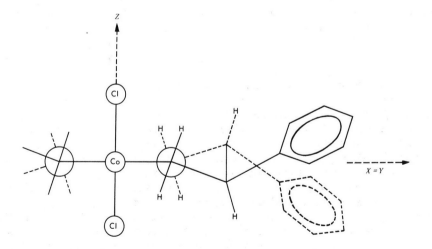

Fig. 14. The preferred λ-conformation of a (R,R)-$(-)$-stilbenediamine chelate ring in the coordinate frame of the octahedral regional rule (4), i.e. Fig. 12(b).

mechanism.[84] The phenyl group has a substantially larger polarizability[85] (10·32 Å³) than a C—C (0·64 Å³) or a C—H group (0·65 Å³), but it is unlikely that the benzene nuclei of a stilbenediamine chelate ring carry a static charge significantly larger than that of the carbon and hydrogen atoms of the ring.

A first-order perturbational treatment of the conformational optical activity encounters the difficulty that the octahedral regional rule [4] requires a large inverse power in the distance, $(R)^{-19}$, for the potential between the chromophore and the perturbing substituent, given that both of these are point-sources, in either the static-field or the dynamic-coupling mechanism. The difficulty may be circumvented in both treatments by proceeding to second order. Sugano and Shinada[27, 28] showed that a static A_{1u} octahedral field is produced by the superposition of the ungerade field [1] and the gerade field [5], with T_{2u} and T_{2g} symmetry, respectively, and that a net second-order rotational strength results in D_3 complexes from these fields. Recently Richardson[81] has extended this approach in detail, formulating sector rules for all of the main structural types of chiral chelated metal complexes.

For the net second-order rotational strength of a perturbed octahedral chromophore, covering the conformational optical activity, the simplest sector rules, with a $(R)^{-12}$ overall distance-dependency, are

$$\sum_r \sum_s Z_r[X_s\,Y_s(X_s^2 - Y_s^2)]\,Q_r\,Q_s \qquad [15a]$$

$$\sum_r \sum_s X_r[Y_s\,Z_s(Y_s^2 - Z_s^2)]\,Q_r\,Q_s \qquad [15b]$$

$$\sum_r \sum_s Y_r[X_s\,Z_s(Z_s^2 - X_s^2)]\,Q_r\,Q_s \qquad [15c]$$

and an analogous set of three rules, obtained similarly by cyclic permutation of the coordinates of each substituent r and s in the first member

$$\sum_r \sum_s [X_r(Y_r^2 - Z_r^2)\,Y_s\,Z_s]\,Q_r\,Q_s \qquad [16]$$

where Q_r and Q_s are the respective charges of the substituents r and s. In [15] and [16] the substituent r gives rise to an ungerade static field, which mixes the d- with p- and f-orbitals, while the substituent s produces a gerade field, mixing the d-orbitals amongst themselves. The general perturbation implied by [15] and [16] is a three-way interaction between the two substituents, r and s, and the metal-ion. For N dis-symmetrically disposed substituents the number of three-way interactions increases as $(N!/2)$, whereas the conformational rotational strength is additive, proportional to N, in good approximation (Table 3). If it is assumed that only the one-centre terms for $r = s$ are important, so producing a proportionality to N, the sum of the conformational rotational strengths governed by the three rules, [15a], [15b] and [15c], vanishes, as do those dependent upon the three rules [16]. However, the one-centre terms, $r = s$, in the higher-order sector rules for the net rotational strength of a perturbed octahedral chromophore, with an overall $(R)^{-16}$ distance-dependency, have a non-zero sum.[81]

(B). Trigonal Optical-Activity; The Configurational Effect

The configurational rotational strength of D_3 or C_3 tris-chelated metal complexes is described by a sextant regional rule (Fig. 12c) based on the functional form of Moffitt's ungerade potential [1] or the equivalent form [2]. The basis of the sextant rule in the potential [1] suggests that it is likely to be strictly valid only for the first-order trigonal rotational strengths accessible through the axial single-crystal CD spectrum of the complex (Table 1). In the form of the sextant rule illustrated (Fig. 12c) substituents in hatched sectors induce a positive configurational rotational strength in the D_3 component $A_1 \to A_2$ and a negative rotational strength in the $A_1 \to E$ component, converse relations between optical activity and substituent-position applying to the unhatched sectors.

The sextant rule indicates that if the L–M–L bond angle is 90° the coordinated ligand atoms lie in a nodal plane and make no contribution to the optical activity, but those atoms make a contribution of the same sign as the non-coordinated atoms of the chelate if the L–M–L ring angle is less than 90° or of opposite sign if that angle is greater than 90°. Thus $R(E)$ is positive and large for Λ-(+)-[Co(en)$_3$]$^{3+}$ (I) where the N–Co–N ring angle is[35] 85·3° but negative and relatively small for Λ-(–)-[Co(tn)$_3$]$^{3+}$ (II) where that angle is[35] 94·5°. In the latter case the negative contribution of the coordinated NH_2 groups outweighs the positive contribution of the σ-bonded CH_2 groups, but where the non-coordinated groups of the chelate rings are unsaturated their contribution outweighs that of the coordinated ligand atoms when the L–M–L ring angle is greater than 90°, as in the cases of Λ-(–)-[Co(acac)$_3$], Λ-(+)-[Cr(mal)$_3$]$^{3-}$, and Λ-(+)-*trans*-[Cr(atc)$_3$] (see section 3.6.3). In general, unsaturated systems have a larger polarizability than analogous saturated molecules, but they are not necessarily more polar. Moreover the stilbenediamine complexes, (+)- and (–)-[Co(*R*,*R*-stien)$_3$]$^{3+}$, with phenyl substituents of large polarizability, have a relatively large configurational rotational strength (Table 3). Thus the available evidence suggests that the more probable origin of configurational optical activity is the dynamic coupling than the static-field mechanism.

A consequence of the trigonal-polar functional form [1] of the sextant rule (Fig. 12c) is the expectation that substituents close to the XY-equatorial plane where $\sin^3 \theta$ has a maximum value make a correspondingly large contribution to the configurational optical activity. In both the five- and the six-membered chelate ring series the alkyl groups of the rings lie closer to the equatorial plane ($\theta = \pi/2$) in the *ob*-conformation, e.g. IV and VI, than in the *lel*-conformation, e.g. III and V. The area of the lowest-energy CD band, or bands where the A_2 and E components are resolved, is generally larger for the *ob* than the *lel* isomer in the five-membered ring series (Figs. 3 and 4) and is some five-times larger in the six-ring series (Fig. 5). The comparison is confined, in the absence of crystal CD studies, to the net rotational strength of the A_2 and E components and necessarily includes the conformational effect.

The first-order perturbation treatment of D_3 complexes, using the static-field model, reproduces the sextant rule for the axial single-crystal CD spectrum with the correct sign if it is assumed that the chiral substituents carry a net positive charge due, e.g. to the incomplete screening of the atomic nuclei.[81] The rotational strength of the D_3 component $A_1 \to E$ is given by[81]

$$R(E) = C \sum_s Q_s \sin^3 \theta_s \sin^3 \phi_s / R_s^4$$

$$= C \sum_s Q_s [3 Y_s X_s^2 - Y_s^3] / R_s^7 \qquad [17]$$

where Q_s is the charge and θ_s, ϕ_s or X_s, Y_s are the coordinates in a trigonal frame of the substituent s, and C is a positive constant. However the corresponding dynamic-coupling treatment carried to first order does not afford the sextant rule. The leading electric multipole moment of the D_3 component $A_1 \to A_2$ is the $[xz(x^2 - 3y^2)]$ component of a hexadecapole which connects with the z-component of an electric dipole through a potential dependent upon the geometric factor[80]

$$[(9Z^2 - R^2)(3XY^2 - X^3)/R^{11}] \tag{18}$$

The geometric relation [18] gives a regional rule with the nodal surfaces $R = \pm 3Z$ lying at an angle of $\pm 19 \cdot 5°$ to the equatorial plane, $Z = 0$, in addition to the three nodal planes of the sextant rule [1]. According to [18] the contributions of the CH_2 groups and the NH_2 groups are opposed in $(+)$-$[Co(en)_3]^{3+}$ but additive in $(-)$-$[Co(tn)_3]^{3+}$, contrary to the implications of the axial single-crystal CD measurements (Table 1).

The static-field treatment carried to second order provides a sector rule for the net rotational strength $R(T_1)$ in the region of the octahedral $A_{1g} \to T_{1g}$ absorption for complex ions randomly orientated in solution[81]

$$R(T_1) = R(E) + R(A_2)$$
$$= c \sum_r \sum_s Q_r Q_s (3 \cos^2 \theta_r - 1)(\sin^3 \theta_s \sin 3\phi_s)/(R_r^3 R_s^7)$$
$$= c \sum_r \sum_s Q_r Q_s (3Z_r^2 - R_r^2)(3 Y_s X_s^3)/(R_r^5 R_s^{10}) \tag{19}$$

where c is a positive constant smaller than C of [17]. The substituents r and s, with the charges Q_r and Q_s, give rise to the gerade [5] and ungerade potential [1], respectively, and by a three-way interaction with the metal ion generate $R(T_1)$. For N substituents $R(T_1)$ is expected to be proportional to $N!/2$, as is observed if each chelate ring is regarded as a substituent (Table 3). However, $R(T_1)$ vanishes if the trigonal-splitting parameter, K [7], is zero, as found[29] for the O—O band of $[Co(en)_3]^{3+}$. This parameter depends upon[81]

$$K = d \sum_r Q_r (3 \cos^2 \theta_r - 1)/R_r^3 \tag{20}$$

where d is a positive constant, so that K is expected to be negative in all cases where the L–M–L ring angle is less than $90°$ and the substituents carry a net positive charge, e.g. $[Co(en)_3]^{3+}$.

(C). Tetragonal Optical Activity

A tetragonal optical activity distinct from the conformational Cotton effects, which are always present in chiral *trans*-bis-diamine complexes, is suggested by the CD spectra of complexes containing the *trans*-$[CoN_4Cl_2]^+$ chromophore, XV–XVII (Fig. 11), where N-methylation produces a change of sign in the Cotton effects due to the two D_4 components, E and A_2, compared with the corresponding complexes containing the $[CoN_6]$ chromophore, IX–XI, where N-methylation has little effect upon the optical activity (Fig. 8). The complex[82] $(-)$-*trans*, *trans*-$[Co(Meen)_2Cl_2]^+$ (XV) has the same absolute stereochemistry as $(+)_{546}$-*trans* $[Co(S\text{-}pn)_2Cl_2]^+$ (XVI),[10] both structures being determined by the anomalous X-ray diffraction method, and the *N*-methyl derivatives[60] of the latter, e.g. XVII, have the same configuration on conformational grounds.[38]

The comparison between XV–XVII and IX–XI suggests that the tetragonal optical activity consists in itself of rotational strengths equal in magnitude but of opposite sign associated with the D_4 components, A_2 and E. The tetragonal effect of the *N*-methyl group in a 1,2-diamine has been analysed in these terms.[86] For complexes containing the *trans*-$[CoN_4Cl_2]^+$ chromophore the tetragonal effect is the least obscured when the conformational effect is weak, as in the case of *trans*-$[Co(R,R$-ptn$)_2Cl_2]^+$ (Fig. 9), and it is largely overlaid where the latter effect is strong, e.g. *trans*-$[Co(RR$-stien$)_2Cl_2]^+$ (Fig. 10). The tetragonal effect is expected to be small when the ligands A and B in a *trans*-$[CoA_4B_2]$ complex are close together in the spectrochemical series, vanishing when A = B.

The comparison between the complexes IX–XI and XV–XVII indicates further that the tetragonal rotational strengths are antisymmetric with respect to the reflection planes of D_{4h} but not to the σ_d planes of the octahedron containing the *N*-methyl groups of a *trans*-bis-*N*-methyl-1,2-diamine complex (Fig. 13). The symmetry behaviour of the tetragonal optical activity under both primary and secondary operations indicates a sector rule based on the lowest D_{4h} pseudoscalar function,[26]

$$[XYZ(X^2 - Y^2)] \qquad [21]$$

which is double-octant[77] or hexadecadal.[80] In the form of the rule depicted (Fig. 12d) the Cotton effect due to the $A_1 \rightarrow A_2$ tetragonal component is positive for substitution in a hatched sector or negative in an unhatched sector, converse relations applying to the corresponding $A_1 \rightarrow E$ component.

Models and the X-ray crystal structures of the complexes XV[82] and XVI[10] indicate that the magnitude of the Z-coordinate in the tetragonal or octahedral frame (Fig. 1) is larger for the carbon atom of the *N*-methyl group than for that of each chelate-ring carbon atom, while the methyl carbon atom of the C-methyl group lies close to the *XY*-plane. The coordinate product $[XY(X^2 - Y^2)]$ is comparable for each carbon atom, so that the function [21] of the tetragonal rule has the largest magnitude for the *N*-methyl group. Analysis of the CD spectra of the complexes XV–XVII, making use of the known conformational or octahedral contribution from the CD spectra of IX–XI, indicates[80, 86] that the specific tetragonal contribution of the *N*-methyl groups is larger than that of the C-methyl and ring alkyl groups (Fig. 11).

The first-order dynamic-coupling treatment, assuming an isotropic polarizability of the chelate ring substituents, reproduces the correct form of the tetragonal rule [21] but with the wrong sign. The A_2 tetragonal component arises from the one-electron transition, $d_{xy} \rightarrow d_{x^2-y^2}$, which has for its leading electric moment the $[xy(x^2 - y^2)]$ component of a hexadecapole in addition to a z-polarized magnetic dipole moment. The product, $[im_{no}^z P_{0n}^{1m} \bar{\alpha}(v_{0n})]$ of [14] is positive and real, and the geometric factor for the potential between the $[xy(x^2 - y^2)]$ component of an electric hexadecapole and the z-component of an electric dipole has the form,

$$[XYZ(Y^2 - X^2)/R^{11}] \qquad [22]$$

giving the incorrect sign for the A_2 tetragonal Cotton effect.

The corresponding static-field treatment, carried to second order,[81] does not distinguish between the individual contribution of the conformational or octahedral effect and the specifically tetragonal effect to the total optical activity of a D_4 complex. The general conclusions emerging from the treatment are the sets of sector rules [15] and [16] and analogous formulations describing three-way interactions between two substituents r and s and the metal ion. Specific conclusions drawn for complexes of the type *trans*-[Co(R-pn)$_2$Cl$_2$]$^+$ with a λ-conformation of the rings are as follows[81]

(i) $d_{xy} \rightarrow d_{x^2-y^2}$, $R(A_2)$ negative and small

(ii) $d_{yz} \rightarrow d_{y^2-z^2}$, R negative and moderate $\left.\right\}$

(iii) $d_{xz} \rightarrow d_{z^2-x^2}$, R positive and large $\left.\right\}$ $R(E)$ positive

for the three components of the octahedral $A_{1g} \rightarrow T_{1g}$ cobalt(III) transition, the net sign of $R(T_1)$ being positive, and

(iv) $d_{xy} \rightarrow d_{z^2}$, $R(A_1)$ zero $\left.\right\}$

(v) $d_{yz} \rightarrow d_{x^2}$, R positive and small $\left.\right\}$ $R(T_2)$ negative

(vi) $d_{xz} \rightarrow d_{y^2}$, R negative and moderate $\left.\right\}$

for the three components of the octahedral $A_{1g} \rightarrow T_{2g}$ transition, $R(T_2)$ being negative. The sum over all components, $R(T_1) + R(T_2)$, is expected to be positive.

These particular conclusions are supported by the observed CD spectrum of the enantiomeric complex, *trans*-[Co(S-pn)$_2$Cl$_2$]$^+$ (XVI), Fig. 11, where $R(A_2)$ is small and positive while $R(E)$ from T_1 is large and negative. However, the splitting of $R(E)$ in (−)-*trans,trans*-[Co(Meen)$_2$Cl$_2$]$^+$ (XV) gives two CD bands of the same sign (Fig. 11). Moreover the expectation[81] that $R(A_2)$, due to $d_{xy} \rightarrow d_{x^2-y^2}$, is always small compared with $R(E)$, is not supported by the CD spectra of the N-methyl complexes XV and XVI (Fig. 11), nor by the CD data[87] for the N-methyl-(S)-(+)-propylenediamine complexes of copper(II) (Table 4). In the case of square-planar bis-diamine complexes with a λ-ring conformation, e.g. [Cu(R-pn)$_2$]$^{2+}$, the expectations are[81] two positive d-electron CD bands, the lower-frequency component having the smaller magnitude, as is observed (Table 3).

(D). *Lower-symmetry d-Electron Optical Activity*

The lowest holohedralized symmetry of an orthoaxial octahedral 6-coordinate complex, with six different ligand atoms in the general case, is D_{2h} for which the lowest-order pseudoscalar function is $[XYZ]$, giving an octant rule for the specific low-symmetry optical activity. It is to be expected, however, that there are additional contributions to the total optical activity from the specific tetragonal, trigonal (configurational), and octahedral (conformational) effects, each following their own individual regional rule. The Cotton effect of a given d-electron transition is likely to follow a regional rule of higher order than the octant rule if one of the senior perturbations in the descent from O_h is strong, and the net rotational strength of the set of d-electron transitions even more probably follows a higher order sector rule, as low-symmetry effects are typically resolved CD bands of opposite sign with a common E or T parentage. There has been an extensive discussion recently as to the octant[75] (D_{2h}) or double-octant[77] (D_{4h}) behaviour of the Cotton effects observed in square-planar amino acid complexes containing the *trans*-[MN_2O_2] chromophore and tripeptide complexes with the [MN_3O] chromophore.[75, 79] It is expected that both types of behaviour are generally superposed and that these types are separable by studies of appropriate model systems, as in the higher-symmetry cases of the complexes XV–XVII, compared with the complexes IX–XI. Detailed sector rules for square-planar complexes of low symmetry have been formulated by the static-field perturbational procedure.[81] It is expected that the net d-electron rotational strengths follow a double-octant rule in these complexes.[81]

3.6.6 The Optical Activity of σ-Electron Charge-transfer Transitions

The hexammine and tris-diamine complexes of cobalt(III) and other transition metal ions give absorption bands of high intensity in the 250–185 nm region (Figs. 2–5), which are generally ascribed to $\sigma(t_{1u}) \rightarrow d(e_g)$ ligand-to-metal charge-transfer excitations. The replacement of the ligands of the hexammine complex by diamine chelate rings shifts the charge-transfer band to the red but produces little intensity-change.

For the five-membered chelate ring complexes the charge-transfer optical activity consists of a major CD band near 210 nm, which is negative for the $\mathit{\Lambda}$-configuration (Figs. 2 and 3) and positive for the Δ-forms (Fig. 4), followed by another large CD band, which is only partly accessible, of opposite sign at higher frequency. From the axial single-crystal CD spectrum of $\mathit{\Lambda}$-(+)-[Co(en)$_3$]$^{3+}$ it is found[22] that the longer-wavelength edge of the negative charge-transfer CD band, and probably the whole band, is due to a transition with E symmetry, polarized perpendicular to the C_3 axis of the complex ion (I). The corresponding $A_1 \rightarrow A_2$ component of the octahedral $A_{1g} \rightarrow T_{1u}$ charge-transfer transition is probably represented by the incom-

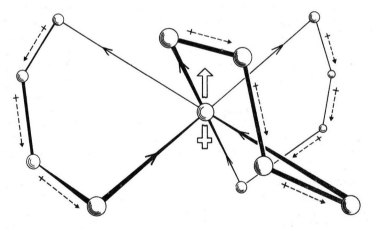

Fig. 15. The phase relationships between the charge displacements along the Co—N bonds (small arrows) of $\mathit{\Lambda}$-(+)-[Co(en)$_3$]$^{3+}$ giving the $A_1 \rightarrow A_2$ component (large arrow) of the $A_{1g} \rightarrow T_{1u}$ ligand to metal charge-transfer transition, and the coulombically-correlated phases of the transient dipoles (broken arrows) induced in the C—C and C—N bonds of the chelate rings by the radiation field.

pletely-accessible positive CD band of Λ-(+)-[Co(en)$_3$]$^{3+}$ appearing below 52 kK (Fig. 2).

A possible origin for the charge-transfer optical activity may be found in the polarizability[72] or dynamic-coupling model.[71] The intensity of the charge-transfer band shows that each of the two D_3 components of the octahedral $A_{1g} \rightarrow T_{1u}$ transition has an intrinsic electric moment (c. 3 Debye per component of T_{1u}) and the coulombic coupling of this moment with transient electric dipoles induced in the C—N and C—C bonds of the chelate rings by the chromophore field produces optical activity. For the Λ-configuration the rotational strength of the $A_1 \rightarrow A_2$ component of the octahedral $A_{1g} \rightarrow T_{1u}$ charge-transfer transition is positive (Fig. 15), and that of the corresponding $A_1 \rightarrow E$ component is negative as observed for Λ-(+)-[Co(en)$_3$]$^{3+}$ (Fig. 2).

In explicit form,[71, 72] the rotational strength of the A_2 component of the charge-transfer transition, $R(A_2)$, with the wave-number, $\bar{\nu}_{CT}$, and electric moment, μ_{CT}, is given by

$$R(A_2) = - \sum_{k} \pi\bar{\nu}_{CT}|\mu_{CT}|^2(\alpha_{\parallel} - \alpha_{\perp})_k[\vec{R}_{ik} \cdot (\vec{e}_i \times \vec{e}_k)]G_{ik} \qquad [22]$$

where $\vec{e}_i$ and $\vec{e}_k$ are unit vectors directed along the C_3 axis of the complex ion and along the bond k, respectively. Each bond k at the frequency ν_{CT} has the polarizability $\alpha_{\parallel}$, parallel and $\alpha_{\perp}$, perpendicular to the bond direction, the sum being taken over all of the non-coordinate bonds. In equation [22], G_{ik} is the geometric factor for the coulombic potential between two point-dipoles,

$$G_{ik} = [(\vec{e}_i \cdot \vec{e}_k)/R_{ik}^3 - 3(\vec{e}_i \cdot \vec{R}_{ik})(\vec{e}_k \cdot \vec{R}_{ik})/R_{ik}^5] \qquad [23]$$

where R_{ik} is the distance between the centre of the bond k and the metal ion.

Values of the anisotropies of bond polarizabilities are not well established,[72, 88-91] although it is generally accepted that the C—H bond and probably the N—H bond are approximately isotropic, whereas the C—C and C—N bonds are strongly anisotropic. Accordingly it is assumed that the C—H and N—H bonds of Λ-(+)-[Co(en)$_3$]$^{3+}$ make no contribution to the charge-transfer rotational strength and that only the C—C and C—N bonds make non-zero contributions to the sum in equation [22]. Values of the anisotropy $(\alpha_{\parallel} - \alpha_{\perp})$ from Denbigh[88] are +1·86 and +1·52 Å^3 for the C—C and the C—N bond, respectively, at the sodium D-line and the corresponding values at 200 nm are estimated to be twice as large. The bond distances and angles determined by Saito and co-workers[6, 10] for the lel-conformation of Λ-(+)-[Co(en)$_3$]$^{3+}$ adopted in the crystal, with the wavelength-corrected bond-anisotropy values, give $R(A_2)$ from [22] the value of +1·9 Debye magneton (1·83 × 10^{-40} c.g.s.).

The corresponding $A_1 \rightarrow E$ component of the charge-transfer transition is expected to have a rotational strength of equal magnitude and opposite sign for the same configuration. The experimental rotational strength of the 210-nm CD band of Λ-(+)-[Co(en)$_3$]$^{3+}$ (Fig. 2) is −1·0 Debye magneton, although this ion does not exist substantially in the lel-form in solution at ambient temperature.[44] The corresponding band of the lel-isomer $\Lambda(\delta\delta\delta)$-(+)-[Co(S-pn)$_3$]$^{3+}$ (Fig. 3) and that of the ob-isomer $\Delta(\delta\delta\delta)$-(−)-[Co(S-pn)$_3$]$^{3+}$ (Fig. 4) have rotational strengths of −1·1 and +0·4 Debye magneton, respectively.

3.6.7 The Optical Activity of Internal Ligand Transitions

In a bis- or tris-chelated dissymmetric complex containing unsaturated ligands the major CD bands are often associated with the absorption due to the $\pi \to \pi^*$ excitations of the ligands (Figs. 16–19). These CD bands are ascribed in the simple excitation treatment[92–95] to molecular electronic transitions resulting from the coulombic

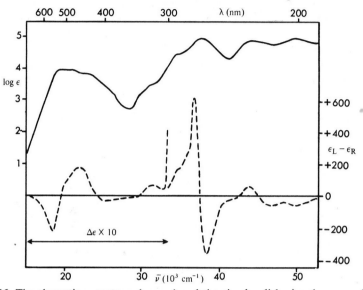

Fig. 16. The absorption spectrum (———) and the circular dichroism (— — —) of Λ-(−)-[Fe(phen)$_3$]$^{2+}$ in water. (From B. J. Peart, Thesis, University of East Anglia, 1970.)

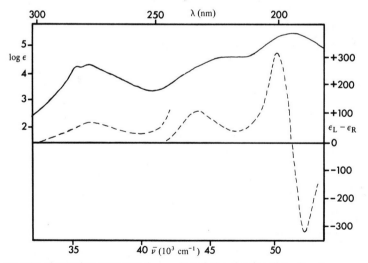

Fig. 17. The absorption spectrum (———) and the circular dichroism (— — —) of Λ-(+)-[As(cat)$_3$]$^{-}$ in aqueous solution. (From B. J. Peart, Thesis, University of East Anglia, 1970.)

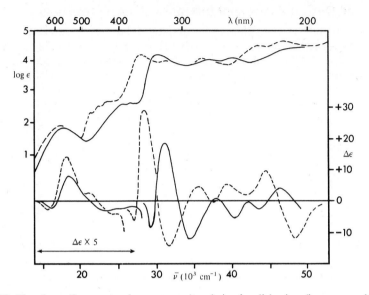

Fig. 18. The absorption spectra (upper curves) and circular dichroism (lower curves) of *trans*-(+)-[Cr(D-hydroxymethylenecamphor)₃] (————) and (+)-[Cr(acac)₃] (———) in ethanol (Fay and Mason[98]).

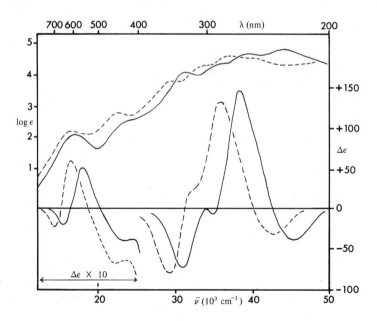

Fig. 19. The absorption spectra (upper curves) and circular dichroism (lower curves) of *Λ*-(−)-[Co(acac)₃]   (———)   and   *trans*-(−)-[Co(D-hydroxymethylenecamphor)₃] (————) in ethanol (Fay and Mason[98]).

coupling of individual $\pi \rightarrow \pi^*$ excitations with the same energy in different ligands of the complex. If the electric moments of the individual $\pi \rightarrow \pi^*$ excitations are long-axis polarized in the free ligand, and so directed along the octahedral edge spanned by a chelate ring in the complex, the coulombic correlation between the moments gives rise to resultant transitions to molecular states with A_2 and E trigonal symmetry (Fig. 20). These resultant transitions have large zero-order rotational strengths which are equal in magnitude but opposite in sign for the A_2 and the E coupling mode.

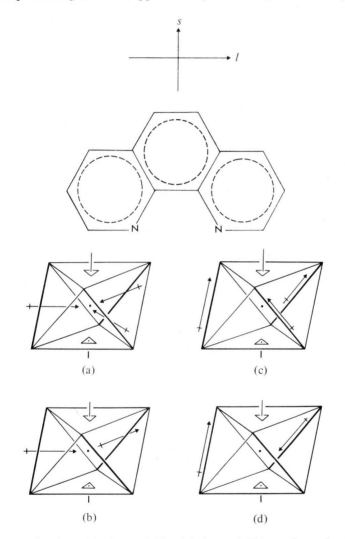

Fig. 20. The directions of the short-axis (s) and the long-axis (l) internal $\pi \rightarrow \pi^*$ excitations of the phenanthroline ligand, and the coupling-modes in the corresponding tris-complex giving resultant molecular transitions with the D_3 symmetry, (a) A_1 and (b) E, from a short-axis excitation, and (c) A_2 and (d) E, from a long-axis excitation. Only one component of each of the doubly-degenerate E coupling modes is illustrated.

An individual $\pi \to \pi^*$ excitation which is short-axis polarized in the free ligand gives, in the corresponding tris-chelated complex, resultant molecular transitions that have no zero-order optical activity as the set of excitation moments are coplanar in both the coupling modes, which have A_1 and E symmetry in D_3 (Fig. 20).

The sign of the CD band due to an A_2 coupling mode reflects directly the chirality of the tris-chelated complex, the rotational strength being negative for the Λ and positive for the Δ-configuration. In the exciton approximation, where it is assumed that there is no electron-exchange between the individual ligands of a complex or between a ligand and the metal ion, the coulombic potential between the ligand excitation moments for octahedral, or near-octahedral, coordination gives the A_2 coupling-mode a higher energy than the corresponding E coupling mode (Fig. 20). Thus the observation of two CD bands with opposed signs and approximately equal areas in the frequency region of a single isotropic ligand absorption band of a complex indicates that the individual ligand excitation is long-axis polarized, lying parallel to an octahedral edge, or nearly so. Further, if the positive CD band of the exciton-pair lies at the higher frequency, the complex has the Δ-configuration or, if that band lies at a lower frequency, the Λ-configuration.

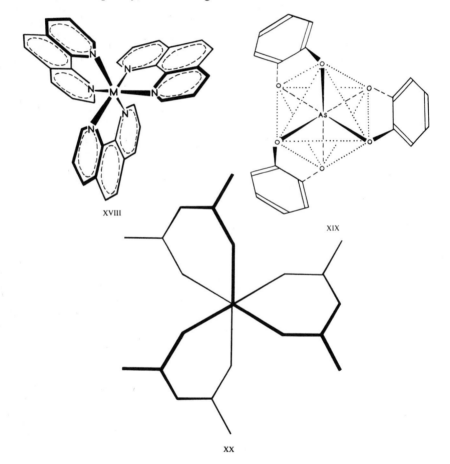

XVIII

XIX

XX

X-ray diffraction studies indicate that the Λ-configuration is common to (−)-[Fe(phen)$_3$]$^{2+}$ (XVIII, M = Fe),[96] (+)-[Ni(phen)$_3$]$^{2+}$ (XVIII, M = Ni),[11] (+)-[As(cat)$_3$]$^-$ (XIX),[97] and (−)-[Cr(bgd)$_3$]$^{3+}$ (XX),[16] in agreement with the exciton analysis of these complex ions, e.g. (Figs. 16 and 17). It has been shown similarly by X-ray methods[13] that (+)-*trans*-tris[(+)-3-acetylcamphorato] chromium(III) has the Λ-configuration, and an exciton analysis of the CD spectrum of the complex[13] and of its analogues[96] (+)-*trans*-tris[(+)-3-formylcamphorato]chromium(III) and (+)-[Cr(acac)$_3$] (Fig. 18) lead to the same configurational assignment. However, the simple exciton treatment is here less clear-cut, and it becomes more tenuous for the corresponding cobalt(III) complexes[98] (Fig. 19), on account of the interaction between the near-degenerate internal-ligand and metal-ligand charge-transfer excitations,[99] although it is known from an X-ray study[14] that (−)-[Co(acac)$_3$] has the Λ-configuration.

The majority of exciton analyses of optical activity due to the internal ligand excitations of metal complexes have been carried out in the strong-coupling approximation where it is assumed that the interaction between the ligand excitations is purely electronic. It has been argued[66] that such analyses are not generally reliable as the electronic coupling energy is small compared with the frequencies of the ligand vibrations which are active in the excitation process, and that the weak or intermediate coupling approximation[100] is the more appropriate. However, as Forster has shown,[101] the distinction between the strong and weak coupling cases vanishes when the sum of the vibronic band widths in an electronic band system equals or exceeds the total electronic band width, and the band is smooth or has only weakly developed vibronic structure, as in the case of relatively large polyatomic ligands, such as 1,10-phenanthroline, 2,2′-bipyridyl, or acetylacetonate.

The trimer intermediate coupling theory of Perrin and Gouterman[102] has been used by Hawkins and co-workers[66] to calculate the rotational strengths of the molecular A$_2$ and E transitions resulting from the coupling of the long-axis polarized excitation of bipyridyl near 300 nm in a tris-complex, [M(bipy)$_3$]$^{n+}$, on the assumption that the electronic interaction energy between the ligand excitations is only 70 cm^{-1}, compared with an active vibration with a frequency of 1400 cm^{-1}. The calculations show[66] that, on this assumption, the rotational strengths $R(A_2)$ and $R(E)$ resulting from the coupling of the ligand excitations in [M(bipy)$_3$]$^{n+}$ substantially overlap on the frequency scale and mutually cancel over 90 % of the band area, so that the observed CD should be no more than 10 % of the theoretical. However, the experimental CD band areas for a range of [M(bipy)$_3$]$^{n+}$ complexes are found[92] to have 30–50 % of the theoretical rotational strength calculated from the observed dipole strength of a monochelate bipyridyl complex in either the weak- or the strong-coupling limit.

In order to account for the observation that the areas of the CD bands due to the A$_2$ and the E coupling modes have some 40 % of the theoretical value, the rotational strengths $R(A_2)$ and $R(E)$ overlapping and mutually cancelling only to the extent of 60 %, it is necessary to assume in the Perrin and Gouterman[102] analysis that the electronic interaction energy has a value in the region of one-half of the active vibration frequency. For the calculated spectra illustrated (Fig. 21), which give the theoretical absorption and circular dichroism quantitatively, the active vibration has a frequency of 700 cm^{-1} and the theoretical electronic energy interval $[v(A_2) - v(E)]$ between the A$_2$ and E transitions of the complex [M(bipy)$_3$]$^{n+}$ is

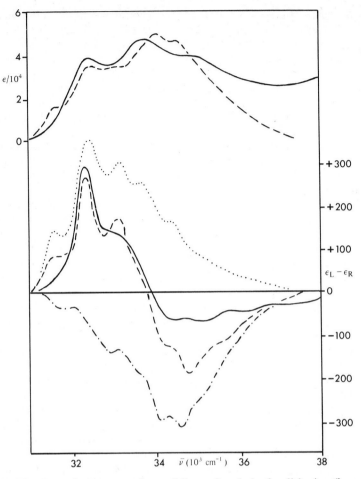

Fig. 21. The absorption spectrum (upper full curve) and circular dichroism (lower full curve) of (+)-[Ni(bipy)$_3$]$^{2+}$ in ethanol, and the theoretical absorption and CD spectra calculated by the method of M. H. Perrin and M. Gouterman, *J. Chem. Phys.* **46**, 1019 (1967), with the parameters (op. cit.), $\lambda = 1$, $\varepsilon = 0.5$ and $\alpha = 0.5$. The net theoretically-observable absorption [$D(A_2) + D(E)$] and circular dichroism [$R(A_2) + R(E)$] are given by the upper and lower dashed curves (————), distinct from the individual components $R(E)$ (.......) and $R(A_2)$ (—·—·—·—).

+1000 cm^{-1}. The theoretical absorption and CD curves show more vibrational structure than is observed in the case of (+)-[Ni(bipy)$_3$]$^{2+}$ (Fig. 21), as the pro-gramme[102] employed in the calculations considers only one active vibrational mode, but the low-temperature spectra of 2,2'-bipyridyl and its mono-chelate complexes show that at least three modes are active in the 300-nm absorption. The simultaneous activity of several modes with different frequencies results in a loss of structure in the absorption and CD curves and almost inevitably ensures that the sum of the vibronic band widths exceeds the electronic band width, when the distinction between the strong, intermediate and weak-coupling cases vanishes in principle.[101]

3.6.8   The Optical Activity of π-Electron Charge-Transfer Transitions

The bipyridyl and phenanthroline complexes of the iron-group metal ions have moderately strong absorption bands in the visible wavelength region due to π-electron charge-transfer between the ligands and the metal ion.[92–95] The transitions are of the $d(t_{2g}) \rightarrow \pi^*$ (ligand) type for the divalent, and of the π (ligand) $\rightarrow d(t_{2g})$ type for the trivalent complexes.[103] In both cases the charge-transfer transitions have no zero-order rotational strength if the coordination is octahedral, and the observed charge-transfer optical activity, e.g. the 18–26 kK region in the spectrum of (–)-[Fe(phen)$_3$]$^{2+}$ (Fig. 16), is ascribed[92, 94, 95] to configurational interaction between the charge-transfer and the internal-ligand excitations.

Like the latter, the charge-transfer excitations are either short-axis or long-axis polarized with respect to an individual ligand, as in a mono-chelate complex. Calculations by the dipole-length method show that only the short-axis charge-transfer excitations have a non-vanishing zero-order dipole strength. The plane-polarized single-crystal spectra of [Fe(bipy)$_3$]$^{2+}$ and [Ru(bipy)$_3$]$^{2+}$ show[104] that in fact the charge-transfer absorption of these ions in the visible region is substantially polarized perpendicular to the C_3 axis of the complex, i.e. short-axis polarized in each ligand.

The long-axis charge-transfer excitations give resultant molecular transitions of A_2 and E symmetry which borrow both dipole and rotational strength from the corresponding internal-ligand transition with the same symmetry. The resultant transitions from the short-axis charge-transfer excitations are to molecular states with A_1 and E symmetry, and only the latter mixes with internal-ligand excited states to acquire a first-order rotational strength, since all $A_1 \rightarrow A_1$ transitions are forbidden in D_3 symmetry. Accordingly, from a zero-order isoenergetic set of six metal-ligand charge-transfer excitations, three long-axis and three short-axis polarized, a pattern of three CD bands with alternating signs is expected. Such a pattern is observed in the 18–26 kK region of the spectrum of Λ-(–)-[Fe(phen)$_3$]$^{2+}$ (Fig. 16) and of analogous complexes of the iron group,[92] although more detailed treatments indicate that two sets of six charge-transfer excitations are active in the visible wavelength region of the spectra of these complexes.[94, 95] A recent SCF calculation[105] of the electronic structure and spectrum of Δ-(+)-[Fe(phen)$_3$]$^{2+}$ gives theoretical absorption and circular dichroism curves closely resembling the experimental spectra in both the visible (charge-transfer) and the ultraviolet (internal-ligand) region.

References

1. A. Cotton, *C.R.H. Acad. Sci.* **120**, 989, 1044 (1895).
2. *Alfred Werner* 1866–1919, *Helv. Chim. Acta*, Commemoration Volume IX ICCC, Zurich, 1966.
3. F. M. Jaeger, *Spatial Arrangements of Atomic Systems and Optical Activity*, George Fisher Baker Lectures, Vol. 7, Cornell University. McGraw-Hill, New York, 1930.
4. J. P. Mathieu, *Les Théories Moléculaires du Pouvoir Rotatoire Naturel*. Gauthier-Villars, Paris, 1946.
5. W. Kuhn and K. Bein, *Z. Phys. Chem., Leipzig* **B24**, 335 (1934).
6. Y. Saito, K. Nakatsu, M. Shiro and H. Kuroya, *Acta Crystallogr.* **8**, 729 (1955).
7. W. Kuhn, *Naturwissenschaften* **26**, 289 (1938).
8. *I.U.P.A.C. Information Bulletin* No. 33, 68 (1968); *Inorg. Chem.* **9**, 1 (1970).
9. J. P. Mathieu, *J. Chim. Phys. Physicochim. Biol.* **33**, 78 (1936).
10. Y. Saito, *Pure Appl. Chem.* **17**, 21 (1968) and references therein.
11. K. R. Butler and M. R. Snow, *J. Chem. Soc. A* 565 (1971).

12. K. R. Butler and M. R. Snow, *Chem. Commun.* 550 (1971).
13. W. DeW. Horrocks, D. L. Johnston and D. MacInnes, *J. Amer. Chem. Soc.* **92**, 7620 (1970).
14. R. B. von Dreele and R. C. Fay, *J. Amer. Chem. Soc.* **93**, 4936 (1971).
15. A. Kobayashi, F. Marumo, Y. Saito, J. Fujita and F. Mizukami, *Inorg. Nucl. Chem. Lett.* **7**, 777 (1971).
16. G. R. Brubaker and L. E. Webb, *J. Amer. Chem. Soc.* **91**, 7199 (1969).
17. Y. Saito, T. Nomura and F. Marumo, *Bull. Chem. Soc. Japan* **41**, 530 (1968).
18. M. Ito, F. Marumo and Y. Saito, *Inorg. Nucl. Chem. Lett.* **6**, 519 (1970).
19. W. Moffitt, *J. Chem. Phys.* **25**, 1189 (1956).
20. S. Sugano, *J. Chem. Phys.* **33**, 1883 (1960).
21. E. Drouard and J. P. Mathieu, *C.R.H. Acad. Sci.* **236**, 2395 (1953).
22. A. J. McCaffery and S. F. Mason, *Mol. Phys.* **6**, 359 (1963).
23. R. E. Ballard, A. J. McCaffery and S. F. Mason, *J. Chem. Soc.* 883 (1965).
24. R. G. Denning, *Chem. Commun.* 120 (1967).
25. R. R. Judkins and D. J. Royer, *Inorg. Nucl. Chem. Lett.* **6**, 305 (1970).
26. J. A. Schellman, *J. Chem. Phys.* **44**, 55 (1966); *Accounts Chem. Res.* **1**, 144 (1968).
27. S. Sugano and M. Shinada, *Abstracts International Symposium on Molecular Structure and Spectroscopy*, Tokyo, 1962.
28. M. Shinada, *J. Phys. Soc. Japan* **19**, 1607 (1964).
29. R. Dingle and C. J. Ballhausen. *Mat. Fys. Medd. Dan. Vid. Selsk.* **35**, No. 12 (1967).
30. C. E. Schäffer, *Proceedings of the VII ICCC*, Vienna, 1964, p. 77.
31. C. E. Schäffer, *Proc. Roy. Soc. A* **297**, 96 (1967).
32. T. S. Piper and A. Karipides, *Mol. Phys.* **5**, 475 (1962).
33. A. Karipides and T. S. Piper, *J. Chem. Phys.* **40**, 674 (1964).
34. A. D. Liehr, *J. Phys. Chem.* **68**, 665 and 3629 (1964); in R. L. Carlin, Ed., *Transition Metal Chemistry*, Vol. 2. Edward Arnold, London, 1966, p. 165.
35. Y. Saito, F. Marumo and M. Ito, *Proc. Jap. Acad.* **47**, 495 (1971).
36. E. C. Lingfelter and R. L. Braun, *J. Amer. Chem. Soc.* **88**, 2951 (1966).
37. J. N. van Niekerk and F. R. L. Schoening, *Acta Crystallogr.* **5**, 499 (1952).
38. E. J. Corey and J. C. Bailar, *J. Amer. Chem. Soc.* **81**, 2620 (1959).
39. T. S. Piper and A. G. Karipides, *J. Amer. Chem. Soc.* **86**, 5039 (1964).
40. F. P. Dwyer, F. L. Garvan and A. Shulman, *J. Amer. Chem. Soc.* **81**, 290 (1959).
41. F. P. Dwyer, T. E. MacDermott and A. M. Sargeson, *J. Amer. Chem. Soc.* **85**, 2913 (1963).
42. F. P. Dwyer and A. M. Sargeson, *J. Amer. Chem. Soc.* **81**, 5272 (1959).
43. K. N. Raymond, P. W. R. Corfield and J. A. Ibers, *Inorg. Chem.* **7**, 842 (1968).
44. J. K. Beattie, *Accounts Chem. Res.* **4**, 253 (1971).
45. L. Harland, S. F. Mason and B. J. Peart. Forthcoming publication.
46. S. F. Mason, A. M. Sargeson, R. Larsson, B. J. Norman, A. J. McCaffery and G. H. Searle, *Inorg. Nucl. Chem. Lett.* **2**, 333 (1966); *J. Chem. Soc. A*, 1304 (1968).
47. R. Larsson, G. H. Searle, S. F. Mason and A. M. Sargeson, *J. Chem. Soc. A*, 1310 (1968).
48. F. Mizukami, M. Ito, J. Fujita and K. Saito, *Bull. Chem. Soc. Japan* **43**, 3973 (1970).
49. K. R. Butler and M. R. Snow, *Inorg. Chem.* **10**, 1838 (1971).
50. P. G. Beddoe, M. J. Harding, S. F. Mason and B. J. Peart, *Chem. Commun.* 1283 (1971).
51. P. G. Beddoe and S. F. Mason, *Inorg. Nucl. Chem. Lett.* **4**, 433 (1968).
52. J. R. Gollogly and C. J. Hawkins, *Chem. Commun.* 689 (1968).
53. S. F. Mason and B. J. Norman, *Proc. Chem. Soc.* 339 (1964); *J. Chem. Soc. A* 307 (1966).
54. H. L. Smith and B. E. Douglas, *J. Amer. Chem. Soc.* **86**, 3885 (1964); L. R. Froebe and B. E. Douglas, *Inorg. Chem.* **9**, 1513 (1970).
55. E. N. Duesler and K. N. Raymond, *Inorg. Chem.* **10**, 1486 (1971).
56. J. E. Sarneski and F. L. Urbach, *J. Amer. Chem. Soc.* **93**, 884 (1971).
57. S. F. Mason and B. J. Norman, *Chem. Commun.* 73 (1965).
58. B. E. Douglas, *Inorg. Chem.* **4**, 1813 (1965).
59. K. Ogino, K. Murano and J. Fujita, *Inorg. Nucl. Chem. Lett.* **4**, 351 (1968).
60. M. Saburi, Y. Tsujito and S. Y. Yoshikawa, *Inorg. Nucl. Chem. Lett.* **5**, 203 1969); *Inorg. Chem.* **9**, 1476 and 1488 (1970).
61. R. S. Treptow, Thesis, University of Illinois, 1966; *Inorg. Chem.* **5**, 1593 (1966).
62. B. E. Douglas and S. Yamada, *Inorg. Chem.* **4**, 1561 (1965).
63. T. Yasui, J. Hidaka and Y. Shimura, *Bull. Chem. Soc. Japan* **39**, 2417 (1966).

64. J. I. Legg, D. W. Cooke and B. E. Douglas, *Inorg. Chem.* **6**, 700 (1967).
65. J. Hidaka and Y. Shimura, *Bull. Chem. Soc. Japan* **40**, 2312 (1967).
66. C. J. Hawkins, *Absolute Configuration of Metal Complexes.* Wiley-Interscience, London, 1971.
67. F. Mizukami, H. Ito, J. Fujita and K. Saito, *Bull. Chem. Soc. Japan* **45**, 2129 (1972).
68. H. Yamatera, *Bull. Chem. Soc. Japan* **31**, 95 (1958).
69. B. E. Douglas, R. A. Haines and J. G. Brushmiller, *Inorg. Chem.* **2**, 1194 (1963).
70. N. K. Hamer, *Mol. Phys.* **5**, 339 (1962).
71. E. G. Höhn and O. E. Weigang, Jr., *J. Chem. Phys.* **48**, 1127 (1968).
72. J. G. Kirkwood, *J. Chem. Phys.* **5**, 479 (1937).
73. D. J. Caldwell and H. Eyring. *The Theory of Optical Activity*, Wiley-Interscience, London, 1971.
74. C. J. Hawkins and E. Larsen, *Acta Chem. Scand.* **19**, 185 (1965).
75. K. M. Wellman, W. Mungal, T. G. Mecca and C. R. Hare, *J. Amer. Chem. Soc.* **89**, 3647 (1967); **90**, 805 (1968); *Chem. Eng. News* Oct. 2, 48 (1967).
76. M. Parris and A. E. Hodges, *J. Amer. Chem. Soc.* **90**, 1909 (1968).
77. R. B. Martin, J. M. Tsangaris and J. W. Chang, *J. Amer. Chem. Soc.* **90**, 821 (1968); **92**, 4255 (1970); *J. Phys. Chem.* **73**, 4277 (1969).
78. K. M. Wellman, S. Bodansky, C. Piontek, C. Hare and M. Mathieson, *Inorg. Chem.* **8**, 1025 (1969).
79. E. W. Wilson, Jr., and R. B. Martin, *Inorg. Chem.* **9**, 528 (1970); **10**, 1197 (1971).
80. S. F. Mason, *Chem. Commun.* 856 (1969); *Pure Appl. Chem.* **24**, 335 (1970); *J. Chem. Soc. A*, 667 (1971).
81. F. S. Richardson, *J. Phys. Chem.* **75**, 692 (1971); *J. Chem. Phys.* **54**, 2453 (1971); *Inorg. Chem.* **10**, 2121 (1971); **11**, 2366 (1972).
82. W. T. Robinson, D. A. Buckingham, L. G. Marzilli and A. M. Sargeson, *Chem. Commun.* 539 (1969).
83. D. A. Buckingham, L. G. Marzilli and A. M. Sargeson, *J. Amer. Chem. Soc.* **89**, 825 (1967).
84. P. L. Fereday and S. F. Mason, *Chem. Commun.* 1314 (1971).
85. Landolt-Börnstein, *Zahlenwerte und Functionen*, Vol. 1, Pt. 3. Springer, 1951, p. 510.
86. C. J. Hawkins, *Chem. Commun.* 777 (1969); J. A. Tiethof and D. W. Cooke, *Inorg. Chem.* **11**, 315 (1972).
87. M. Morita and S. Yoshikawa, *Chem. Commun.* 578 (1972).
88. K. G. Denbigh, *Trans. Faraday Soc.* **36**, 936 (1940).
89. R. P. Smith and E. M. Mortensen, *J. Chem. Phys.* **32**, 508 (1960).
90. R. J. W. Le Fevre, B. J. Orr and G. L. D. Ritchie, *J. Chem. Soc. B* 273 (1966).
91. J. N. Murrell and M. J. P. Musgrave, *Trans. Faraday Soc.* **63**, 2849 (1967).
92. S. F. Mason, *Inorg. Chim. Acta. Rev.* **2**, 89 (1968).
93. B. Bosnich, *Accounts Chem. Res.* **2**, 266 (1969).
94. I. Hanazaki and S. Nagakura, *Inorg. Chem.* **8**, 654 (1969).
95. N. Sanders, *J. Chem. Soc. A* 1563 (1971).
96. D. H. Templeton, A. Zalkin and T. Ueki, *Acta. Crystallogr.*, *Suppl.* **21A**, 154 (1966).
97. T. Ito, A. Kobayashi, F. Marumo and Y. Saito, *Inorg. Nucl. Chem. Lett.* **7**, 1097 (1971).
98. R. C. Fay and S. F. Mason. Forthcoming publication.
99. I. Hanazaki, F. Hanazaki and S. Nagakura, *J. Chem. Phys.* **50**, 265 and 276 (1969).
100. A. S. Davydov, *Theory of Molecular Excitons* (translated by M. Kasha and M. Oppenheimer). McGraw-Hill, New York, 1962.
101. T. Forster, in O. Sinanoglu, Ed., *Modern Quantum Chemistry*, Part III. Academic Press, London, 1965, p. 131.
102. M. H. Perrin and M. Gouterman, *J. Chem. Phys.* **46**, 1019 (1967).
103. P. Day and N. Sanders, *J. Chem. Soc. A* 1530 and 1536 (1967); 2303 (1969); 1190 (1970).
104. R. A. Palmer and T. S. Piper, *Inorg. Chem.* **5**, 864 (1966).
105. N. Sanders, *J. Chem. Soc. Dalton* 345 (1972).

Exciton Circular Dichroism in Metal Complexes

B. BOSNICH

Lash Miller Chemical Laboratories
80 St. George St.
University of Toronto
Toronto

3.7.1 Introduction

Circular dichroism is a property associated with the spectroscopic transitions of optically active molecules. In electronic spectroscopy, two important types of transitions may occur which, in essence, are connected with the way the electrons are promoted during the absorption of light. The two types which we need to consider here are those which are said to be electric-dipole allowed and those which are magnetic-dipole allowed. In a classical sense, the former involve a translation of electronic charge to produce an electric transition dipole moment while the latter involve a circulation of charge to produce a magnetic transition dipole moment. This physical analogy is meant to represent the transformation properties of the transitions and should not be taken too literally. The purpose of the analogy is to fix a model of the processes for subsequent discussion. For an electronic transition to be optically active, both these transitions must, as it were, occur simultaneously in a special way which is seen from the definition of the rotational strength, R[1]

$$R = \mathrm{Im} \langle a|\mu_e| b\rangle \cdot \langle b|\mu_m| a\rangle$$

where a and b are the stationary states for the transition a → b, and μ_e and μ_m are the electric and magnetic transition dipole moment operators respectively. Thus the part $\langle a|\mu_e| b\rangle$ is the expectation value of the transition dipole moment and the part $\langle b|\mu_m|a\rangle$ is the expectation value of the transition magnetic dipole moment. The dot between them indicates that the (pseudo) scalar product is taken in the sense that, if the electric and magnetic vectors are orthogonal, the rotational strength will vanish, and for other inclinations the cosine between them is taken. Thus if the $\langle a|\mu_e| b\rangle$ involves a translation of charge and the $\langle b|\mu_m|a\rangle$ involves a circulation of charge and if the two must have collinear components, optically active transitions involve helical displacements of charge (a rotation superimposed on a collinear translation). A right-hand helical displacement generates positive circular dichroism and a left-hand displacement produces negative circular dichroism. Thus if we could ascertain the sense of the helical displacement for a given electronic transition for a particular hand of the molecule, we should be able to obtain the absolute configuration from the circular dichroism associated with the transition.

This connection between the chirality of the electronic motion and the handedness of the molecule was recognized long ago by Drude,[2] Born[3] and Kuhn[4] who formulated the problem classically. Thereafter, with the advent of quantum mechanics, the problem was rigorously defined and attempts at calculation were begun. The two main approaches viewed the problem as either a one-electron[5] or a multi-electron[6] phenomenon. These early attempts were not particularly successful, not because they were unrealistic, but rather because the necessary spectroscopic information was not available. The subsequent development of molecular spectroscopy is now at a stage where, at least for certain classes of compounds, these theories may be tested. The multi-electron approach in particular is now a standard way of determining absolute configurations but it had to be preceded by the concepts derived from exciton interactions in crystals[7] and was reformulated in this way by Moffitt[8].

3.7.2 Exciton Approach to the Determination of the Absolute Configurations of Metal Complexes

For inorganic complexes the approximation which is used depends on the transitions which one looks at in order to elicit the absolute structural information. The d-d transitions and charge transfer bands of these molecules are only slightly modified by the dissymmetry of the molecular environment and are generally treated in terms of the one-electron theory of the transitions. There are, however, certain classes of inorganic compounds which are susceptible to the exciton formulation. In particular the circular dichroism associated with certain conjugated ligands such as o-phenanthroline (phen) and 2,2'-bipyridyl (bipy) can be used to determine the absolute configurations on a purely spectroscopic basis. There are others but we will concentrate on these ligands since the basic principles are contained in a study of them. The discussion which follows on the exciton approach to the determination of the absolute configurations of metal complexes will be given in a pictorial way so that the basic mechanism can be seen clearly. The reader who is interested in the quantum-mechanical formalism and the details of the calculations may find them in references 9 and 10.

The $\pi \to \pi^*$ transitions of the phen and bipy ligands are electric dipole allowed in the molecular plane and, in a pictorial sense, involve the oscillation of the electrons, during the absorption of light, in the plane to produce transient linear displacements of charge which give rise to transition dipole moments. These transient displacements of charge can be either concentrated (polarized) along the long (x) or short (z) axes of the molecules[9, 10] (Fig. 1). Upon complex formation these transitions appear to remain largely unmodified in themselves but special effects occur when two or more are bound to a metal atom. Consider the case of the optically active complex [Co en^2 phen]$^{3+}$ (where en = 1,2-diaminoethane) which contains only one π-electron ligand. It is found[11] that the circular dichroism associated with both the long- and short-axis polarized transitions of the (complexed) phen molecule is exceedingly weak. This is what might be expected since the $\pi \to \pi^*$ transitions are only electric dipole allowed in the zero order, that is the $\langle a|\mu_e|b \rangle$ part is the predominant constituent of the transition. The fact that the transitions show any circular dichroism at all is due to higher order dissymmetric perturbations which generate a very small collinear magnetic transition dipole moment to the transitions. Thus the rotational strength consists largely of the $\langle a|\mu_e|b\rangle$ part and very little of the $\langle b|\mu_m|a\rangle$ part of the transition. If we consider the optically active complex [Co phen$_3$]$^{3+}$ the circular dichroism under the short-axis polarized transitions of the complex remains weak, but that under the long-axis polarized transitions is very strong and consists of two components of nearly equal and opposite sign. Thus a special effect is involved when the three phen molecules are brought together and it is clear that this effect must generate strong electric and collinear magnetic transition dipole moments in

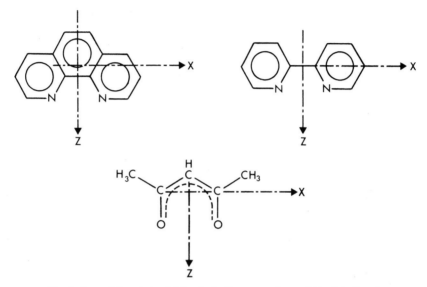

Fig. 1. Long (x) and short (z) polarization axes of some bidentate ligands.

the long-axis polarized transitions. In the language of stationary state theory we can see how this comes about as follows.

Let us assume that a photon of light is capable of interacting with not one of the phen molecules in the complex but with all three. Then the characteristics of the absorption which occurs is determined by the properties of the assembly and not of one phen molecule independently of the others although the spectroscopic character-istics of each phen is retained as a contributing part of the assembly. In the case of the $\pi \rightarrow \pi^*$ transitions of the phen ligands in the [Co phen$_3$]$^{3+}$ complex, the way in which the excitations can occur is limited by the ways in which each individual excitation can combine with its neighbours. These are the so-called coupling modes of the system which, in essence, are the (orthogonal) phase combinations of the individual excitations; the number of phase combinations is equal to the number of transitions associated with each ligand. In Fig. 2 we show the coupling modes for the long- and short-axis polarized transitions of the [M phen$_3$]$^{n+}$ system. We now show how the exciton circular dichroism arises and we consider first the long-axis polarized transitions.

The coupling mode designated as $\Psi_0 \to \Psi_{A_2}$ is a single electronic transition of the assembly and the arrows are meant to represent the phase relationships between the (electric) transition dipoles of the individual phen molecules. (It should be noted that for all the diagrams in Fig. 2 if *all* the arrows in each mode were reversed the nature of the coupling mode would remain the same since the dipoles are oscillating

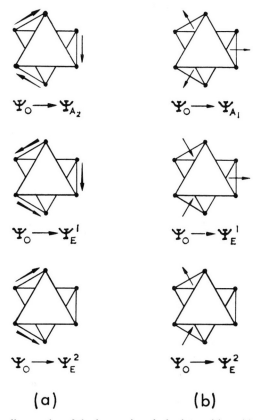

Fig. 2. The coupling modes of the long-axis polarized transitions (a) and the short-axis polarized transitions (b) of a tris-bidentate metal complex.

but retaining the phase relationships.) If the arrows are vectorially added for the $\Psi_0 \to \Psi_{A_2}$ transition, it will be evident that there is a net linear displacement along the three-fold axis of the molecule: but because the vectors are slanted with respect to the three-fold axis their combined effect is to impart tangential components to a circulation of charge about the three-fold axis. Thus by Lenz's law a magnetic moment is produced along the axis. The $\Psi_0 \to \Psi_{A_2}$ coupling mode involves a helical displacement of charge along and about the three-fold axis giving rise to the collinear electric and magnetic moments necessary for the appearance of circular dichroism. For the particular absolute configuration given in Fig. 2, the twist sense of the $\Psi_0 \to \Psi_{A_2}$ transition is left-handed and thus should give negative circular dichroism. (The reader may satisfy himself that in the opposite absolute configuration the situation is identical in all respects except that the twist sense is right-handed.) Despite their appearance, the two other coupling modes are of the same energy, and calculation shows that each carries equal rotational strength which is contributed to the 'total' $\Psi_0 \to \Psi_E$ transition. The pictorial arguments are more easily perceived if we consider the $\Psi_0 \to \Psi_E^2$ component. This component involves only the excitation of two phen molecules (at a time) which, if the vector sums are made, involves a linear displacement along one of the two-fold axes of the molecule. In addition a rotation of charge is involved about this same axis. But unlike the $\Psi_0 \to \Psi_{A_2}$ coupling mode, the helical displacement is right-handed for the same absolute configuration and should give rise to positive circular dichroism. Calculation shows that the 'total' $\Psi_0 \to \Psi_E$ transition will give positive circular dichroism which is equal in magnitude to the negative circular dichroism produced by the $\Psi_0 \to \Psi_{A_2}$ transition. It then follows that if the two transitions were of the same energy, the exciton rotational strength would disappear. In order to see that this does not happen we need to consider the interactions of the dipoles in each of the coupling modes.

Since the transition vectors can be regarded as oscillating dipoles, the interaction energy between them will be different for the various coupling modes. Consider the two transitions $\Psi_0 \to \Psi_{A_2}$ and $\Psi_0 \to \Psi_E^2$; the latter is the same energy as the $\Psi_0 \to \Psi_E^1$ component. For the $\Psi_0 \to \Psi_{A_2}$ transition the vectors are essentially 'head to head', whereas the vectors are in a 'head to tail' arrangement for the $\Psi_0 \to \Psi_E^2$ transition. Simple electrostatic arguments will suggest that the 'head to head' combination will be of higher energy than the 'head to tail' combination. It turns out that these intuitive arguments are correct in this case but care should be taken in using them to predict exciton splitting. Having determined that the $\Psi_0 \to \Psi_{A_2}$ transition is of higher energy than the $\Psi_0 \to \Psi_E$ excitation we have to determine where the centre of gravity of the exciton splitting should be. It will be clear that both the ground- and excited-state energy of the isolated phen molecule will be different from a phen molecule in a complex where it can interact with its neighbours; for the same reason that a gaseous phen molecule is different in energy from a phen molecule in the crystal. This effect is usually assumed to be small and is set to zero but will generally shift the isolated phen absorption slightly to lower energies. For the present purposes we assume that the two exciton components will be displaced from the energy of the isolated phen molecule.

We have shown that, apart from a frequency term which appears in the total rotational strength expression,[1] the exciton rotational strength should appear positive at lower energies and equally negative at higher energies relative to the energy of absorption of the isolated phen molecule if the [M phen$_3$]$^{n+}$ system is in the absolute configuration shown in Fig. 2. For the opposite absolute configuration the energies of the two components will be identical but the sign of the two exciton transitions will be identically reversed. The intensity of the normal absorption is determined by the total number of phen molecules in the complex and is three times as intense for the [M phen$_3$]$^{n+}$ system than for the isolated phen molecule. We may assume that the total observed intensity is almost completely determined by the dipole strength. The dipole strength of a transition is proportional to the square of the quantity $\langle a | \mu_e | b \rangle$. The magnitude and direction of the transition electric dipole moment is clearly related to the nature of the coupling modes and the geometry of the complex. It turns out that, of the total dipole strength of the [M phen$_3$]$^{3+}$ complex, twice as much is distributed into the $\Psi_0 \rightarrow \Psi_{A_2}$ transition as is distributed in the $\Psi_0 \rightarrow \Psi_E$ transition. Thus we have an additional criterion for identifying the exciton components in that the higher-energy component should be twice as intense as the lower-energy exciton component.

We now turn to the short-axis polarized transitions. As in the case of the long-axis transitions there are three coupling modes for the short-axis transitions of the [M phen$_3$]$^{n+}$ complex. The exciton transitions are $\Psi_0 \rightarrow \Psi_{A_1}$ and $\Psi_0 \rightarrow \Psi_E$, the last one consisting of two degenerate components (Fig. 2). It will be seen that the vectors of the $\Psi_0 \rightarrow \Psi_{A_1}$ transition involve an 'outward' linear displacement but there is no circulation of charge and thus there can be no zero-order exciton rotational strength associated with the transition. (As it turns out there is also no net linear displacement because the vector sum cancels and the transition is electric-dipole forbidden.) It will be seen that the vector sum of the $\Psi_0 \rightarrow \Psi_E^1$ transition involves a net linear displacement of charge along the two-fold axis and the other component, $\Psi_0 \rightarrow \Psi_E^2$, involves a net linear displacement at right angles to the two-fold axis. But in neither case is any circulation of charge involved and so no exciton circular dichroism is possible although this transition is electric-dipole allowed. The conclusion is that short-axis polarized transitions should show no exciton circular dichroism.

In Fig. 3 we show the absorption and circular dichroism spectra of (+)-[Ru phen$_3$] (ClO$_4$)$_2$ in water solution. The fairly intense set of bands in the 19,000 to 27,000 cm^{-1} region are charge transfer bands involving excitation of the metal d-electrons into the anti-bonding π^* orbitals of the ligand. Transitions in the 27,000 to 35,000 cm^{-1} energy range are mainly the short-axis polarized transitions of the phen molecules and the intense band centred around 38,000 cm^{-1} represents the long-axis polarized transitions of the phen molecules. It will be seen that the short-axis polarized transitions show weak circular dichroism and that the long-axis polarized transition shows exceedingly strong circular dichroism displayed as an equal and opposite couplet. This is precisely the result we would expect if the exciton coupling was the important factor in determining the circular dichroism in this region of the spectrum. In addition the sign pattern under the long-axis polarized transition indicates that the absolute configuration of (+)-[Ru phen$_3$]$^{2+}$ is a left-handed three blade propeller. The corresponding (−)-[Fe phen$_3$]$^{2+}$ and the (+)-[Ni phen$_3$]$^{2+}$ ion also show a plus–minus pattern under the 38,000 cm^{-1} transition, and absolute crystal structure determinations have confirmed the predictions of the exciton theory.[12, 13] Similar patterns are observed for the corresponding [M bipy$_3$]$^{n+}$ complexes.[14]

However, in both the [M phen$_3$]$^{n+}$ and [M bipy$_3$]$^{n+}$ systems the dipole-strength criterion for assigning the exciton components can be misleading because the long-axis polarized transitions of the ligands are overlayed by both short-axis polarized transitions and charge transfer bands involving both the ligands and the metal d-electrons. The result is that when the metal is changed both the absorption and circular dichroism spectra show variations although the basic exciton pattern is retained.

The (+)-tris-acetylacetonatesilicon (IV) ion, {(+)-[Si(acac)$_3$]$^+$}, shows only the long-axis polarized $\pi \rightarrow \pi^*$ transition in the accessible regions of the spectra and the complications that arise in the phen and bipy transition metal complexes are not

B. Bosnich

present. Figure 4 shows the absorption spectrum of the acac ion, and the absorption and circular dichroism spectrum of the (+)-[Si(acac)$_3$]$^+$ ion.[15] It will be seen that the absorption spectrum of [Si(acac)$_3$]$^+$ is split into a more intense higher-energy component and a less intense lower-energy component and that this total band is three times stronger than the absorption spectrum of the acac ion. In addition, the circular dichroism shows the expected exciton pattern.

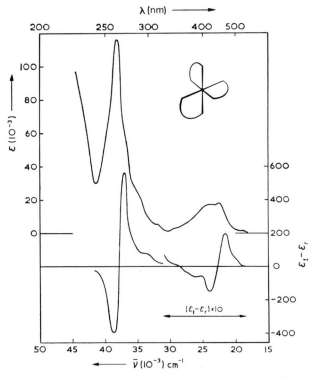

Fig. 3. The absorption and circular dichroism spectrum of the (+)-[Ru phen$_3$]$^{2+}$ ion in water.

We now turn to the case of the *cis*-[M phen$_2$ X$_2$]$^{n+}$ complexes which have only two phen molecules. There are only two coupling modes, one of which is polarized along the two-fold axis and the other at right angles to it. The coupling modes are shown in Fig. 5 and, by similar arguments[16] to the ones used for the tris-bidentate molecules, we expect a strong positive circular dichroism band at lower energies and an equal negative band at higher energies in the regions of the long-axis polarized transitions, provided the molecule has the absolute configuration related to (−)-[Fe phen$_3$]$^{2+}$. In Fig. 6 we show the spectra of the (+)-[Ru phen$_2$ py$_2$]$^{2+}$ ion (py = pyridine) where it will be seen that the expected exciton pattern is observed, except that the higher energy component of the couplet is weaker than the lower energy component. **Apart** from instrumental insensitivity, there are two main reasons for this. First, the bands are heavily overlapped by other transitions which although weaker will tend to diminish one component if these other bands are of the same sign in the relevant energy region. The second reason, which is of more general theoretical interest, is that we have assumed that only the long-axis polarized transition in the 38,000 cm^{-1} region is responsible for the exciton circular dichroism. In principle, however, the two exciton components can mix with all other transitions of the system

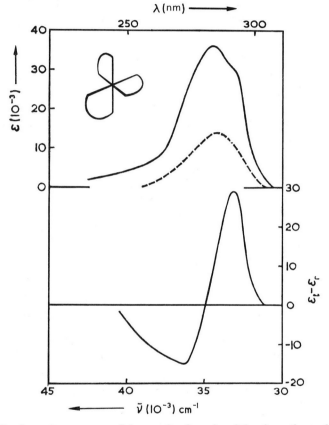

Fig. 4. The absorption spectrum of the acac ion (----) and the absorption and circular dichroism spectrum (———) of the (+)-[Si(acac)$_3$]$^+$ ion in water.

which are of the same symmetry. The amount of mixing will depend on the energy separation, being less as the energy increases from the band in question and on the sign and intensity of the other circular dichroism bands which are involved. These effects would be relatively unimportant in these complexes were it not that there probably is another ligand long-axis polarized transition in the vacuum ultraviolet which can mix with the 38,000 cm^{-1} band. In order to show this effect clearly we consider the complex *cis*-[M phen bipy X$_2$]$^{n+}$ where the long-axis polarized transitions of the phen and bipy ligands occur at 38,000 cm^{-1} and 34,500 cm^{-1}, respectively.

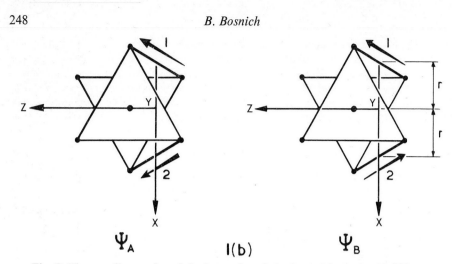

Fig. 5. The coupling modes of the long-axis polarized transitions of a bis-bidentate complex.

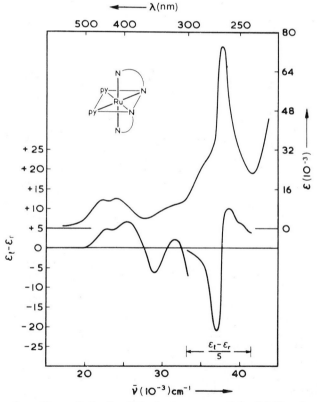

Fig. 6. The absorption and circular dichroism spectrum of the (+)-[Ru phen$_2$ py$_2$]$^{2+}$ ion in water.

As far as the coupling modes are concerned, exactly the same result is obtained for the mixed system as was obtained for the *cis*-[M phen$_2$ X$_2$]$^{n+}$ system (Fig. 5). However, there is a difference in that the magnitudes of the rotational strengths will diminish as the energies between the two transitions increase but, as in the case of

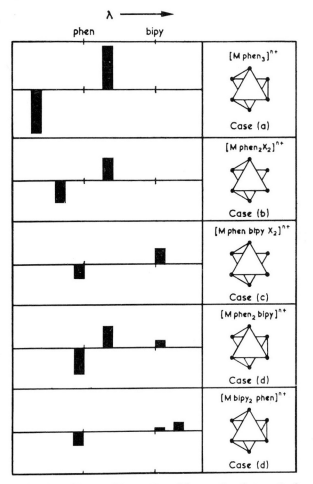

Fig. 7. The predicted positions and intensities of the rotational strengths for complexes containing various permutations of phen and bipy molecules in the absolute configurations shown.

the identical coupling scheme, the sum of the rotational strengths resulting from exciton coupling will be zero. In addition the coupling mode which was associated with the higher energy component in the degenerate system will be the one associated with the higher-energy ligand transition (the phen molecule in *cis*-[M phen bipy X$_2$]$^{n+}$ complex) and similarly for the lower-energy coupling mode. The exciton interaction still occurs in the non-identical system and has the effect of 'repelling' the two

transitions of the ligands to higher and lower energies. Thus the result for the
cis-[M phen bipy X_2]$^{n+}$ system is that the rotational strength will appear positive
in the regions of the long-axis polarized transitions of bipy and (equally) negative
in the regions of the long-axis polarized transitions of the phen, provided the complex has the absolute configuration related to (−)-[Fe phen$_3$]$^{2+}$. This result has been
confirmed for the (+)-[Cr bipy phen ox]$^+$ (ox = oxalate) complex.[17]

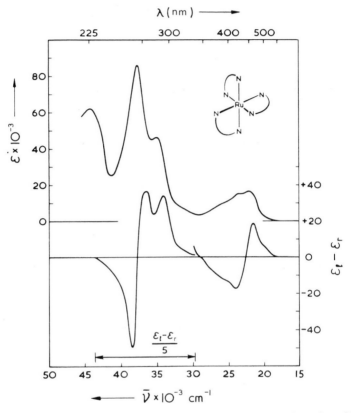

Fig. 8. The absorption and circular dichroism spectrum of the (+)-[Ru phen$_2$ bipy]$^{2+}$
ion in water.

Similar arguments can be used in order to determine the absolute configurations
of mixed systems of the type [M phen$_2$ bipy]$^{n+}$ and [M bipy$_2$ phen]$^{n+}$. The results,[10]
together with those we have already discussed are shown diagrammatically in Fig. 7.
The absorption and circular dichroism spectra of the (+)-[Ru phen$_2$ bipy]$^{2+}$ ion are
shown in Fig. 8 where it will be seen that the predicted +, +, − pattern is observed
under the bipy and phen absorptions. The (+)-[Ru bipy$_2$ phen]$^{2+}$ ion shows only
two circular dichroism bands (Fig. 9) although the analogous Os complex[18] does
show the predicted pattern. This, however, does not preclude the determination of
the absolute configuration of the complex.

We now turn briefly to somewhat more complicated systems where both the short- and the long-axis polarized transitions can couple to produce exciton circular dichroism. The simplest examples occur with the binuclear complexes of the type [M phen$_2$ (OH)$_2$ phen$_2$ M]$^{n+}$, where each metal atom has two *cis*-disposed phen molecules and the OH groups provide a *cis*-bridge between the two metal atoms. In the dissymmetric configuration the molecule belongs to the point group D$_2$ and a consideration of the coupling which results between the short-axis polarized transition of phen molecules on different metals leads to the conclusion that exciton

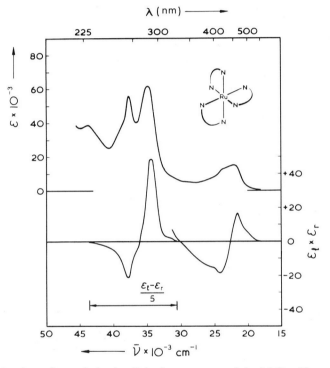

Fig. 9. The absorption and circular dichroism spectrum of the (+)-[Ru bipy$_2$ phen]$^{2+}$ ion in water.

circular dichroism should occur. In addition the long-axis polarized transitions give exciton circular dichroism by coupling between the excitation moments of phen molecules on the same metal and also between the moments of phen molecules in different metals. This situation is further complicated by the possible large coupling between the short- and long-axis transitions as well as the difference in interaction energies between the excitation moments of neighbouring phen molecules and those on different atoms. We will not discuss these systems further except to note their absolute configurations can be derived from the circular dichroism.[14]

The arguments which have been given above can be used to derive the absolute configurations of other metal complexes with different ligands. Thus, for example, the (−)-[As cat$_3$]$^−$ ion (cat = 1,2-benzenediolate) shows the typical exciton pattern in the 45,000 to 55,000 cm^{-1} region and the predictions of the exciton theory and an absolute crystal structure determination are in agreement.[19] Because of the general agreement between theory and experiment a general rule may be formulated for monomeric complexes with symmetrical ligands; namely, that in the regions of the long-axis polarized transitions the circular dichroism will appear strongly positive at lower energies and strongly negative at higher energies if the complex has the absolute configuration related to (−)-[Fe phen$_3$]$^{2+}$. This rule is shown diagrammatically in Fig. 7.

3.7.3 Final Remarks

In all the above discussion we have ignored a number of factors which could lead to ambiguity in the interpretation. There seems little doubt that the exciton interpretation of the circular dichroism spectra is correct but a crucial element involves the determination of the sense of the exciton splitting in the identical chromophore cases. There are a number of methods of calculating this exciton splitting[10, 14] and in the more sophisticated method using coulombic monopole interactions, the agreement between experiment and theory is generally good. This, perhaps, is a surprising result in view of the number of factors which can affect the splitting. The first of these, which is peculiar to transition metal complexes, is the perturbation that interaction between d$_\pi$ orbitals of the metal and the π^* orbitals of the ligands can cause to the sense of the splitting. A certain amount of effort[14, 20] has been put into this problem and the more sophisticated approach[14] concludes that, although some perturbation of the splitting does occur, the sense of the exciton splitting is retained. The same applies if the overlap between neighbouring ligands is considered.[14] Within the present limitations of theory these conclusions are firm although it is doubtful that they are sufficiently precise to be applicable to all cases. A second, and more serious, problem which can be raised[21] is related to vibronic interactions. Indeed, this factor has seldom been considered in the calculation of exciton circular dichroism of these or any other systems. The problem arises when the vibronic intervals are of comparable magnitude to the exciton splitting and the arguments[22] which are used to determine the nature of the transitions are more complicated than those which have been used here. Our assumption has been that the sense of the exciton splitting is determined by the interactions of the transition dipole moments of the ligands. A rigorous test of this hypothesis in the present series of complexes is made extremely difficult by the poorly resolved absorption manifolds which are heavily overlaid by transitions of varying provenance and intensity. Despite the approximations, there is no case where the simplified theory has been shown unambiguously to give the incorrect absolute configuration.

References

1. E. U. Condon, *Rev. Mod. Phys.* **9**, 432 (1937).
2. P. Drude, *Lehrbuch der Optik*. Hirzel, Leipzig, 1900.
3. M. Born, *Phys. Z.* **16**, 251 (1915); *Ann. Phys. Leipzig* **55**, 177 (1918).
4. W. Kuhn, *Z. Phys. Chem. B*, **4**, 14 (1929).
5. E. U. Condon, W. Alter and H. Eyring, *J. Chem. Phys.* **5**, 753 (1937).
6. J. G. Kirkwood, *J. Chem. Phys.* **5**, 479 (1937).
7. R. Sibey, J. Jortner and S. A. Rice, *J. Chem. Phys.* **42**, 1515 (1965).

8. W. Moffitt, *J. Chem. Phys.* **26**, 467 (1956).
9. B. Bosnich, *Inorg. Chem.* **7**, 2379 (1968).
10. B. Bosnich, *Accounts Chem. Res.* **2**, 266 (1969).
11. J. Hidaka and B. E. Douglas, *Inorg. Chem.* **3**, 1180 (1964).
12. D. H. Templeton, A. Zalkin and T. Ueki, *Acta Crystallogr.* **21**, A154 (1966).
13. K. R. Butler and M. R. Snow, *Chem. Commun.* 355 (1971).
14. S. F. Mason, *Inorg. Chim. Acta Rev.* **2**, 89 (1968).
15. E. Larsen, S. F. Mason and G. H. Searle, *Acta Chem. Scand.* **20**, 191 (1966).
16. B. Bosnich, *Inorg. Chem.* **7**, 178 (1968).
17. S. Kaizaki, J. Hidaka and Y. Shimura, *Bull. Chem. Soc. Jap.* **43**, 3024 (1970).
18. S. F. Mason and B. J. Norman, *Chem. Phys. Lett.* **2**, 22 (1968).
19. T. Ito, A. Kobayashi, F. Marumo and Y. Saito, *Inorg. Nucl. Chem. Lett.* **7**, 1097 (1971).
20. J. Ferguson, C. J. Hawkins, N. A. P. Kane-Maguire and H. Lip, *Inorg. Chem.* **8**, 771 (1969).
21. R. G. Bray, J. Ferguson and C. J. Hawkins, *Aust. J. Chem.* **22**, 2091 (1969).
22. M. H. Perrin and M. Gouterman, *J. Chem. Phys.* **46**, 1010 (1967).

Induced Optical Activity

B. BOSNICH

Lash Miller Chemical Laboratories
80 St. George St.
University of Toronto
Toronto

3.8.1 Introduction

The enantiomorphs of an optically active substance are identical in their physical and chemical properties provided they exist in a symmetrical chemical or physical environment and provided their properties are observed by an achiral probe. Since the two differ from each other as object and mirror image they can only be differentiated by physical and chemical interactions which themselves differ in the same way. It then follows that the interaction between any set of chiral entities is the same as the interaction of the same set of chiral entities viewed enantiomorphically. This last statement is true because the transference, as it were, from the object to the mirror world only involves a change from a right- to a left-hand coordinate frame. We illustrate this, often confused, point with two examples, one physical and the other chemical. Suppose we measure the extinction coefficient of a particular absorption band of a given optical isomer using right-hand circularly polarized light: then the same experiment carried out in the mirror world will give the same value for the extinction coefficient for the reason that, in going to the mirror world, the optical isomer becomes its enantiomorph and right-hand circularly polarized light becomes left-hand circularly polarized light. Similarly the resolution of a D optical isomer using, for example, an L resolving agent carried out in the object world will occur with equal facility in the mirror world because the latter is the resolution of the L isomer with the D resolving agent. The principle can be illustrated more generally by considering a number of chemical interactions and we take first the interactions between the D and L forms of the same molecule.

Three possible interactions may occur namely L with L, D with D and D with L. The first two sets of interactions are identical since they are the mirror image of each other, the third, namely D with L, is different from the other two. These facts are manifested in, for example, the observation that the boiling and melting points of the optical isomers of a compound are identical but differ from those of the racemic isomers of the same compound. It is perhaps interesting to note that it is generally assumed that, for example, the NMR spectra of the optical isomers will be the same as the racemic isomer. This of course will be true if the solvent is achiral and the molecules of the solute exist as monomers. However if dimers or polymers are formed between the solute molecules, the NMR spectrum will, in principle, be different in the two cases because, if we take the dimer as an example, the L,L and D,D dimers will have the same signal but the D,L dimer will be different.

Consider now the interactions between the optical isomers of two different chiral molecules A and B. The possible interactions that can occur are shown below. The

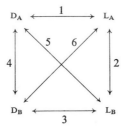

problem of deciding which of the interactions is the same is less obvious than before. If, however, we follow the principle that object and mirror image interactions are identical, it follows that, $2 = 4 \neq 5 = 6 \neq 3 \neq 1$, because $D_A D_B(4)$ is the mirror image of $L_A L_B(2)$ and $D_B L_A(6)$ is the mirror image of $D_A L_B(5)$. This last case is, in fact, well known when optical resolutions are carried out using diastereoisomers and the reader may convince himself of the relationships by imagining that A is an acid and B a base and working out the identical diastereomers. We may, of course, extend this problem to any number of interacting chiral entities where in any case the mirror image principle will reveal the identical interactions.

It is perhaps amusing, though not trivial in the present context, to pose the question Lewis Carroll posed when Alice was about to step into the comic world behind the looking-glass. Alice turned to the cat and inquired, 'How would you like to live in Looking-Glass House, Kitty? I wonder if they'd give you milk in there? Perhaps Looking-Glass milk isn't good to drink ...' This is probably as complex a situation as we need to pursue and the answer to the question about the nature of Looking-Glass milk depends on whether a Looking-Glass cat or an object cat is drinking it. As is well known, both Alice's cat and the milk contain molecules which are optically active and to some extent the question as to whether milk is good to drink depends on the optical isomers present in the milk and the cat. If object milk is good to drink for the object cat, then by the mirror image principle, mirror milk drunk by a mirror cat is just as good; but an object cat drinking mirror milk or, what is the identical situation, a mirror cat drinking object milk would certainly find the milk different whether 'good to drink' or otherwise. Thus the mirror principle would instruct Alice that looking-glass milk is good to drink provided her cat drinks it in the Looking-Glass House and not in the object house.

3.8.2 Asymmetric Transformations of the First Kind

In an achiral medium, the D and L forms of an optically active substance are in equilibrium, which, if there is no association between the enantiomorphic entities, may be written

$$D \underset{k_{-1}}{\overset{k_1}{\rightleftharpoons}} L$$

We note that the two rate constants, k_1 and k_{-1}, are identical since the reaction rates of the two forms must be identical. It then follows that the equilibrium constant, K, which is equal to the ratio of the two rate constants, is unity and hence the free energy for the process, ΔG, is zero. This of course does not mean that the activation energy is zero but that the energies of the factor and product are the same.

Suppose that a chiral influence is impressed upon this equilibrium and, for the purposes of being specific, imagine the addition of the D* form of another molecule to the system. Without being precise about the mechanism involved, we now have a new equilibrium situation:

$$\text{DD*} \underset{k_{-1}^*}{\overset{k_1^*}{\rightleftharpoons}} \text{LD*}$$

where DD* and LD* are meant to represent the interaction of the D* molecule with the D and L molecules respectively. It will be clear that the chemical potentials of the D and L forms will no longer be the same, and hence it follows that, $k_1^* \neq k_{-1}^*$, that, $K \neq 1$ and that $\Delta G \neq 0$ at least in principle. The effect is to shift the enantiomeric equilibrium so that one or other of the optical forms predominates. Such a process was called by Kuhn[1] an 'asymmetric transformation of the first kind', whereas inorganic chemists refer to it as the 'Pfeiffer effect' after Pfeiffer who observed and studied the effect in inorganic systems.[2] We prefer to call the process of shifting the enantiomeric equilibrium as *enantiomerization* which has the advantage of defining the process rather than the phenomenon. The enantiomerization process has been found to occur extensively in organic systems[3] which, for practical reasons, are optically labile, but perhaps the more spectacular observations are found among inorganic complexes and we will discuss some of these as examples.

When two or more of the bidentate ligands, *o*-phenanthroline (phen) or 2,2′-bipyridine (bipy), are coordinated to an octahedral metal ion, potentially optically active complexes are formed. The optical stability of these complexes varies enormously as the metal ion is changed giving complexes of Zn^{2+} and Cu^{2+} which are so labile that they cannot be resolved to the Ru^{2+} and Os^{2+} species which are so stable that fused caustic soda is required to racemize them. The complexes of Ni^{2+} and Fe^{2+} are of intermediate stability, being just stable enough to permit resolution but racemize at a convenient rate at room temperature. It was with the complexes of high medium lability that Pfeiffer observed his effects.

Pfeiffer found that, when phen was added to a solution of zinc D-camphor-π-sulphonate, there was a large and rapid change in rotation which was not observed when pyridine or ammonia were added to the solution. He interpreted this behaviour as being due to the potentially optically active zinc phen complex undergoing enantiomerization which could not occur with the symmetrical pyridine or ammonia complexes. Perhaps the most thoroughly studied of Pfeiffer's systems is the [Ni phen$_3$]$^{2+}$ ion.[4]

The addition of L-malic acid to an aqueous solution of racemic [Ni phen$_3$]$^{2+}$ causes the rotation to change at a rate which is *roughly* equal to the rate of racemization of the [Ni phen$_3$]$^{2+}$ in water. The rotation reaches a maximum which does not represent the total resolution of the complex. After freeze-drying the equilibrated solution the nickel complex is found to be optically active. There is therefore no doubt that L-malic acid had caused the complex to enantiomerize. Furthermore, it has been found that the rates of racemization of the D and L forms of [Ni phen$_3$]$^{2+}$

are different in the presence of large optically active ions.[5] This differential racemization has also been observed in organic systems.[6] The origin of the enantiomerization process, at least for inorganic systems, appears to be connected with the association between the D and L forms and the added optically active molecules. Whether differential association or some other mechanism is involved has not been established.[7]

All these enantiomerization reactions can be viewed in a more rigorous and quantitative way by considering the thermodynamics of the process.[8, 9] If the D and L forms of a substance are crystallized from an achiral solvent under identical conditions the two crystals will have identical chemical potentials and thus their solubilities will be identical in an achiral solvent. Suppose, however, that dissolution is carried out in a chiral medium, which can be either a chiral solvent or an achiral solvent containing optically active molecules dissolved in it, then, in principle, the D and L crystals will have different solubilities which are related to the different solvation energies. We take the specific example for which the experiment has been carried out in order to illustrate the principle. The system involved the solubilities of (−), (+) and (±) *cis*-[Co en$_2$ Cl$_2$]ClO$_4$ (en = 1,2-diaminoethane) in (−)-2,3-butanediol. The solubility data are shown in Table 1.

Table 1[a]

Compound	Solubility (mole l^{-1})	Solubility product
(±)*cis*-[Co en$_2$ Cl$_2$]ClO$_4$	0·6 × 10^{-3}	0·35 × 10^{-6}
(+)*cis*-[Co en$_2$ Cl$_2$]ClO$_4$	2·6 × 10^{-3}	7·0 × 10^{-6}
(−)*cis*-[Co en$_2$ Cl$_2$]ClO$_4$	1·25 × 10^{-3}	1·5 × 10^{-6}

[a] Temperature = 30°.

The solubility product, $K_{SP(\ )}$, and the standard chemical potentials, $\bar{\mu}^0$, involved in the solubility measurements are typified by

$$\{(\ )cis\text{-}[\text{Co en}_2\text{Cl}_2]\text{ClO}_4\}_{solid} \rightleftharpoons \{(\ )cis\text{-}[\text{Co en}_2\text{Cl}_2]^+\}_{solution}$$
$$\bar{\mu}^0_{S(\ )} \qquad\qquad\qquad\qquad \bar{\mu}^0_{(\ )}$$
$$+\{\text{ClO}_4^-\}_{solution}$$
$$\bar{\mu}^0{}_{\text{ClO}_4}$$

$$K_{SP(\ )} = \{(\ )cis\text{-}[\text{Co en}_2\text{Cl}_2]^+\}_{solution}\{\text{ClO}_4^-\}_{solution}$$

Hence

$$-RT\ln K_{SP(\ )} = -\bar{\mu}^0_{S(\ )} + \bar{\mu}^0_{(\ )} + \bar{\mu}^0_{\text{ClO}_4}$$

Thus the appropriate equations which relate the chemical potentials and the solubility products for the (+) and (−) forms are

$$-RT\ln(K_{SP(-)}) = -\bar{\mu}^0_{S(-)} + \bar{\mu}^0_{(-)} + \bar{\mu}^0_{\text{ClO}_4}$$

$$-RT\ln(K_{SP(+)}) = -\bar{\mu}^0_{S(+)} + \bar{\mu}^0_{(+)} + \bar{\mu}^0_{\text{ClO}_4}$$

Subtracting these last two equations gives

$$-RT\ln\left(\frac{K_{SP(-)}}{K_{SP(+)}}\right) = \bar{\mu}^0_{(-)} - \bar{\mu}^0_{(+)}$$

This last relationship follows because the chemical potentials, $\bar{\mu}^0_{S(-)}$ and $\bar{\mu}^0_{S(+)}$, of the two solids are identical as are of course those referring to ClO_4^- ion. The enantio-merization reaction, specified by the enantiomerization constant K, is

$$(+)cis\text{-}[Co\,en_2Cl_2]^+ \rightleftharpoons (-)cis\text{-}[Co\,en_2Cl_2]^+$$
$$\bar{\mu}^0_{(+)} \qquad\qquad\qquad \bar{\mu}^0_{(-)}$$

and hence

$$-RT\ln K = \bar{\mu}^0_{(-)} - \bar{\mu}^0_{(+)} = \Delta G^0 = -RT\ln\left(\frac{K_{SP(-)}}{K_{SP(+)}}\right)$$

Thus the enantiomerization constant is related to the ratio of the solubility products. This is quite a general result and its physical significance is readily seen. If the solvent is achiral then the solubilities of the two enantiomers are the same and hence, $\Delta G^0 = 0$, since the two chemical potentials must be equal: an observation which we have already asserted. If, however, the solvent is chiral, the chemical potentials of the two crystals will of course be identical but, in principle, the two solution chemical potentials will no longer be the same and will reflect the difference in dissymmetric free energy of solvation for the two enantiomorphs.

Using the relationships just derived and the solubility data in Table 1, the free energy of enantiomerization is +0·9 kcal.mole^{-1} in the sense that at equilibrium, 80% of (+)-cis-[Co en$_2$Cl$_2$]$^+$ and 20% of (−)-cis-[Co en$_2$Cl$_2$]$^+$ would be present in (−)-2,3-butanediol. This result has been confirmed by the dissolution of intimate mixtures of the solid (+) and (−) complexes where it was found that the equilibrated solution contained the (+) and (−) forms in the ratio of 4:1 respectively. The actual experiment of allowing the racemic compound to enantiomerize cannot be done because of other complicating factors.[9] Other experiments of this kind have been carried out in water containing optically active ions and differences in solubility have been observed[10] although the thermodynamics were not recognized.

The derived relationships allow us to make certain observations about the possibility of resolving molecules by crystallizing from optically active solvents or achiral solvents containing chiral molecules. In the absence of any enantiomerization, fractional crystallization from an active solvent will only work if the chemical potential for the crystals containing equal numbers of (+) and (−) forms (racemic compound) is greater than the crystals which contain exclusively the (+) or (−) forms, i.e. crystals belonging to enantiomorphic space groups. In other words the (+) or (−) crystals must be less soluble than the (±) crystals. It will be seen in Table 1 that this is not the case here where the (±) crystals are less soluble. A proper survey has not been done, but it seems that generally (±) crystals tend to be more stable than enantiomorphic crystals although there have been some successful resolutions from optically active solvents.[11,12] Allowing the enantiomerization to occur before the crystallization does not help because the increment in concentration of one form over the other exactly compensates the differential solubility; that is the solution stabilized form is also the more soluble.

3.8.3 Asymmetric Transformations of the Second Kind

Asymmetric transformations of the second kind are in essence heterogeneous enantiomerization reactions. As an example, consider the two diastereomers formed between [Fe phen$_3$]$^{2+}$ and the antimonyl-(+)-tartrate ion [Sb(+)tart]$^-$, namely (+)-[Fe phen$_3$][Sb(+)tart]$_2$ and (−)-[Fe phen$_3$][Sb(+)tart]$_2$. These two crystalline salts have different chemical potentials because the anion–cation interactions in their respective crystals will be different. It then follows that their solubilities even in achiral solvents will be different. This of course is the principle on which chemical resolutions are based.

In solution the following equilibrium exists

$$(+)\text{-[Fe phen}_3]^{2+} \rightleftharpoons (-)\text{-[Fe phen}_3]^{2+}$$

which in this case is reasonably rapid; total racemization occurs in about four hours in water at room temperature. For this system the (−)(+) diastereomer is less soluble than the (+)(+) diastereomer. When an excess of Sb(+)tart is added to a water solution containing the racemic iron complex, an immediate precipitate of the (−)(+) diastereomer is formed. But if this solution is allowed to stand for a day the solution contains practically no iron complex and the precipitate consists of a *chemically* quantitative yield of the (−)-[Fe phen$_3$][Sb(+)tart]$_2$ salt. The reason for this is that, after initial precipitation of the (−)(+) diastereomer, the (+)-[Fe phen$_3$]$^{2+}$ remaining in solution racemizes to give (−)-[Fe phen$_3$]$^{2+}$ which, when its concentration is equal to the solubility product of the (−)(+) diastereomer, again precipitates. This process goes on continuously until all the complex is out of solution as the (−)(+) diastereomer. These types of resolutions will only occur under conditions where the compound to be resolved is optically labile. It is, however, quite a common phenomenon.[3]

3.8.4 Asymmetric Induction

The circular dichroism associated with particular electronic transitions usually involves chromophores which are inherently symmetric. The circular dichroism is induced into the transition because of the dissymmetric perturbations exerted by some group or groups belonging to the dissymmetric molecule to which the chromophore is attached. It is then reasonable to suppose that circular dichroism could be induced in a chromophore belonging to a symmetrical molecule which is surrounded by a chiral chemical environment.

The first experiment[13] of this kind was carried out with the square coplanar [PtCl$_4$]$^{2-}$ ion dissolved in (−)-2,3-butanediol. Figure 1 shows the absorption and circular dichroism spectra of the ion in the chiral solvent. The bands seen are d-d transitions involving, at 390 nm the spin-allowed excitation d$xy \rightarrow$ d$x^2 - y^2$ and, at 335 nm the spin-allowed dxz, d$yz \rightarrow$ d$x^2 - y^2$ (degenerate) transition. The bands at lower energies involve singlet-triplet transitions within the d-electron manifold. It will be seen that only the d$xy \rightarrow$ d$x^2 - y^2$ transition involving an electronic displacement in the molecular plane and a magnetic moment polarized in the z-direction gives detectable circular dichroism.

It is well known that square planar complexes such as the $[Pt\,Cl_4]^{2-}$ ion form weak bonds in the tetragonal sites ($+z$ and $-z$ axes) and presumably the induced circular dichroism is in some way associated with the weak coordination of the chiral solvent at these sites. However, the two orbitals involved in the transition which shows circular dichroism cannot interact with the solvent donor atoms, whereas the dxz, dyz orbitals, involved in the other spin-allowed transition which does not show detectable circular dichroism, can interact with donor atom orbitals of the solvent. Thus it appears that the induced activity is not directly connected with the bonding between the ion and the solvent. The intensity of these transitions is undoubtedly

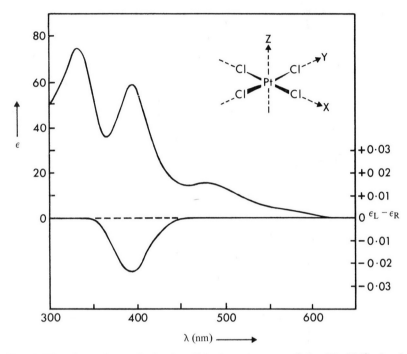

Fig. 1. The absorption and circular dichroism spectrum of the $[Pt\,Cl_4]^{2-}$ ion in (−)-2,3-butanediol.

due to a vibronic mechanism[14] and the intriguing observation is that there is no vibrational mode in D_{4h} which produces an electric moment in the z direction to the d$xy \rightarrow$ d$x^2 - y^2$ transition. Thus the mechanism which engenders a collinear electric moment to the optical activity of this transition is even more subtle than the intensity-giving mechanism of the achiral $[PtCl_4]^{2-}$ ion.

Induced optical activity has also been observed in the magnetic dipole transitions of organic molecules. The first recorded cases were observed in the $n \rightarrow \pi^*$ transitions of benzil and benzophenone dissolved in (−)-2,3-butanediol.[15] The two spectra are shown in Fig. 2. These results can be interpreted in either of two ways; either that the molecules exist in some preferred dissymmetric conformation in the chiral solvent or that the optical activity is induced by the solvent without the presence of preferred dissymmetric conformations. Subsequent work[16] has shown that induced activity is found in systems which cannot adopt dissymmetric conformations. In addition, while hydrogen bonding between the lone-pair electrons of the carbonyl chromophore and the protic solvent may be an important factor in these cases, it is not a necessary condition because induced activity has been observed in systems where formally no hydrogen bonding is possible.[16]

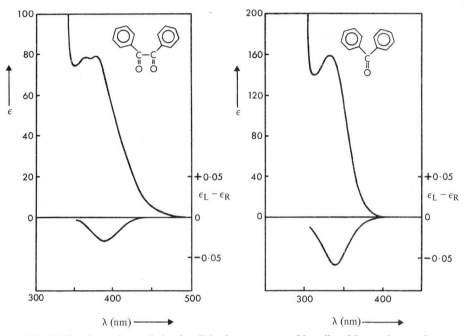

Fig. 2. The absorption and circular dichroism spectrum of benzil and benzophenone in (−)-2,3-butanediol.

We should point out that, in principle, optical activity will be induced in any chromophore surrounded by chiral molecules even if there is a completely random distribution of the chiral molecules about the chromophore. The reason for this is simply that no matter how the chiral molecules distribute themselves, randomly or otherwise, the chromophore will be in a dissymmetric environment. This is not to say that special preferred orientations will not alter the magnitude of the effect, indeed they will, but it is not a necessary condition.

There are situations where the optical activity of a symmetric molecule can be observed with a fixed orientation of the perturbing chiral molecule. This is most easily achieved in the crystal. The $[Co(NH_3)_6]^{3+}$ ion is symmetrical except in special rotamers of the ammine groups and when it is precipitated as the tris[(+)-α-bromo-camphor-π-sulphonate ion] [(+)BCS] salt, $[Co(NH_3)_6]$ $[(+)BCS]_3$, the solid in a **KBr** disc shows circular dichroism in the regions of the d-d transitions of the cobalt atom.[17] Figure 3 shows the spectra where the lower energy band is the magnetic dipole allowed $^1A_{1g} \rightarrow {}^1T_{1g}$ transition. This effect is observed in other ions with different optically active anions or cations.[17] In this particular case it will be noted that the circular dichroism maximum and the solution absorption spectrum maximum are displaced by about 1000 cm^{-1} and, furthermore, the solid absorption spectrum shows evidence of splitting. These observations suggest that the

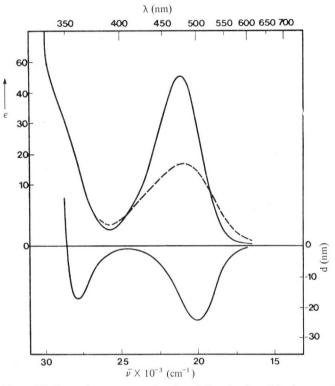

Fig. 3. The solid absorption spectrum (---) and the circular dichroism spectrum of [Co(NH$_3$)$_6$](BCS)$_3$ in a KBr disc and the absorption spectrum of the [Co(NH$_3$)$_6$]$^{3+}$ ion in water.

[Co(NH$_3$)$_6$]$^{3+}$ is not exactly octahedral in the crystal because of anion–cation interactions. It is thus possible that the main part of the induced activity arises from chiral distortions of the Co—N bonds which adjust themselves to the chiral interactions of the neighbouring anions. Whether this is the case or not, the Co chromophore will experience a dissymmetric perturbation even if there are no dissymmetric donor atom distortions or the molecule does not adopt a dissymmetric conformation.

Circular dichroism spectra provide valuable spectroscopic information[18,19] and the above result presents the intriguing possibility that the technique can be applied to all molecules whether they are optically active or not. Indeed work has begun on the circular dichroism of such species as [Co(H$_2$O)$_6$]$^{2+}$ and [Cu(H$_2$O)$_6$]$^{2+}$ doped in the uniaxial enantiomorphic crystal α-Zn(H$_2$O)$_6$SeO$_4$.[20]

3.8.5 Asymmetric Photosynthesis

The D and L forms of an optically active molecule in an achiral environment will absorb achiral light in identical amounts and hence any photochemical reactions which the two isomers may undergo will proceed at identical rates. If, however, circularly (or elliptically) polarized light of one chirality is passed into a mixture of D and L molecules one of the optical isomers will absorb a particular hand of light more than the other. Thus, for example, if right-circularly polarized light (^+hv) is used the following two reactions have different rates

$$D \xrightarrow{\ ^+hv\ }$$

$$L \xrightarrow{\ ^+hv\ }$$

Two types of reactions can occur. A racemic compound may photochemically react to give products which are optically inactive. This process leads to the preponderance of one of the starting optical isomers over the other. A second type of asymmetric photosynthesis may occur where the starting material is optically inactive but the product is optically active. The first process is sometimes called photodestruction and the second photo-synthesis although both involve the creation of optical activity.

The most carefully studied[21] example of the first process was concerned with the $[Cr\ ox_3]^{3-}$ ion (ox = oxalate dianion). This species can be resolved into optical isomers which slowly racemize both thermally and photochemically. Thus when right-circularly polarized light (at 546 nm) was passed into a solution containing racemic $[Cr\ ox_3]^{3-}$ the chemical composition of the solution remained constant but the rotation of the solution slowly rose to a maximum value. Leaving aside the concomitant thermal racemization, four possible photochemical equilibria are set up with ^+hv

$$D \underset{2}{\overset{1}{\rightleftharpoons}} D \quad K_{DD}$$

$$D \underset{4}{\overset{3}{\rightleftharpoons}} L \quad K_{DL}$$

$$L \underset{6}{\overset{5}{\rightleftharpoons}} D \quad K_{LD}$$

$$L \underset{8}{\overset{7}{\rightleftharpoons}} L \quad K_{LL}$$

The equilibrium constants K_{DD} and K_{LL} are identical and equal to unity and are unobservable processes even though the rate constants 1 and 2 are different from 7 and 8. The constants K_{DL} and K_{LD} are also identical but are not equal to unity because the rate constants are different namely, $3 \neq 4$ and $5 \neq 6$ although $6 = 3$ and $5 = 4$. Thus although the process is identical to photoracemization, when circularly polarized light is used, there will be a build-up of one enantiomer over the other. It is perhaps amusing to speculate whether the assumed rate constant relationships, $1 = 2 = 4 = 6 \neq 4 = 5 = 7 = 8$ hold exactly. In other words does, for example, a D isomer after absorbing ^+hv have an identically equal chance of producing either D or L isomers? One can envisage certain excited-state profiles which might lead to an uneven distribution of products. This effect is likely to be small but has not been checked.

The second type of asymmetric photosynthesis has recently been observed in the production of active helicenes from optically inactive starting materials.[22,23] The first reported example involved the ultraviolet illumination of either 1-(β-naphthyl-2-(3-phenanthryl) ethylene or 1-(2-benzo[c] phenanthryl)-2-phenylethylene to produce hexahelicene in low, *c*. 0·3%, optical yield. The reactions were shown to be genuine asymmetric photosynthetic reactions and not photodestruction reactions as had been observed by Kuhn[24] and in other systems.

Apart from trivial complications, photochemically induced activity will only be observed if the left- and right-circularly polarized light is differentially absorbed at the irradiation wavelength. It then follows that in all cases the substrate must be chiral. The extent of photochemical induction depends on the dissymmetry factor, $(\varepsilon_L - \varepsilon_R)/\varepsilon$, where ε is the normal extinction coefficient of the absorption band at the wavelength of irradiation and the maximum optical yield that can be obtained is equal to this ratio. Thus, in general, the amount of chiral photochemical induction will be small because the circular dichroism represents only a small fraction of the total absorption process. It is clear that maximum yields will be obtained in regions where the circular dichroism is large and the normal absorption is small. The second condition for chiral photosynthesis, namely that the substrate must be chiral, is important because it has sometimes been assumed that chiral photosynthesis may be observed in systems where the primary photochemical activation involves only a symmetric molecule, e.g. Br_2. We emphasize this point with an example.

Consider the photochemically induced $2 + 2$ addition between ethylene and *trans*-butene to give the chiral *trans*-1,2-dimethylcyclobutane molecule. (Other reactions occur in this system which are not relevant to the point we wish to make.) It will be noted that both ethylene and *trans*-butene are achiral molecules and hence will absorb left- and right-circularly polarized light to the same extent. Thus if the photochemical reaction involves the excitation of either of the separated molecules, the subsequent cycloaddition cannot lead to the production of an optically active product since, as it were, the excited molecule cannot (quantitatively) remember whether it was excited by left- or right-circularly polarized light. However, asymmetric photosynthesis can occur in this system if the two molecules are associated with each other when the photochemical excitation occurs. The reason for this is that the associated dimer will be chiral. For example, the dimer where the two molecules are associated with their molecular planes parallel gives rise to D and L forms depending on whether the ethylene is associated with the 'top' or 'bottom' (enantiotopic) face of the trans-butene. Such a chiral eximer will distinguish left- and right-circularly polarized light and in principle can give asymmetric photosynthesis. The general conclusion is that for asymmetric photosynthesis to occur the chiral light must excite a chiral molecule involved in the reaction either as an intermediate or as the starting material.

References

1. R. Kuhn, *Ber.* **65**, 49 (1932).
2. P. Pfeiffer and K. Oruehl, *Ber.* **64**, 2667 (1931).
3. E. E. Turner and M. M. Harris, *Quart. Rev. Chem. Soc.* **1**, 299 (1947).

4. S. Kirschner and N. Amad, *J. Amer. Chem. Soc.* **90**, 1910 (1968).
5. N. R. Davies and F. P. Dwyer, *Trans. Faraday Soc.* **50**, 24 (1954).
6. M. M. Harris, *Progress in Stereochemistry*, Vol. 2. London, Butterworths, 1958, p. 157.
7. V. Landis, Thesis, University of Minnesota, Minneapolis, 1956.
8. W. R. Fitzgerald, A. J. Parker and D. W. Watts, *J. Amer. Chem. Soc.* **90**, 5744 (1968).
9. B. Bosnich and D. W. Watts, *J. Amer. Chem. Soc.* **90**, 6228 (1968).
10. F. P. Dwyer, E. C. Gyarfas and M. F. O'Dwyer, *J. Proc. Roy. Soc. N.S. Wales*, **89**, 146 (1956).
11. G. Buchanan and S. H. Graham, *J. Chem. Soc.* 500 (1950).
12. J. Glazer, M. M. Harris and E. E. Turner, *J. Chem. Soc.* 1753 (1950).
13. B. Bosnich, *J. Amer. Chem. Soc.* **88**, 2606 (1966).
14. D. S. Martin and C. A. Lenhardt, *Inorg. Chem.* **3**, 1368 (1964).
15. B. Bosnich, *J. Amer. Chem. Soc.* **89**, 6143 (1967).
16. L. D. Hayward and R. N. Totty, *Can. J. Chem.* **49**, 624 (1971).
17. B. Bosnich and J. MacB. Harrowfield, *J. Amer. Chem. Soc.* **93**, 4086 (1971).
18. B. Bosnich, *J. Amer. Chem. Soc.* **90**, 627 (1968).
19. J. S. Rosenfield and A. Moscowitz, this volume, Chapter 2.2.
20. K. D. Gailey and R. A. Palmer, *Chem. Phys. Lett.* **13**, 176 (1972).
21. K. L. Stevenson and J. K. Verdieck, *J. Amer. Chem. Soc.* **90**, 2974 (1968); *Mol. Photochem.* **1**, 271 (1969).
22. A. Moradpour, J. F. Nicoud, G. Balavoine, H. Kagan and G. Tsoucaris, *J. Amer. Chem. Soc.* **93**, 2353 (1971).
23. W. J. Bernstein, M. Calvin and O. Buchardt, *J. Amer. Chem. Soc.* **94**, 494 (1972).
24. W. Kuhn and E. Knopf, *Z. Phys. Chem. B*, **7**, 292 (1930).

Use of ORD and CD in Conformational Analysis

CHAPTER 4.1

Generalities on Low-molecular-weight Organic Compounds

M. LEGRAND

Department of Physics
Roussel-Uclaf
Romainville, France

4.1.1 Introduction

When molecular theories began to be applied in organic chemistry, chemists were especially interested in the relations between the atoms of molecules. In order to explain the properties of chemical compounds it became necessary to consider the tridimensional aspect. Similarly, in the pharmaceutical field, the tridimensional structure is probably the most important characteristic of a molecule in relation to its pharmaceutical properties. This fact, well-known to chemists involved in this field of research, has gained strength in recent years with the work on the geometric complementarity between substrates and enzymes.

4.1.2 Theoretical Conformational Analysis

A molecule is not completely defined by the nature of its atoms and their mode of linking. Free rotations, around the single bonds, allow different forms to be taken up without modifying the configuration of the molecule. The apparently infinite possibilities are greatly limited by considerations of energy, such as Baeyer and Pitzer strains and nonbonded interactions. Baeyer strain (E_B) corresponds to the increase in energy when bond lengths and bond angles are different from the characteristic values of a given atom. For small deviations around the normal values, and if restoring forces are assumed, Hooke's law is valid and the energies of deformation introduced by these factors are given by:

$$E_r = (1/2)k_r(\Delta_r)^2 \qquad [1]$$

$$E_\alpha = (1/2)k_\alpha(\Delta_\alpha)^2 \qquad [2]$$

k_r and k_α are deduced from infrared and Raman spectra.

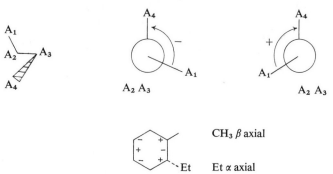

Fig. 1 (modified from reference 4).

Pitzer, or torsional strain (E_P), is related to the dihedral angle formed by four atoms (Fig. 1). It has been shown experimentally that in a simple molecule such as ethane, the eclipsed conformers are about 3 kcal higher in energy than the staggered ones.[1] The potential function accounting for torsional strain is of the form:

$$E(\Phi) = q(1 - \cos 3\Phi) \tag{3}$$

for a three-fold barrier as in ethane. Not all authors agree about the value to give to q.[2] A set used in our laboratory can be found in reference 3. It should be noted that with this type of function the nonbonded interactions are not taken into account, that is the torsional energy is independent of the atoms A_1, A_4 (Fig. 1).

Nonbonded interactions (E_{nb}) are of two sorts, an attractive one (London forces) and a repulsive one (van der Waals' forces). Repulsive forces become preponderant at short distances. No good mathematical functions are as yet available for describing these effects correctly. The most commonly used are [4] and [5]

$$V(d) = a/d^{12} - b/d^6 \tag{4}$$

$$V(d) = a' \exp(-b'd) - c'd^6 \tag{5}$$

These are the three most important types of interactions and are always present in an organic molecule. Others should sometimes be taken into account, for instance dipole–dipole interaction $(E_{dd}$ when strongly polar groups are close together in the molecule.

Finally, any conformation of a molecule will have an energy of deformation given by the sum

$$E_d = \sum E_B(r,\alpha) + \sum E_P(\Phi) + \sum E_{nb}(d) + \sum E_{dd} \tag{6}$$

where the sums are extended to all atoms and all pairs of atoms of the molecules.

Consequently, the different conformers of a given molecule can be classified with respect to their energies of deformation. Then, the conformational analysis becomes a thermodynamic problem since the second more stable conformer can only be observed together with the first one, if the thermal energy of the medium, RT, is of the same order of magnitude as the difference in strain energy E_d of the two conformers.

Mathematically, the ratio between the two conformers is given by

$$A_2/A_1 = \exp(-\Delta G/RT) = \exp(-\Delta H/RT + \Delta S/R) \qquad [7]$$

ΔH and ΔS being the differences in enthalpy and entropy of the two conformers and ΔG the free energy. If $\Delta S = 0$, the ratio A_2/A_1 is directly related to $\Delta E_d = \Delta H$. If not, ΔS should be calculated independently, but this is a rather difficult problem, rarely solved.

When the difference in energy of deformation is much higher than RT, only one species can be observed. Otherwise, both conformers in equilibrium are present in the medium. This result can be extended to equilibria between more than two conformers. With cyclic molecules, rarely more than two species are observed at room temperature and frequently only one. With non-cyclic compounds, a mixture of three or more conformers is more usual.

The search for conformers in relation to their energy for a given molecule is called conformational analysis and is an indispensable step in the use of experimental methods for the determination of conformation (except by X-rays). This can be done in a qualitative way using molecular models such as Dreiding's. Generally with this model only Baeyer strain is taken into account since by definition bond angles and bond lengths are kept constant. Pitzer strain and non-bonding interactions can only be roughly estimated. But despite the approximations, these molecular models allow a first selection of possible conformations. They are always the first step in more sophisticated evaluations.

Semi-quantitative methods are a little more refined. Having selected the more probable conformations from molecular models, the results of calculations or measurements on simple molecules such as cyclopentane, cyclohexane, etc. are applied to these models, taking into account as well the deformations introduced by ring fusion and the non-bonded interaction energies due to substituents. This leads to approximate values of ΔE, thus allowing a classification of the conformers according to their stability.

Some factors facilitating a qualitative and semi-quantitative analysis of conformation will now be given:[4]

(1) Torsional angles formed by four consecutive atoms of the molecules as indicated on the Newman projections of Fig. 1 are said to be either positive or negative, that is, the angle is positive if the shortest rotation to bring the bond situated in front of the figure over the remote one is clockwise and negative in the other case.

This is the convention of Klyne and Prelog.[5] Unfortunately the reverse one is also used.[6]

(2) The sequence of sign and the value of the torsional angles characterize the conformation of a ring. For instance, in Fig. 2 the sequence of signs corresponds to a chair conformation.

(3) An axial group substituted on a ring is β if the ring atom bearing it is preceded by a positive torsional angle and followed by a negative one in a clockwise direction $(+ -)$. It is α axial if the sequence is $- +$ (Fig. 1).

(4) At a *trans* junction between two rings, the dihedral angles are of opposite signs (Fig. 2). The substituents at the junction are always axial. If one

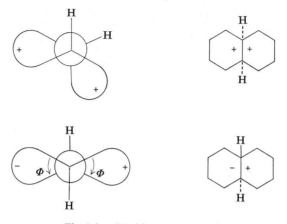

Fig. 2 (modified from reference 4).

of the torsional angles at the junction decreases, that of the other ring increases, in such a way that the sum $\phi + \phi' = 120°$.

(5) At a *cis* junction, the torsional angles are of the same sign (Fig. 2). Each substituent at the junction is axial for one ring and equatorial for the other.

   The torsional angles at the junction decrease or increase together. Consequently the sign at the junction can be reversed without modifying the configuration, which is not the case with a *trans* junction.

(6) A junction between two rings is possible only if the torsional angles at this junction are not too different from the normal values after the ring fusion has been made.

(7) The most stable conformer in a cyclic system possesses the maximum number of rings with the conformation of lower energy, the minimum of non-bonded interactions and the least deformed torsional angles at the junctions.

If some of these conditions are contradictory, at least a semi-quantitative evaluation of the energy implied is necessary. Such an analysis is facilitated by a knowledge of the different parameters for the most simple rings.

In cyclohexane (Fig. 3), the chair form is the more stable one. It is characterized by a sequence of equal torsional angles of inversed signs amounting to 54°.[7] In Fig. 3 only one form is given; the inverted chair is obtained by simply changing all the signs. Among the flexible forms the twist is the most stable, but nevertheless is 5 kcal above the chair. It is characterized by a symmetry in the signs and the values of the torsional angles with respect to a line linking two opposite corners of the ring. This line represents the axis of the twist.

At a slightly higher energy, we find the boat with four small torsional angles of antisymmetric sign with respect to the plane of symmetry of the boat and a plane perpendicular to this latter. In the same figure, information is given about cyclohexanone because of the interest of this chromophore in optical activity. Here also, the more stable form is the chair. The sequence of signs is the same as in cyclohexane but the values of the angles are slightly different.

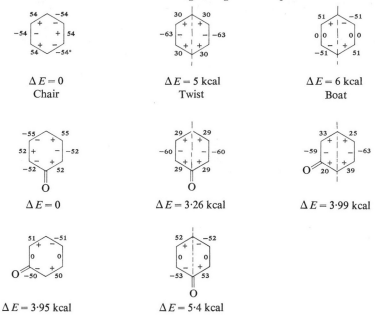

$\Delta E = 0$
Chair

$\Delta E = 5$ kcal
Twist

$\Delta E = 6$ kcal
Boat

$\Delta E = 0$

$\Delta E = 3\cdot26$ kcal

$\Delta E = 3\cdot99$ kcal

$\Delta E = 3\cdot95$ kcal

$\Delta E = 5\cdot4$ kcal

Fig. 3 (modified from reference 7).

The next two forms are the twist ones with the carbonyl along and off the axis. It can be seen that the difference in energy from the chair is less than in cyclohexane. The first boat form with the carbonyl outside the plane of symmetry has practically the energy of the twist forms and can compete with them. However, the second boat form with the carbonyl in the symmetry plane is higher in energy, practically at the same level as the boat form in cyclohexane itself.

Figure 4 displays more succinctly the same analysis for cyclopentane[8] and cycloheptane.[9] In these rings many conformations of almost equivalent energy exist because of the pseudo-rotation phenomenon. We have only given the symmetric forms in the figure.

From the application of the rules given above and the use of the data presented in Figs. 3 and 4 and others found in the literature on non-bonded interaction,[10] an inventory of the more probable conformers can be made. The result is at best semi-quantitative and the classification of a series of conformers is rather difficult when the differences in strain energy are small.

Improved methods are more and more often used following Westheimer's pioneer work.[11] Not only do they permit the total energy of deformation of the model of the given conformer to be obtained by expressions such as [6], they also modify the parameters of the entire molecule step by step until the form of lowest energy is reached.

In fact, it should be recalled that the well known forms for the rings, such as chair, twist, half-chair, etc. are limiting forms rarely encountered as such in real molecules. As the X-ray diagrams point out, the exact form of molecules is somewhere intermediate between limiting forms. These new methods minimizing the

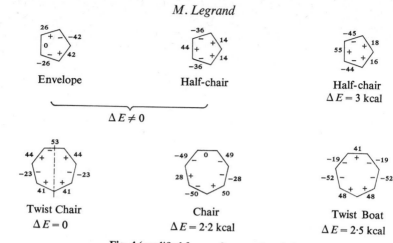

Envelope   Half-chair   Half-chair
$\Delta E = 3$ kcal

$\Delta E \neq 0$

Twist Chair   Chair   Twist Boat
$\Delta E = 0$ $\Delta E = 2\cdot2$ kcal $\Delta E = 2\cdot5$ kcal

Fig. 4 (modified from references 8 and 9).

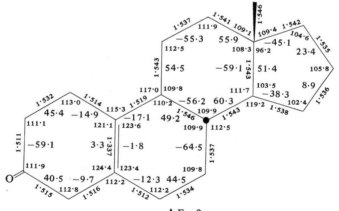

$\Delta E = 0\cdot9$ kcal/mole

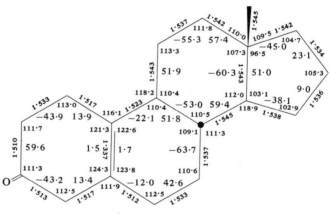

$\Delta E = 0$

Fig. 5 (redrawn from reference 3).

energy of deformation by distributing it over the bond lengths and angles, the dihedral angles and the non-bonded interactions, give intermediate forms which are closer to the reality.

With these techniques the result is heavily dependent on the functions chosen to describe the different types of strain energy. Also, the starting formula, necessary in order to begin the computations, influences the final result. This is common to all these types of method. The minimum obtained is not necessarily the minimum minimorum but one corresponding to a conformation closest to that initially given. In practice, molecular models give a first selection, and the parameters leading to an energy minimum for each proposed conformer are computed by machine.

Figure 5 shows an example of such a calculation. The only reasonable conformers following Dreiding's models are inverted half-chairs for ring A, but it is difficult to say which of the two is the more stable. The computation allows a classification which is confirmed by chemical results. The search for the optimum took 10 minutes with an IBM 360-75 and necessitated the evaluation of 5000 intermediate conformations.

4.1.3 Experimental Conformational Analysis

The physical methods applicable to the study of conformations are numerous and among them X-ray diffraction deserves special mention. When applicable, this method gives a tridimensional image of the whole molecule, which is not the case with other methods. But it can only be used with crystalline material so that the molecule is observed in a crystalline field and its conformation could be very different from that in solution. However, it should be pointed out that the agreement is generally good between X-ray determination, theoretical calculations and experiments when there is a large difference in strain energy between the two most stable conformers.

The other physical methods usually applied in conformational analysis are circular dichroism and optical rotatory dispersion, NMR and sometimes dipole measurements. When applying optical activity, the approaches are essentially the same as for configuration determinations,[12] but more attention must be given to small variations of wavelength or amplitude.

A. Direct Comparison

The first possible method is to compare directly products having the same chromophore, the same configuration around it and a similar surrounding. If these conditions are fulfilled, the method is straightforward: when two compounds give superimposable curves they probably have the same conformation around the chromophore.

One example drawn from a work on the configuration of oxindolic alkaloids illustrates this approach.[13] I, II, III have the same configuration at the spiro junction and at the junction between the rings C and D. By comparing the CD curves given in Fig. 6, it can be seen that the ring closure which differentiates I from II has little effect on the spatial distribution of atoms around the chromophore, here the oxindole; on the other hand, the inversion of the ethyl group substituted on the ring D modifies the CD curves more profoundly, which probably indicates that rings

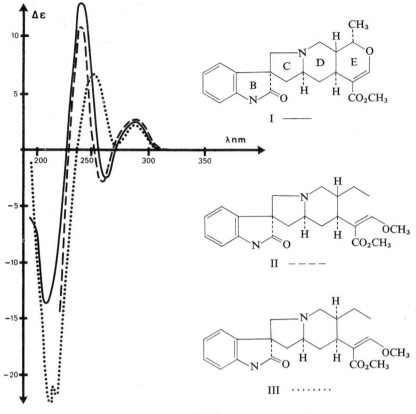

Fig. 6

C and D have not the same conformation in II and III. This can be easily understood with molecular models which show strong steric hindrance around the spiro junction: in III, the ethyl group can only be axial, which adds to the strain.

This approach is limited in use because only identity or non-identity can be detected. Nothing can be said about the real conformations and the nature of possible differences. It is however frequently applied to chromophores for which no reliable rules relating the optical activity to the structures are available. In these cases, configurations and conformations are very often examined together and, when the curves of a series of products are superimposable, it can be deduced that their configuration and conformation are the same or similar for all of them.

B. Semi-quantitative Estimation

The second approach is more complex. Firstly, by conformational analysis, the most stable conformers are selected by the usual criteria; that is a species is neglected if its difference in conformational energy from the most stable conformer is much higher than RT. Secondly, by applying the known rules concerning the chromophore the optical activity of the selected conformers is estimated taking into account their different concentrations in the medium at the selected temperature. From the comparison with experimental data, the results of the conformational analysis can be tested.

The validity of the test and the possibility of distinguishing between two conformers of close strain energy depend on the quality of the conformational analysis and on the exactness of the quantitative estimation of the optical activity. At first, only qualitative analyses were made, as in the example given in Fig. 7 taken from work by Djerassi and Klyne.[14]

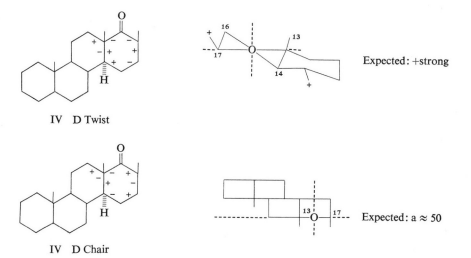

IV   D Twist

Expected: +strong

IV   D Chair

Expected: a ≈ 50

Found experimentally: a = +150°

Fig. 7 (modified from reference 14).

In the D homosteroid IV, the 17- and 18-methyl are in a strong non-bonded interaction if the D ring has a chair conformation. The straightforward means to release this strain energy is to get the D ring in twist form, since as the sequence of signs shows the 17-methyl is now equatorial. Cyclohexanones in this conformation give very strong amplitudes as two carbons of the ring are in octants of same sign (Fig. 7). On the other hand, the value of the ORD amplitude of the chair form can easily be anticipated: the same D homosteroid without 17-methyl has practically no Cotton effect. So, only the contribution of the axial 17-methyl should be expected, that is a = +50. The experimental value of +150 is more in agreement with the hypothesis of a twist conformation. In such a case, the Cotton effect is so characteristic that the qualitative analysis is quite sufficient.

When differences are less evident, especially if equilibrium between conformers is suspected, a semi-quantitative or even a quantitative analysis is required.

A series of B homosteroids studied by Snatzke and a team from Belgrade University, and partially represented in V and VI, is a good illustration of this situation.[15] For the different configurations at the AB junction, the only reasonable conformations of the B ring are the twist chairs given in Tables 1 and 2. The number following 'twist chair' indicates the position of the axis in the ring. Other conformations are

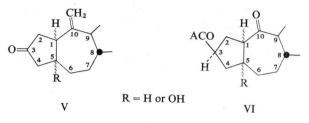

R = H or OH

incompatible either with the junctions between B and A and C and/or add strong non-bonded interactions. The difference in strain energy of the different conformations is estimated following the indications given by Hendrickson.[9]

It can be seen from Tables 1 or 2 that when R = H an equilibrium between nearly equal quantities of the different conformers can be expected, except for the series $1\alpha, 5\beta$, where twist chair 6 is predominant.

Table 1
Five-membered Ring Ketones (Modified from Reference 15)

Configuration	Conformation	ΔE		$\Delta\varepsilon$ expected		$\Delta\varepsilon$ found	
		R = H	R = OH	R = H	R = OH	R = H	R = OH
$1\alpha,5\alpha$	Twist chair 5	0·4	0·4	0·4	4·2	—	2·7
	Twist chair 1	0·2	2·17				
$1\beta,5\alpha$	Twist chair 9	0·1	0·1	2·5	2·7	—	3·34
	Twist chair 10	0·5	1·80				
$1\alpha,5\beta$	Twist chair 6	1·6	1·6	1·1	1·3	—	—
	Twist chair 7	0·4	0·7				
$1\beta,5\beta$	Twist chair 1	0·1	0·1	0	−0·4	−1·92	—
	Twist chair 5	0·8	0·8				
	Twist chair 8	0·5	1·2				

Table 2
Seven-membered Ring Ketones (Modified from Reference 15)

Configuration	Conformation	ΔE		$\Delta\varepsilon$ expected		$\Delta\varepsilon$ found	
		R = H	R = OH	R = H	R = OH	R = H	R = OH
$1\alpha,5\alpha$	Twist chair 5	0·4	0·4	0	−0·2	—	−0·06
	Twist chair 1	0·2	2·17				
$1\beta,5\alpha$	Twist chair 9	0·1	0·1	6	4·2	—	3·52
	Twist chair 10	0·5	1·8				
$1\alpha,5\beta$	Twist chair 6	1·6	1·6	0·3	−0·5	—	—
	Twist chair 7	0·4	0·7				
$1\beta,5\beta$	Twist chair 1	0·1	0·1	2·1	1·8	3·18	—
	Twist chair 5	0·8	0·8				
	Twist chair 8	1·2	1·2				

The second and perhaps more difficult part of this approach involves computing the optical activity, in this case the circular dichroism, of each conformation. In the absence of an effective method of calculation, approximate values, obtained from more or less similar compounds are used. Finally, a weighted sum of the contribution of the different conformers gives the expected values shown in Table 1 for the five-membered ring ketones and in Table 2 for the seven-membered ones.

Not all the isomers studied have been chemically prepared; but with perhaps the exception of the cyclopentanone-$1\beta,5\beta$, the concordance is relatively good in spite of the approximations introduced.

As already pointed out, the real conformations of rings are intermediate between the limiting forms such as chair, twist, boat, etc. used in qualitative analysis, since the molecule accommodates strong non-bonded interactions or difficult junctions by small deformations of the limiting forms. This situation has been demonstrated by Allinger with 3 keto A/B *trans* steroids methylated in positions 2 and 4.[16] The results are summarized in Table 3. Only the most stable conformations are indicated for each compound and the corresponding strain energy computed by Allinger is reproduced in the third column of the table.

In all cases, the flattened chair is the more stable form, except for the 2β-methyl compound (VII, $R_1 = CH_3$, $R_2 = H$) where some equilibrium could be present. For this latter and the corresponding 2-gem-dimethyl (VIII, $R_1 = CH_3$, $R_2 = H$) the ORD confirms the conclusion of the conformational analysis, since among the more stable forms the flattened chair alone can produce in sign and amplitude the experimentally found ORD. For the 4-methyl and the gem-dimethylated compounds at the same position (VII and VIII, $R_1 = H$, $R_2 = CH_3$) the ORD does not contradict

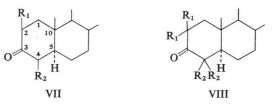

VII   VIII

Table 3
(Modified from Reference 16)

Compound	Conformation	ΔE calc.	a expected	a observed
VII $R_1 = CH_3$	Twist axis 1·4	4·4	W sign?	
$R_2 = H$	Boat 2·5	3·7	W neg.	+73
	Flattened chair	3·8	M pos.	
VII $R_1 = H$	Twist 1·4	6·9	W sign?	
$R_2 = CH_3$	Flattened chair	5·4	M.W. pos.	+11
VIII $R_1 = CH_3$	Twist 1·4	5	S neg.	
$R_2 = H$	Boat 2·5	9·7	S neg.	+80
	Flattened chair	4·1	M.S. pos.	
VIII $R_1 = H$	Twist 1·4	7·7	W. sign?	
$R_2 = CH_3$	Flattened chair	6·2	M.W. neg.	−14

W = weak; M = medium; S = strong.

the result of conformational analysis but a second experimental method is necessary to confirm it. Allinger used the dipole moment technique.

When more than one or two species are present in the solution the conformational analysis is much more difficult. However, Ouannes and Jacques have obtained good results with substituted monocyclopentanones (IX to XII[17] see Table 5).

In a ring of such a low symmetry, there are many possible conformations which are readily interconvertible via pseudo-rotation, each carbon of the ring being successively situated in the plane of symmetry of the molecule (envelope) or along the symmetry axis (half-chair: Fig. 8). If substituents are present, all these symmetric forms are no longer equivalent in energy. During a pseudo-rotation, 20 symmetrical conformations are encountered. For each of them, the strain energy has been computed, and equilibrium concentrations deduced.

For 3-methyl cyclopentanone, Fig. 9 shows the 10 more stable conformations in order of increasing energy. The diagram corresponds to octant projections. Table 4 gives the calculated strain energy for each of the conformations and the percentage

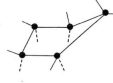
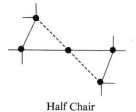

Envelope   Half Chair

Fig. 8

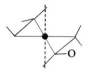
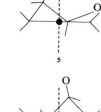
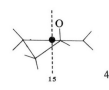
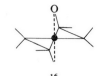

6   5   15   4   16

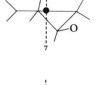
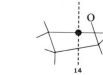
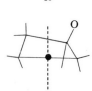

7   17   14   4

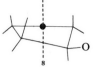
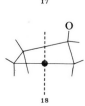

8   18

Fig. 9 (modified from reference 17).

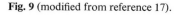

Table 4
(From Reference 17)

Confor- mation number	4	5	6	7	8	14	15	16	17	18
E	9·75	9·01	8·78	9·26	10·21	9·64	9·00	9·03	9·60	10·45
P%	4·4	16·2	23·4	10·25	1·95	5·3	16·2	15·2	5·75	1·3
a	+80	+80	+220	+80	+80	−80	−80	−220	−80	−80
a_p	+3·5	+12·9	+51·5	+8·2	+1·6	−4·2	−12·9	−33·4	−4·6	−1·1

Table 5
(From Reference 17)

Compound	a expected	a found
IX	21·5	86
X	−49	−69
XI	−141	−80
XII	Weak	−17

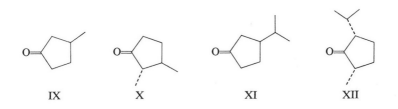

IX   X   XI   XII

present at 20° at room temperature. The second steps again involve estimating the optical contribution of the different conformers. Ouannes and Jacques adopted as a first approximation a value of ±200 for projections such as 6 or 16 and ±80 for all the others. These values are obtained from ORD results on 1 and 2 hydrindanone, and are indicated with their sign for each conformer of Table 4. By multiplying rows 2 and 3 of the table, the contribution of each conformer is calculated (row 4) and the summation of all of them gives the value of +21·5 for the mixture.

Computations have been made for compounds IX–XII and the expected values of a, together with the experimentally found ones, are given in Table 5. The agreement can be considered good, given the approximations used.

The carbonyl chromophore is not the only symmetric chromophore which can be utilized for conformational analysis. Studies have been effected with lactones, acids and esters, peptides, nitro derivatives, azoalkanes, aromatics, sulphoxides, sugars, indolic alkaloids and even very complex molecules such as tetracyclines. But it should be pointed out that in certain of these cases, so little is known about the optical activity of the chromophore, that the approach adopted looks more like the first one described than the second.

All the chromophores previously cited are of the symmetric type. Their use is often critical because the Cotton effect is the resultant of the contribution of the atoms or groups of atoms distributed around them. Inherently dissymmetric chromophores should be, *a priori* easier to use since a simple relation generally exists between their geometry and the sign of the Cotton effect but they generally allow the determination of only one parameter.

In complex molecules, this is not sufficient to establish the general conformation, but it often gives a very good idea. In conjugated ketones, for instance, the sign of the Cotton effect is related to the sign of the torsional angle between the carbonyl group and the double bond if this angle is sufficiently different from zero.[18] When the conjugated ketones are embedded in a polycyclic system, knowledge of the sign of this angle is often sufficient for determining the conformation of the ring.

Table 6

Compounds	$\Delta\varepsilon_{n\to\pi^*}$(ET OH)	$\Delta\varepsilon_{\pi\to\pi^*}$(ET OH)	Sign of Φ deduced
XIII	−1·44	+4·93	−
XIV	+1·50	−19·19	+
XV	−2·18	+19·60	−
XVI	$\neq 0$	$\leqslant 0$	?
XVII	+4·08	−25·60	+
XVIII	−1·93		−
	(Dioxane)		

Compounds XIII–XVIII are steroid conjugated ketones differently substituted in 1 and 11.[19] From Table 6, it can be concluded that all of them belong to the group of inherently dissymmetric chromophores since the sign of their n → π^* and $\pi \to \pi^*$ transitions are opposite and the amplitude of their $\pi \to \pi^*$ is strong. (The non-substituted 11-ketone, XVI, is an exception.) Applying Moscowitz's rule for conjugated ketones, the sign of the torsional angle ϕ can be deduced (Table 6).

The limiting forms of the conformer corresponding to negative and positive signs are half-chair (a) and (b) with inverted signs for A ring torsional angles; form (a) is the more stable conformer for testosterone (not represented here). It is adopted by the non-substituted products and the compounds axially substituted. For the others, XIV and XVII, the steric hindrance between the 1β-methyl group and the position 11, is such that the ring adopts the less privileged form (b).

No exact conformational analysis has yet been made but in a simple way, one can see that in the b form, the 1β-methyl group is axial but is not in strong interaction with the other groups since the 10-methyl is now equatorial to the A ring, as the sequence of signs of the torsional angles shows (Fig. 10).

In most of the examples given in this paper, emphasis has been laid on the necessity for good theoretical conformational analysis for interpreting the optical activity of the conformers studied. We have, now, at our disposal, methods which seem to give a close approximation to the reality. Although not yet perfect, they are constantly being improved, both in their facility of use and their reliability. On the other hand, the success of a study of conformers by optical activity is conditioned by the possibility of computing the rotational strength of the conformers selected. At present,

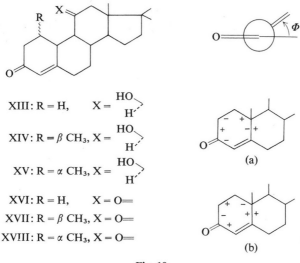

XIII: R = H,   X = $\overset{HO}{\underset{H}{\diagdown}}$

XIV: R = β CH$_3$, X = $\overset{HO}{\underset{H}{\diagdown}}$

XV: R = α CH$_3$, X = $\overset{HO}{\underset{H}{\diagdown}}$

XVI: R = H,   X = O=

XVII: R = β CH$_3$, X = O=

XVIII: R = α CH$_3$, X = O=

Fig. 10

no effective method exists and this is certainly the principal drawback in conformational analysis.

Allinger was very conscious of this problem when he made some criticisms about Djerassi's article concerning the conformation of the 17-acetyl chain in 20-ketone steroids.[20] To quote: 'The qualitative usefulness of Cotton effect curves has been tremendous, but until they can be calculated quantitatively, one must use caution in making predictions about systems which contain groups in both positive and negative octants.' This was in 1966, and we are not much more advanced now.

The same author with Chow-Tai made an attempt at a semi-empiric quantum mechanical method for determining rotational strength induced in a ketone.[21] It required the experimental determination of two parameters for each group inducing optical activity using molecules of known geometry including the group. The calculation of rotational strength involved the computation of the overlapping integral between the group X and n and π* orbitals of the carbonyl group.

This method seems to have only been tried with methyl groups on cyclohexanone and ketosteroids. The agreement between the estimation and the experiment was fairly good, but apparently, some speculations have been necessary to adjust some of the parameters, and it is not at all certain that this procedure can be extended to more complex cases.

On the other hand, dissymmetric solvation such as Coulombeau and Rassat encountered with some terpenes can be a severe disturbance in quantitative and sometimes qualitative work[22] and it is a wise precaution to make measurements in different solvents to detect such solvent effects. If there are any, one must be very careful in the conclusions of the analysis.

A first consequence of all these imperfections is that the resolution of the conformational analysis by optical activity is not very high for distinguishing the right conformer among different possibilities. On the other hand, this is a very sensitive method which can be used advantageously to detect small changes in a family of similar products.

A second consequence is that, as far as possible, other experimental methods should be applied jointly with ORD or CD. For complex molecules, the more frequently used are NMR and dipole moment. Both of them give information similar to that obtained with inherently dissymmetric chromophores; that is one parameter of the conformation is given, generally a torsional angle by NMR or the relative orientation of two polar groups in the molecule by dipole moment measurement.

By adding together the information obtained by these methods, the optical activity and the theoretical analysis of conformations, a fairly good image of the molecule is generally reached.

Finally, when an equilibrium of conformers is present in solution or is easily obtained by warming the solution, more information can be obtained either by varying the nature of the solvent and/or the temperature. This possibility will be developed in Chapter 4.2.

Thanks are due for permission to reproduce the following material in this chapter:

Figure 5 (ref. 3) by permission of Robert Maxwell & Co. Tables 4 and 5 (ref. 17) by permission of Masson et Cie, Paris.

References

1. J. D. Kemp and K. S. Pitzer, *J. Amer. Chem. Soc.* **59**, 276 (1937).
2. J. E. Williams, P. J. Stang and P. Von R. Schleyer, *Ann. Rev. Phys. Chem.* **19**, 531 (1968).
3. N. C. Cohen, *Tetrahedron* **27**, 789 (1971).
4. R. Bucourt, *Bull. Soc. Chim. Fr.* 2080 (1964); R. Bucourt and D. Hainaut, *Bull. Soc. Chim. Fr.* 1366 (1965); *Bull. Soc. Chim. Fr.* 501 (1966).
5. W. Klyne and V. Prelog, *Experientia* **16**, 521 (1960).
6. J. B. Hendrickson, *J. Amer. Chem. Soc.* **83**, 4537 (1961).
7. R. Bucourt and D. Hainaut, *Bull. Soc. Chim. Fr.* 4562 (1967).
8. R. Bucourt. Private communication.
9. J. B. Hendrickson, *Tetrahedron* **19**, 1387 (1963).
10. Y. L. Chow, C. J. Colon and J. N. S. Tam, *Can. J. Chem.* **46**, 2821 (1968); R. Pauncz and D. Ginsburg, *Tetrahedron* **9**, 40 (1960).
11. F. H. Westheimer, in M. S. Newman, Ed., *Steric Effects in Organic Chemistry*. John Wiley, New York, 1956, p. 523.
12. L. Velluz, M. Legrand and M. Grosjean. *Optical Circular Dichroism, Principles, Measurements and Applications*. Verlag Chemie, Academic Press, 1965.
    P. Crabbé, *Optical Rotatory Dispersion and Circular Dichroism in Organic Chemistry*. Holden Day, 1965.
    P. Crabbé, *Application de la Dispersion Rotatoire et du Dichroïsme Circulaire Optique en Chimie Organique*. Gauthier Villars, Paris, 1968.
    L. Velluz and M. Legrand, *Bull. Soc. Chim. Fr.* 1785 (1970).
13. J. L. Pousset, J. Poisson and M. Legrand, *Tetrahedron Lett.* 6283 (1966).
14. C. Djerassi and W. Klyne, *Proc. Natl. Acad. Sci. U.S.A.* **48**, 1093 (1962).
15. M. Lj. Mihailovic, Lj. Lorenc, J. Forsek, H. Nesovic, G. Snatzke and P. Trska, *Tetrahedron* **26**, 557 (1970).
16. N. L. Allinger and M. A. DaRooge, *J. Amer. Chem. Soc.* **84**, 4561 (1962).
17. C. Ouannes and J. Jacques, *Bull. Soc. Chim. Fr.* 3611 (1965).
18. C. Djerassi, R. Records, E. Bunnenberg, K. Mislow and A. Moscowitz, *J. Amer. Chem. Soc.* **84**, 870 (1962).
19. D. Bertin and J. Perronnet, *Bull. Soc. Chim. Fr.* 2782 (1964).
20. N. L. Allinger, P. Crabbé and G. Perez, *Tetrahedron* **22**, 1615 (1966).
21. J. Chow-Tai and N. L. Allinger, *J. Amer. Chem. Soc.* **88**, 2179 (1966).
22. C. Coulombeau and A. Rassat, *Bull. Soc. Chim. Fr.* 2673 (1963).

Use of Solvent and Temperature Effects

M. LEGRAND

Department of Physics
Roussel-Uclaf
Romainville, France

4.2.1 Introduction

As seen in the previous Chapter, when ΔG, the difference in free energy between two conformers, is not too much higher than RT in the range of usable temperatures, a mixture of both conformers can be expected in solution. Consequently, at least for some values in the range of variations of ΔG or T, modifications of the experimental conditions lead to a change in the measured rotational strength, following the relation [1].

$$R_{obs} = (R_1 C_1 + R_2 C_2)/(C_1 + C_2)$$
$$= [R_1 + R_2 \exp(-\Delta G/RT)]/[1 + \exp(-\Delta G/RT)] \qquad [1]$$

In this expression R_1 and R_2 are the rotational strengths of the pure conformers and C_1 and C_2 are their concentrations.

For more than two conformers, similar equations can be written:

$$R_{obs} = \left(\frac{R_1 + R_2 \exp(-\Delta G_{12}/RT) + \cdots + R_i \exp(-\Delta G_{1i}/RT)}{1 + \cdots + \exp(-\Delta G_{1i}/RT)} \right) \qquad [2]$$

where ΔG_{1i} is the free energy difference between the more stable conformer and the conformer i. The factor $\Delta G/RT$ can be varied by acting on ΔG or on T or on both.

4.2.2 Variations of ΔG

(a) Chemical modifications of the molecule are a means of changing ΔG, but it can no longer be said that both molecules are conformers. However, this case is cited here because the method is frequently used to freeze molecules in a given form. For instance, *trans*-2-bromo-4-methyl cyclohexanone, I, gives an equilibrium between equatorial (Ie) and axial (Ia) forms;[1] the introduction of a bulky *tert.*-butyl group at position 5 freezes the equatorial isomer II, because the high steric hindrance exhibited by this group in the axial position, considerably increases ΔG between the two inverted chairs.[2] To a first approximation, the contribution of the *tert.*-butyl group is not very different from that of a methyl group and from this point of view II can be considered as the equatorial conformer of I.

Table 1 shows that the axial isomer in I imposes its sign on the Cotton effect, the bromine atom being in a negative octant in this isomer, and that a change in the polarity of the solvent modifies the equilibrium. With II, the Cotton effect is positive as expected from the octant rule for the equatorial isomer and insensitive to the solvent.

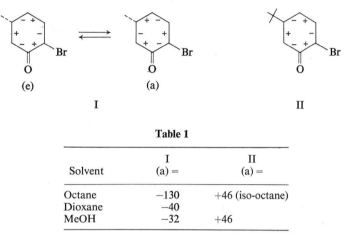

Table 1

Solvent	I (a) =	II (a) =
Octane	−130	+46 (iso-octane)
Dioxane	−40	
MeOH	−32	+46

When the bulky group is introduced into a molecule in order to freeze out one conformer, it could be thought that the optical activity of the new compound would be a good approximation of the rotational strength of the remaining isomers. But distortions of the skeleton can be caused by the bulky group, even in the equatorial position, and these modify the expected value of the rotational strength.[3]

(b) Other means of changing ΔG are physical in nature and apparently the only possibility so far used for the study of small molecules is the modification of the polarity of the medium by changing the solvent. In order to be sensitive to a change of solvent the molecule should possess either an internal hydrogen bond or strongly polar groups in interaction.

A. Internal Hydrogen Bonding

If some conformers of the molecules have the right spatial disposition to give an internal hydrogen bond while others cannot do so, then a competition is possible between the solvent and the groups forming the H bonds in the molecule. If the solvent is a donor or acceptor stronger than the corresponding groups of the molecule it breaks the bonding so that the stabilizing energy brought by the H bond is lost. Indeed, this case could be almost classified with the chemical modifications of ΔG, since a bond is modified inside the molecule. But generally, such a transformation is not considered as a chemical one by chemists. Several cases of this type have been described in the literature, concerning generally hydroxyketones.[4] 17α-OH,17β-Acetylsteroid, for example, studied by Danilewicz[5] and by us,[6] is a good illustration of this effect.

The conformation of a 17β-acetyl chain when no hydroxyl group is present in α (IIIa), has been thoroughly studied by Djerassi[7] and confirmed by Allinger *et al.*[8] applying theoretical conformational analysis and verifying the results by dipole moment measurements. A summary of Allinger's analysis is given in Table 2.

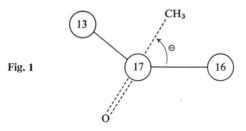

III(a): X = H
III(b): X = OH

Table 2

Pregnan-20-one. (Modified from Reference 8)

Θ	ΔE 17α-H	ΔE 17α-OH
0	6·8 Kcal	6·4 Kcal
60	4·4	4·2
120	10·5	10·3
180	1·0	0·9
210	0·7	0.7
240	1·3	2·2
300	1·9	1·9

θ is the torsional angle formed by the carbons 16, 17, 20 and 21 (Fig. 1). From the second column of Table 2 it can be concluded that the stable conformer corresponds to an angle of about 210°. ORD estimations through the octant rule are in agreement with the experimental results and dipole measurements also confirm the conformational analysis. The introduction of a 17-OH, when only strain energy is taken into

Fig. 1

account, does not perturb the situation very much as can be seen from Table 2 in the last column. The non-bonded interactions O ... O, O ... H and O ... C were estimated from Dreiding's models using values given by Scott and Sheraga.[9] Only for $\theta = 240°$ is the interaction between the 17-OH and the 21-CH$_3$ noticeable. For the other values of θ, a small stabilization is apparent, due to London's dispersion forces.

Now, to give a complete picture of the situation, one must take into account the possibility of a hydrogen bonding for $\theta = 60°$. No exact values of energy are known for this type of bond but from Pimentel's review[10] it can be assumed that in this case the H bond has an energy of between 2 and 5 kcal. Consequently, the conformer with $\theta = 60°$ has a ΔG which should be of the same order of magnitude as that of the conformer with $\theta = 210°$.

Fig. 2 shows the circular dichroism of the 3α-acetoxy-17β-acetyl-17α-hydroxy-5α-androstane in cyclohexane. The curve is easily explained on the basis of the conformational analysis given above. The positive maximum corresponds to the nonbonded isomer, $\theta = 210°$ and the negative one to the isomer with hydrogen bonds. The octant projection of both conformers given in the same figure additionally confirms this. The wavelength shift observed between the two maxima is due to the well-known effect of hydrogen bonding on the carbonyl chromophore. As expected, an equilibrium between both conformations is observed at room temperature.

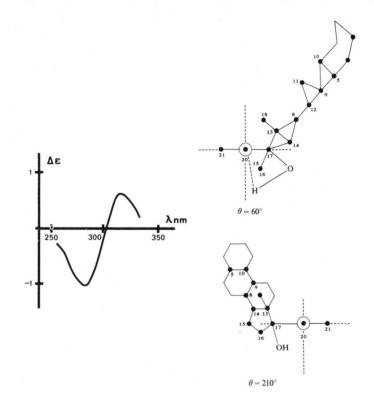

Fig. 2

If cyclohexane is replaced by solvents such as ethanol, capable of forming a hydrogen bond, the conformer with $\theta = 60°$ is no longer stabilized and we revert to the situation of the non-hydroxylated products. Only one positive maximum is then observed experimentally (Fig. 3), comparable to that of the 17β-acetyl without an OH group.

B. Dipolar Interaction

This type of interaction is especially encountered in halogeno-ketones where a strong interaction exists between the carbonyl group and the C—X bond. The interaction energy is related to the dipole moments μ_1 and μ_2 of the groups, some geometrical parameters such as the distance r between the two dipoles and angular terms χ, α_1 and α_2 defining the relative orientations of the groups and the dielectric constant D.

The mathematical expression is given by [3].

$$V_D = \frac{\mu_1 \mu_2}{Dr^3}(\cos X - \cos \alpha_1 \cos \alpha_2) = V/D \qquad [3]$$

In the simplified expression, V groups all the geometric parameters and the values of the dipoles, that is all the terms independent of the solvent.

Fig. 3

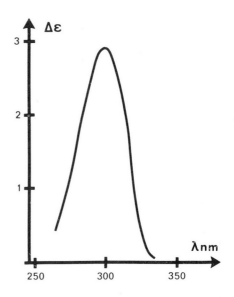

Between two conformers, we have a difference in strain energy given by:

$$\Delta G = \Delta E_s + \Delta V/D \qquad [4]$$

ΔE_s is the difference of energy of deformation and ΔV the difference in electrostatic repulsion for $D = 1$. A change of solvent modifies ΔG through the dielectric constant D. A polar solvent (D high) decreases the repulsion giving more stability to conformers with the two dipoles in the same plane.

The case of the bromocyclohexanone, previously treated, is an example of this situation. Another well-characterized one is found in an article by Kuriyama.[11] The compound studied is a 6β-bromo-3,8-dimethyldecahydroazulen-5-one (IV). A conformational analysis applying the principles given in Chapter 4.1 shows that the most stable isomer is the twist chair form with axis in position 10 (IVe), if the dipole interaction is not taken into account. The other possible form is a twist chair with axis in 6 (IVa) in which the bromine atom is pseudo-axial.

It can be guessed that, if the strain energy and the dipole repulsion energy are of the same order of magnitude, an equilibrium dependent on the polarity of the solvent will be obtained. Circular dichroism curves given by Kuriyama show that this is so

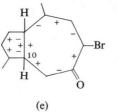 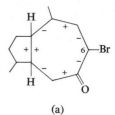

(e)   (a)

IV

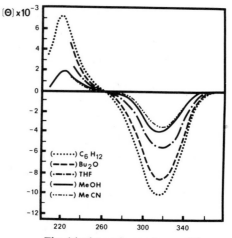

Fig. 4 (redrawn from reference 11).

(Fig. 4). The axial halogen effect at 325 nm is very characteristic in cyclohexane (dotted line) and much less in MeCN. It may be noted that the sign of the dichroism is in agreement with the octant projections (Fig. 5).

A quantitative interpretation has been attempted. By rearranging formula [1], the following expression is obtained:

$$\Delta G = RT \log \left[(R_{obs} - R_a)/(R_e - R_{obs}) \right] \qquad [5]$$

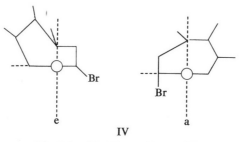

IV

Fig. 5 (modified from reference 11).

where R_a and R_e are the rotational strengths of IVa and IVe. Using expressions [4] and [5], a relation between the dielectric constant of the solvent and R_{obs} is obtained:

$$y = \log \{(R_{obs} - R_a)/(R_e - R_{obs})\} = \Delta E_s/RT + (V/RT) \times Y/D \qquad [6]$$

A value deduced from measurements of the parent ketone without bromine has been tentatively given to R_e and, by trial and error, a value of R_a has been found leading approximatively to a straight line when y is plotted versus $1/D$. Figure 6 shows the result obtained with $R_e = 4 \times 10^{-40}$ c.g.s. and $R_a = -30 \times 10^{-40}$ c.g.s.

From the slope and the intercept, $\Delta E = 0.8$ kcal and $\Delta V = -0.7$ kcal are deduced. They are only approximate values because of the hypothesis made on R_e and possibly asymmetric solvation effects. Nevertheless, they reflect that the equatorial form would be more stable than the axial one, which was confirmed by an X-ray analysis.

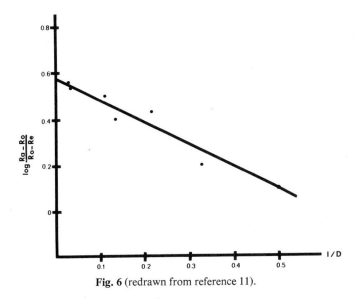

Fig. 6 (redrawn from reference 11).

These two examples might lead us to think that analysis of a solvent effect is straightforward. This is not always the case because other effects not related to conformation modifications can induce changes in optical activity. Asymmetric solvation is probably the most important of them. This phenomenon described for the first time by Coulombeau and Rassat[12] is as yet incompletely elucidated and it is difficult to say when it is effective and when not. In certain cases, a tremendous modification of the optical activity is observed leading sometimes to the inversion of the Cotton effect. Occasionally, associations between molecules of the product studied are observed in certain solvents but this effect can be traced out by a dilution study.

4.2.3 Temperature Effects

The variation of optical activity due to the effect of temperature on the equilibrium between several conformers is more general than the solvent effect. For practical reasons, the range of temperatures experimentally used at present is limited to between −190°C (liquid nitrogen) and around 100°C. Consequently, this method is applicable to conformers with a difference of strain energy in the range of 0·5 to about 3 kcal, but, as already pointed out, a ΔS different from zero could modify this range.

In most cases, studies have been made at low temperatures and for experimental reasons, only in circular dichroism. Many attachments have been described and Fig. 7 shows the one we use in our laboratory which can give any temperature between 37°C and −190°C with an accuracy of ±0·5°C inside the cell.

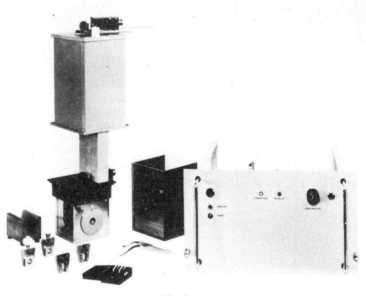

Fig. 7

Solvents generally used at low temperatures are mixtures of methylcyclohexane and isopentane (MI) for work in a non-polar medium, and mixtures of ether, iso-pentane and alcohol (EPA) for a polar medium. These mixtures of solvents have the advantage of giving transparent glasses at low temperatures without any cracking, even if the temperature is rapidly lowered. Other mixtures are possible but these two are the most frequently used. At higher temperatures the choice is greater; decalin is a good solvent for working with a non-polar medium.

Important corrections have to be made to take into account the contraction and expansion of the solvent with the temperature, which change the concentration of the solute.[13]

In general, circular dichroism varies with temperature for four different principal reasons:

(1) The ratio of conformers varies causing a modification of the amplitude of the circular dichroism. This is the effect which we require.

(2) Equilibrium between solvated and non-solvated forms can be changed and new solvated forms can become apparent at low temperatures.

(3) The population of some excited levels of rotational modes or of low energy vibrations can vary, thus inducing a modification of the borrowed rotational strength. This effect is especially important with symmetric chromophores such as the carbonyl group.[14]

(4) Aggregations and micro-crystallizations lead sometimes to unexpected, strong modifications of the optical activity.

This last phenomenon has not very often been cited. However, Horwitz *et al.* described it in detail about two years ago with regard to an *N*-acetylphenylalanyl-amide.[15] It can very often be traced by slowly decreasing the temperature or gently rewarming the solution after a rapid decrease at −190°C. In these conditions germs develop and a visible crystallization becomes apparent, with a fading of the circular dichroism as a whole.

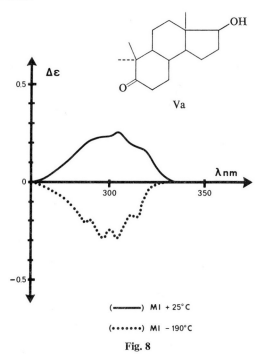

(————) MI + 25°C

(••••••) MI − 190°C

Fig. 8

Solubility plays an important role in aggregation and this trouble can be avoided either by diluting the solution, if this is possible, or by changing the solvent, or even by modifying the molecule at a position far from the chromophore in order to increase its solubility.

We encountered the phenomenon with product Va and Fig. 8 shows the tremendous modification of the CD with temperature. By substitution (Fig. 9) of methoxyl for the hydroxyl at position 17 (Vb) we get an optical activity which does not change much with temperature.

VI is a particularly interesting case because its structure is very close to that of a previously described 11-ketosteroid VII[16] for which the observed inversion of the circular dichroism at low temperature had been related to a flexibility of ring C. We obtained with VI a curve at low temperature very similar to that of VII (Fig. 10). By applying the tests previously described, we were able to conclude that the inversion is due to micro-crystallization: Fig. 11 shows flakes of crystallized product after 20 minutes of rewarming at −140°C. No conclusion can be drawn for VII since the experimental conditions and the structure are not exactly the same. However, the similitude between the curves leads us to assume that the inversion has the same origin in both cases.

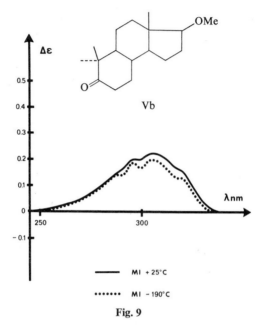

Fig. 9

There are probably some other products whose circular dichroism at various temperatures has been published, which are in the same situation and it is wise to make aggregation tests before correlating large changes in CD to variation in conformation.

Discrimination between the three other effects is not so easy. Vibrational and rotational effects are generally not very important and only give trouble for CD of small amplitude. Solvation is more troublesome because the amplitude of the changes caused by it can be of the same order of magnitude as those issued from a change in conformation. On the other hand, no reliable tests are at present available to distinguish between both effects. Some broadening of a vibronic structure can give an indication. Also, with chromophores capable of forming H bonds with the solvent, the solvated form does not display a CD maximum at the same wavelength as the free form. These two phenomena give information but a general test is not yet available.

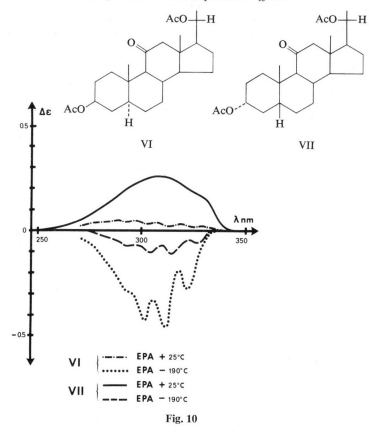

Fig. 10

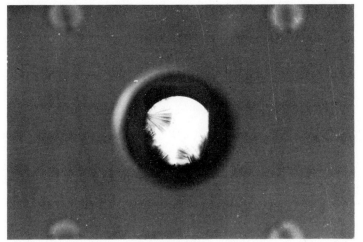

Fig. 11

A. Determination of the Thermodynamic Constants

If the secondary effects described above have a negligible influence, temperature experiments in circular dichroism should be a good method of estimating the thermodynamic constants of the equilibrium between two conformers. In fact, as R_1 and R_2, the rotational strengths of the pure conformers in formula [1], are generally not known, four parameters, R_1, R_2, ΔH and ΔS, must be deduced from the experimental data, which is not an easy operation.

When it can be safely supposed that ΔS is close to zero a simplified method described by Moscowitz can be applied with good results. If $\Delta S = 0$, ΔG is independent of T. So by rearranging [1] as follows:

$$R_{\text{obs}} = (R_1 - R_2)/[1 + \exp(-\Delta G/RT)] + R_2 \qquad [7]$$

and if a good constant value is attributed to ΔG, a straight line should be obtained when R_{obs} is drawn with respect to $[1 + \exp(-\Delta G/RT)]$ as abscissa. ΔG is found by trial and error in such a way that the best fit is reached. Slope and intercept give R_1 and R_2.

Figure 12 shows the example presented by Moscowitz et al.[17] It can be seen that for $\Delta G = 1 \cdot 72$ kcal/mol, almost a straight line is obtained. This value seems plausible for the studied equilibrium.

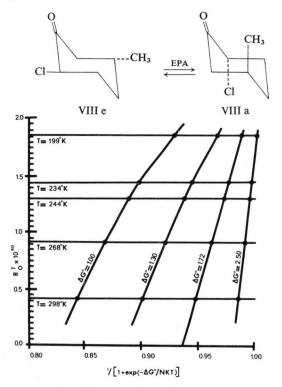

Fig. 12 (redrawn from reference 17).

When ΔS cannot be neglected, iterative methods should be applied. Starting from initial values of the parameters, the latter are adjusted in such a way that a given criterion, generally the sum of the square differences between the experimental and the calculated value of R, is minimized. The use of a computer is necessary. The results obtained with this method are not always satisfactory because the measurements are often not sufficiently accurate. Consequently, even if the mathematical expression [1] does not exactly describe the experimental results, because of solvation

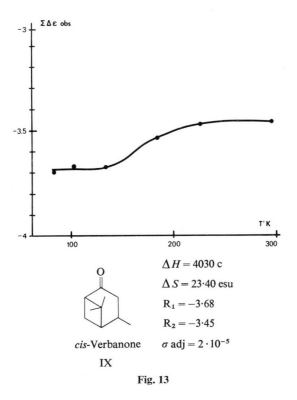

$\Delta H = 4030$ c

$\Delta S = 23 \cdot 40$ esu

$R_1 = -3 \cdot 68$

$R_2 = -3 \cdot 45$

cis-Verbanone σ adj $= 2 \cdot 10^{-5}$

IX

Fig. 13

or for some other reason, it is nevertheless possible to find a set of four parameters for which the error of adjustment is inside the experimental error. Evidently, in these conditions the values of the parameters are without physical significance.

For instance, for the terpene ketone IX the experimental values of $\sum \Delta \varepsilon_{obs}$ at different temperatures are given by the black points in Fig. 13. The curve in full line was computed from equation [1] with the parameters indicated on the figure. The σ obtained for the adjustment is not significantly different from the σ of measurement $(1 \cdot 4\%)$.

However, the values of ΔH and ΔS do not seem realistic; indeed, a value of $\Delta S = 23$ e.s.u. leads us to suppose that we are in the presence of a solvation of the type

$$AS_n \rightleftharpoons A + nS \qquad [8]$$

since $A + nS$ has more degrees of freedom than AS_n. But $\Delta H = 4$ kcal appears far too great for a solvation with a solvent so little polar as MI. A disturbing vibronic effect must be responsible for this situation.

Many other thermodynamic calculations of this type have led to deceptive results. Moreover, it seems that all three causes previously mentioned for the action of temperature are always mixed together and this prevents thorough calculations. Consequently, so long as we have not at our disposal a good mathematical expression and much more accuracy in the measurements, the coefficient:

$$I_{T_0}^T = \frac{T_{\max} - T_{\max}^0}{T_{\max}^0} \times 100 \ (\%)$$

can be used.

However, it should be noted that such a relative coefficient magnifies the effect for CD of small amplitude. Now, some of the causes of variations—for example, solvent equilibrium and possibly vibronic contribution—are not proportional to the average amplitudes and can add or subtract a more or less constant value in a family of compounds of largely different $\Delta\varepsilon_{\max}$, leading to false conclusions for compounds with small amplitudes.

B. Applications

(a) If a compound in solution at room temperature gives an equilibrium between several conformers, the determination of the configuration by optical activity can be misleading when the less preponderant species have much stronger rotational strength.

We were faced with such a difficulty during a total synthesis of steroids with compounds X and XI.[18] Both belong to the cyclopentanone series. As already pointed out in Chapter 4.1, several conformations are possible for this ring of low symmetry, some of them having a positive Cotton effect and the others a negative one. In Fig. 14, which concerns the hydroxy compound X, the negative forms are more stable because in the positive ones two 1,3-diaxial interactions are present instead of one, so we can expect a constant sign with temperature. Indeed, except for an increase in fine structure, the CD is practically invariant (Fig. 15).

The situation is not the same with XI as Fig. 16 shows, since two 1,3 non-bonded interactions are always present because of the ethylene ketal. Consequently, the difference in energy between the negative and positive forms should not be very important. For the first ones, the interaction is between one of the oxygens of the ketal and the methyl group and for the others, it is between the chain and the other ketal oxygen.

Preference is to be given to the negative forms but the difference should be small in energy. In this example the contribution of each conformer to the Cotton effect of the mixture has not been calculated. From the experimental results (Fig. 17), it can be deduced that the negative forms are the more stable but that the intrinsic $\Delta\varepsilon$ values of the positive forms are higher, since at room temperature the net result is positive. As expected, at low temperature circular dichroism is very similar to that of X. This is an example where the wrong enantiomer could have been chosen if measurement has been made only at room temperature.

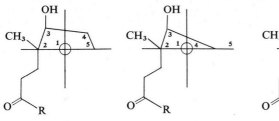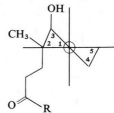

(a)

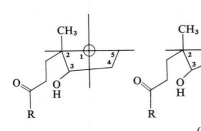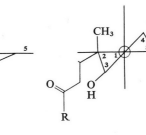

(b)

Fig. 14

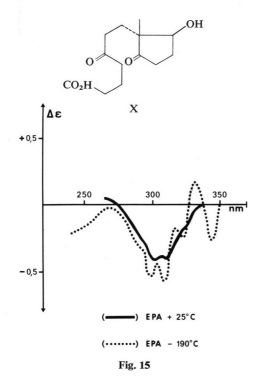

X

(———) E PA + 25°C

(·········) EPA − 190°C

Fig. 15

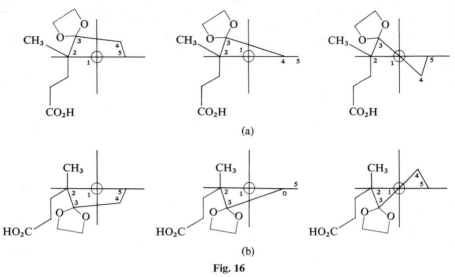

(a)

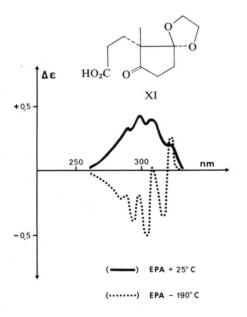

(b)

Fig. 16

(b) When the configuration of the compound is known, temperature experiments are more specially used to confirm a thorough conformational analysis or to decide which conformer is the more stable when the conformational analysis is only qualitative.

Ouannes and Jacques' paper on substituted cyclopentanones described in Chapter 4.1, shows how a temperature study can confirm a rather difficult theoretical analysis. For XII, XIII and XIV (Table 3) the variation of the rotational strength is in agreement with the expected displacement of the equilibrium.[19] For XV no

Fig. 17

conclusion can be drawn because a detailed conformational analysis has not been possible. XVI is an exception and the unexpected stability of the optical activity with temperature is not yet understood.

Table 3. $R \times 10^{-40}$ c.g.s.

(Modified from Reference 19)

	Equilibrium expected	Temperature of room			
		25°	−29°	−74°	−192°
XII	56% Forms +	6·02	—	—	9·88
XIII	56% Forms +	3·35	—	—	4·31
XIV	99% Forms −	−5·22	—	−5·69	−5·27
XV	—	0·849	0·988	1·25	0·506
XVI	65% Forms −	−5·92	—	—	−6·04

Temperature variation of the CD is also frequently used to verify conclusions obtained by other means. We have seen before that in the bromo derivative IV, studied by Kuriyama *et al.*[11] the solvent effect led to the conclusion that the equatorial form was more stable. However the difference between the strain energy added in the axial conformer and the increased stabilization due to the decrease of the dipole interaction is so small (0·1 kcal) that an independent confirmation was desirable. Figure 18 shows the variations of θ_{max} with T. The change from negative to positive values of θ and the fact that this change occurs at very low temperature is in agreement with the preceding conclusions.

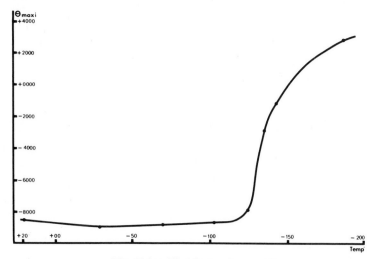

Fig. 18 (modified from reference 11).

Circular dichroism at low temperature may lead to very subtle interpretations. 1-Stercobilin (XVII),[20] an urobilinoid member, was demonstrated to form, at least

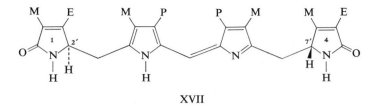

XVII

partially, helices of a single chiral sense, stabilized by intramolecular H bonding (Fig. 19). In a solvent which can form hydrogen bonds such as a mixture of methanol and glycerol, a competition between internal and external H bonding can be expected. In the uncoiled form a definite chirality is not imposed. However, the existence of chiral centres in 2′ and 7′ favours the excess of forms of one chirality over the other. A complex equilibrium between the coiled form and the uncoiled forms of both chiralities is possible. At low temperature, the equilibrium will be shifted towards the more stable form. In this particular case, the experiment showed that it was towards the uncoiled form, exhibiting an optical activity opposite to that of the coiled form (Fig. 20). In a solvent which cannot form strong H bonds, the uncoiled form is now unfavoured and at low temperature the equilibrium is shifted towards

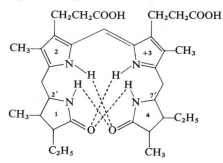

Fig. 19

the coiled form. Consequently, the negative circular dichroism, characteristic of this form in 1-stercobilin increases (Fig. 21).

These few examples were chosen from those whose interpretation is reliable, but very often artefacts make the interpretation difficult. One example will illustrate some of these difficulties.

Low solubility of the compound excludes the use of certain solvents such as MI. This can prevent the examination of products exhibiting an internal hydrogen bond

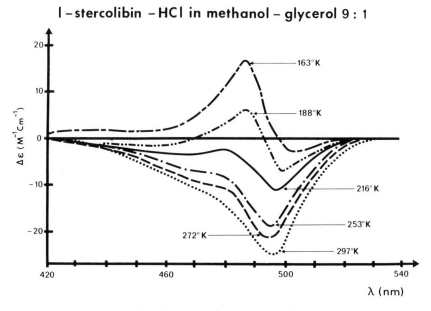

Fig. 20 (redrawn from reference 20).

or at least make this difficult. This was the case with the 17β-acetyl-17α-hydroxy steroid (IIIb) which aggregates before the change in CD with temperature is well on its way.

M. Legrand

When the temperature is lowered, first the CD amplitude of the free form decreases and the negative one (bonded form) increases, which would indicate that the latter is more stable (Fig. 22). But at −190°C a positive maximum is again obtained due to microcrystallization. In fact, the curve at −190°C can only be obtained by a rapid cooling. If the temperature is slowly decreased then dichroism fades out and small crystals become apparent.

More troublesome, because more difficult to detect are the effects of solvation and the vibronic effects. Sometimes changes with temperature can be misleading because

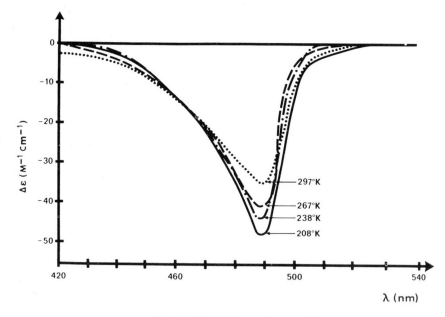

Fig. 21 (redrawn from reference 20).

of them, especially if a quantitative theoretical analysis of conformation is not made.

As for the solvation effect, it is probably always present and authors often admit that they cannot accurately distinguish between this effect and the conformational one. The possible presence of artefacts in temperature studies, and in solvent studies as well, is a severe disadvantage and limits the usefulness of these methods in conformational analysis. This is probably the reason why so many publications are only descriptive without definite conclusions. So long as we have no certain means of distinguishing the solvation effects from the conformation ones, it will often be necessary to apply other methods as a help to the interpretation.

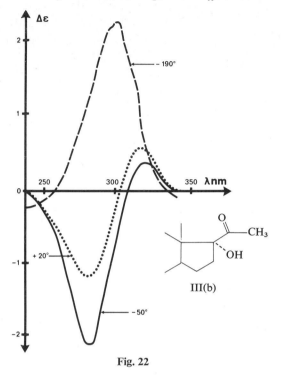

Fig. 22

Thanks are due for permission to reproduce the following material in this chapter:

Figures 4 and 6 (ref. 11) by permission of The Chemical Society, London. Figure 12 (ref. 17) by permission of the American Chemical Society. Figures 20 and 21 (ref. 20) by permission of the National Academy of Sciences, Washington D.C.

References

1. C. Djerassi and L. E. Geller, *Tetrahedron* **3**, 319 (1958); C. Djerassi, L. E. Geller and E. J. Eisenbraun, *J. Org. Chem.* **25**, 1 (1960).
2. C. Djerassi, E. J. Warawa, R. E. Wolff and E. J. Eisenbraun, *J. Org. Chem.* **25**, 917 (1960).
3. C. Beard, C. Djerassi, J. Sicher, F. Sipos and M. Tichy, *Tetrahedron* **19**, 919 (1963).
4. K. M. Wellman, W. S. Briggs and C. Djerassi, *J. Amer. Chem. Soc.* **87**, 73 (1965); T. Suga, T. Shishibori and T. Matsuura, *J. Org. Chem.* **32**, 965 (1967); T. Shishibori, T. Suga, S. Watanabe and T. Matsuura, *Bull. Chem. Soc. Jap.* **42**, 3284 (1969); J. R. Bull and P. R. Enslin, *Tetrahedron* **26**, 1525 (1970); L. Bartlett, D. N. Kirk, W. Klyne, S. R. Wallis, H. Erdtman and S. Thoren, *J. Chem. Soc. C* 2678 (1970).
5. J. C. Danilewicz, Thesis, London, 1963.
6. M. Legrand and V. Delaroff. Unpublished.
7. K. M. Wellman and C. Djerassi, *J. Amer. Chem. Soc.* **87**, 60 (1965).
8. N. L. Allinger, P. Crabbé and G. Perez, *Tetrahedron* **22**, 1615 (1966).
9. T. Ooi, R. A. Scott, G. Vanderkool and H. A. Scheraga, *J. Chem. Phys.* **46**, 4410 (1967).
10. G. C. Pimentel and A. L. McClellan, *The Hydrogen Bond.* Freeman and Co., 1950.
11. K. Kuriyama, T. Iwata, M. Moriyama, M. Ishikawa, H. Minato and K. Takeda, *J. Chem. Soc. C* 420 (1967).
12. C. Coulombeau and A. Rassat, *Bull. Soc. Chem. Fr.*, 2673 (1963).
13. R. Passerini and I. G. Ross, *J. Sci. Instrum.* **30**, 274 (1953).
14. O. E. Weigang, Jr. *J. Chem. Phys.* **42**, 2244 (1965).
15. J. Horwitz, E. J. Strickland and C. Billups, *J. Amer. Chem. Soc.* **91**, 184 (1969).

16. K. M. Wellman, R. Records, E. Bunnenberg and C. Djerassi, *J. Amer. Chem. Soc.* **86**, 492 (1964).
17. A. Moscowitz, K. Wellman and C. Djerassi, *J. Amer. Chem. Soc.* **85**, 3515 (1963).
18. L. Velluz and M. Legrand, *C.R.H. Acad. Sci. Ser. C*, **265**, 663 (1967).
19. C. Djerassi, R. Records, C. Ouannes and J. Jacques, *Bull. Soc. Chim. Fr.* 2378 (1966).
20. D. A. Lightner, E. L. Docks, J. Horwitz and A. Moscowitz, *Proc. Natl. Acad. Sci. U.S.A.*, **67**, 1361 (1970).

Recent Advances in Optical Activity Investigation of Nucleic Acids and Polynucleotides

J. BRAHMS

Institut de Biologie Moléculaire de la Faculté des Sciences de
l'Université de Paris
Paris 5°

4.3.1 Introduction

The aim of this chapter is to correlate the optical properties and particularly the data on the optical activity of polynucleotides and nucleic acids with their macromolecular conformation in solution. The structural parameters of nucleic acids, obtained from the studies on fibres and films by X-ray diffraction and infra-red dichroism, are presented briefly.

Recent refinement of the DNA structure by the King's College group by X-ray analysis supports the double helical model with base pairs of the Watson–Crick type.[1,2]

In Table 1 are summarized structural parameters characterizing different forms of DNA and RNA. The main differences between B-DNA and A-DNA, and also RNA, can be summarized in the following structural parameters:

(1) The arrangement of the base pairs is perpendicular to the helical axis in B-DNA, while tilting of about 20° or of 16° characterizes the A form and RNA. Also in the B form the axis of the helix passes centrally through the base pairs while in the A-form or in RNA the bases are 5 Å or 4·3 Å further away from the axis. The rise per residue along the helix axis is 3·37 Å in the B form, whereas 2·56 Å and 2·8 Å characterizes the A-DNA and RNA, respectively.

(2) Important differences in the orientation of the phosphate residues were detected by infrared dichroism studies of B-DNA and A forms and also of RNA and polynucleotides.[3–5]

(3) The configuration of the sugar residue varies in different forms of DNA and in RNA. This will be considered below in more detail.

The structural parameters shown in Table 1 obtained on films and fibres provide the necessary basis for understanding the ordered structures of some nucleic acids.

J. Brahms

Table 1
Structural Parameters of Nucleic Acids (Investigation of films and fibres)

	A-DNA	B-DNA Na salt	C-DNA Li salt	A-RNA	A'-RNA	Method	References
Residues/turn	11	10	11	11	12	X-ray	80(b), 81
Pitch (Å)	28·2	34·6	31	30·9	36·2	X-ray	
Translation/residue	2·56	3·37	3·3	2·8	3·0	X-ray	82
Angle between bases and the perpendicular to helical axis	20°	0°	6°	14°	9°	X-ray	
Angle of phosphate with helix axis							
θ_{1090} OPO bisector	45°	70°	—	40°		Infrared	4, 5
θ_{1230} O–O line	65°	56°	—	70°		Infrared	3
Sugar pucker	C_3-endo	C_2-endo	C_2-endo	C_3-endo			6, 7
χ_{CN}	82°	143°	139°	62°	82°	X-ray	1, 2
ϕ_{CN}	−14°	−86·7°	−75°				83
Dihedral angle between base planes	16°	5°	10°			X-ray	
Distance between helical axis and base pairs (in Å)	5	0	1·5	4·3		X-ray	1, 2

The investigation of optical activity in the ultraviolet region presents two main advantages: the conformations of biopolymers in solution and particularly in aqueous dilute solution can be studied, and different partially disordered conformations of polynucleotides can be detected which are not attainable by the X-ray diffraction method.

The optical activity of nucleic acids and polynucleotides under investigation occurs in the near-UV region, i.e. in the region of base absorption where the sugars or the phosphate have no absorption bands.

The mononucleotides properties also will be reviewed which appear to be important both for the knowledge of geometry and of optical properties of polynucleotides. In fact, recent comparison of numerous X-ray diffraction results for mononucleotides and nucleosides obtained on single crystals showed that their conformational angles related to nucleic acids are restricted to a few narrow ranges.[6, 7]

4.3.2 Mononucleotides

A. Purine and Pyrimidine Bases

The relatively small optical activity of all mononucleotides or nucleosides can be explained on the following grounds. The bases have a π electron system with planar symmetry and consequently cannot be optically active. The assignment of the electronic origin of the transitions was made by Clark and Tinoco[8] on the basis of correlation with benzene bands and also by Pullman and Pullman.[9] It is now accepted that purine and pyrimidine bases can be correlated with the B_{1u}, B_{2u} and E_{1u} band of benzene; this allowed $\pi \rightarrow \pi^*$ transition in heterocyclic bases characterized by a large extinction coefficient. Furthermore Kasha[10] and Mason[11] indicated that the non-bonding electrons of nitrogen heterocycles give rise to an $n \to \pi^*$ transition of non-allowed character of relatively weak intensity. In adenine spectra the $n \to \pi^*$ longer wavelength transition was recently experimentally resolved[12] in agreement with theoretical prediction. Stewart and Davidson[13] found in crystals of adenine a perpendicularly polarized band. The $\pi \to \pi^*$ transitions of strong intensities are polarized in the plane of the bases.

B. Nucleosides and Nucleotides

The origin of small optical activity in nucleotides and nucleosides must be caused by the perturbation of the base by the asymmetric field of the sugar. The sign and the magnitude of the near Cotton effect must be governed by the orientation of the base relative to the sugar.

Comparison of α-anomers versus β. The proposed rule by Ulbricht and co-workers[14, 15] indicates that the configuration of the sugar affects the sign of the Cotton effect. They attempted to correlate the sign of the Cotton effect with the configuration of the sugar that is with either the presence of β-D-ribose or deoxyribose, as in natural nucleic acids, or α-D-anomers. The reversion of the sign of the Cotton effect allows them to assign the existence of an α or β anomeric configuration.[14] This inversion can be understood easily by molecular model construction, according to which the sugar is placed on the opposite side of the base in an α and β configuration.

Ulbricht and co-workers[14] have observed that pyrimidine-β-nucleoside has a positive Cotton effect while purine-β-nucleoside has a negative one. This empirical rule has also been suggested in several subsequent papers.[16] Recently, Miles et al.[17] investigated a series of uridine and cytidine anomers which, in contrast to the above, give a negative Cotton B_{2u} effect for β anomers and a positive B_{2u} Cotton effect for α anomers.

In conclusion one must emphasize that basic correlation should relate ϕ_{CN} and the rotational strength.

The puckering of sugars was recently thoroughly studied by crystallographic X-ray diffraction.[1, 2, 7, 18(a)] The sugars ribose and deoxyribose exhibit puckers that are either C-2′ endo or C-3′ endo.

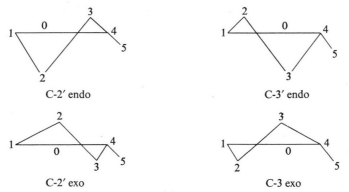

C-2′ endo   C-3′ endo

C-2′ exo   C-3 exo

The conformation is designated endo if the atom most-out-of-plane is on the same side as C-5′ otherwise the designation is exo.

In monomers only two sets C-3' endo and C-2' endo are commonly found. Deoxyadenosine is the sole example of a furanose ring with C-3' exo. The conformation of sugar in B-DNA is C-2' endo; in A-DNA, RNA and polynucleotides it is C-3' endo (see Table 1). At present there is no direct indication that the sugar puckering may significantly influence the optical activity and the optical properties in the spectral region of base absorption.

C. The Torsional Angle ϕ_{CN}

The most important aspect of mononucleotide conformation is the torsional angle ϕ_{CN}. The important feature determining the sign of the Cotton effect is related with nucleoside conformation and is measured by the torsional angle ϕ_{CN}.

The definition of the angle of rotation about the glycosidic bond between $C_{1'}$ of the sugar and N of the base[18(b)]-[20] is shown in Fig. 1. Here the angle is $-50°$ 'anti'.

The torsion angle ϕ_{CN} is the dihedral angle between the plane of the base and the plane formed by the $C_{1'}$—$O_{1'}$ bond of the furanose ring and the $C_{1'}$—N bond. The angle is zero when $O_{1'}$ lies directly in front of C_6 pyrimidine and C_8 for purine; positive angles are measured when C_1—O_1 is rotated in a clockwise direction when viewing from C to N.

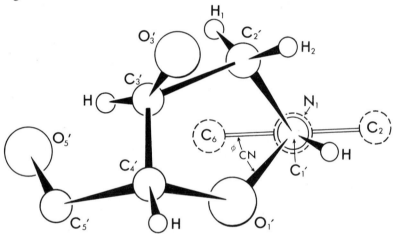

Fig. 1. Illustration of the ϕ_{CN} torsion angle between the plane of the base and the C_1—O bond of the sugar in pyrimidine deoxyribonucleoside (for explanations see the text).

Donohue and Trublood[18] concluded from studies of molecular models that the rotation about the glycosidic bond is restricted mainly by the hydrogen atom bound to $C_{2'}$. They concluded that the base could exist in two conformations differing approximately by 180° which they called *syn* and *anti*. The *anti* range is centred at about $\phi_{CN} = -30°$ and the other at about $+130°$ (the syn range).

Haschemeyer and Rich[19] have computed the steric barriers to rotation about the glycosidic bond with the consideration of sugar puckering. They showed that in pyrimidine nucleoside crystals only the *anti* range is allowed ($-80°$ to $-25°$). In purine nucleoside adenine is in anti conformation, but deoxyguanosine ($C_{2'}$ endo) can form two stable isomers: anti ($\phi_{CN} = -85°$ to $-60°$) and syn ($\phi_{CN} = +110°$) and the barriers of interconversion are not too high.

Several calculations of potential energy associated with the rotation of the base with respect to the sugar around the glycosidic bond indicated that in purine nucleosides the free energy difference between the syn and anti forms is small.[18(a), 21-23]

Crystallographic studies have indicated the almost exclusive presence of the *anti* conformation.[7, 18(a)] However one can enumerate various exceptions: deoxyguanosine, which is *syn* in a mixed crystal with 5-bromodeoxycytidyne;[24] 3′,5′-cyclic AMP, which can exist simultaneously in the anti and syn conformation in the same crystal;[25] 8-bromoadenosine;[26] and 3′-O-acetyl adenosine. More recently, thiouridine was found in the *syn* conformation in the crystalline state.[27] This was also found for uridine by evaluation of conformational energies using molecular orbital calculations.[21]

Finally, several NMR studies have suggested that the anti conformation predominates in solutions.[28-30]

Ulbricht and co-workers[14, 15] have proposed an empirical rule relating the conformation about the glycosidic bond (ϕ_{CN}) of β-D-pyrimide and the sign of the long wavelength Cotton effect,[15] according to which the positive Cotton effect will characterize ϕ_{CN} angles from $-75°$ to $0°$ and to $+105°$.

However, the use of cyclic compounds has been questioned, since the transition dipole moments may be changed by substitution. There are some exceptions to this rule for azapyrimidine and compounds containing chromophores other than the bases.

According to Miles *et al.*[31] the rotational strength depends primarily on the interaction of the B_{2u} transition moment of the base with the pentose ring. The recent calculations of Miles *et al.*[17] of B_{2u} rotational strength as a function of torsional angle by the bond–bond coupled oscillator theory (see below) are in agreement with this empirical rule of Ulbricht.

D. Theoretical Investigations

A substantial effort has been made by Eyring, Miles *et al.* in examining an extensive series of purine and pyrimidine nucleosides and their derivatives in order to assign different electronic transitions. The theoretical work on mononucleosides has been carried out principally by the Eyring and Miles group. The recently published theory of Inskeep *et al.*[32] differs from earlier work. The theoretical basis of their approach is an extension of the coupled oscillator theory of Kuhn–Kirkwood–Tinoco. The $\pi \rightarrow \pi^*$ transition of the base (B_{2u}) can develop significant rotatory power by coupling with intense far-UV bands of the sugar which are approximated by Kirkwood polarizabilities.

The Kirkwood coupled-oscillator theory gives the rotational strength as:

$$R_a = \sum_{b \neq a} \frac{2\pi v_a \, v_b \, \mu_a^2 \mu_b^2}{hc(v_b^2 - v_a^2)} GF$$

where

$$GF = \left[\hat{e}_a \cdot \hat{e}_b - 3 \frac{(\hat{e}_a \cdot \vec{R}_{ab})(\hat{e}_b \cdot \vec{R}_{ab})}{R_{ab}^2} \frac{\hat{e}_a \times \hat{e}_b \cdot \vec{R}_{ab}}{R_{ab}^2} \right]$$

$\hat{e}_b \hat{e}_a$ is the unit vector in the direction of the electronic transition moment of the chromophore, transition $O \rightarrow a$, $\vec{R}_{ab}$ is the distance between the two groups.

The Inskeep theory is based on coupling of bond-centred oscillators. The $\pi \rightarrow \pi^*$ transition moments of the base were calculated using a gradient version of the transition dipole-moment vector into bond contributions and couples each chromophoric band component with the far-UV transitions of the vicinal bonds by their dipole–dipole interactions.

Miles *et al.*[17] prepared and examined a great number of pyrimidine nucleosides many of which are capable of rotation about the glycosidic bond. Their experimental results are in agreement with theoretical predictions and provide evidence for the correctness of their diagram. For the calculation of cytosine and uracil and guanosine derivatives, the authors selected the B_{2u} base transition which may be correct for cytosine and uracil. The conclusion was reached that the main effect is the interaction of the furanose ring with the base that is the dependence on the torsion angle ϕ_{CN}. The ring puckering has a small effect as shown by the diagram in which Miles *et al.* compared the changes of R as a function of ϕ_{CN} for 2′-endo and 3′-endo cytidine and uridine (Fig. 2).

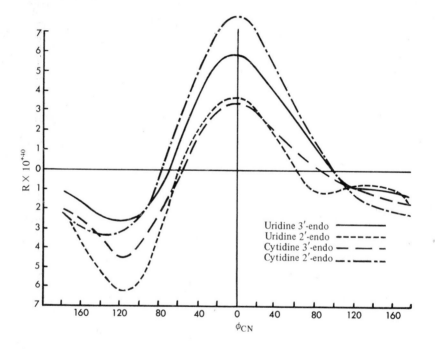

Fig. 2. The dependence of the rotational strength of the B_{2u} transition in uridine and cytosine nucleosides on the torsion angle, ϕ_{CN}, after theoretical computation according to Miles *et al.*[17] and Inskeep *et al.*[32]

Dr. Bush has presented the results of calculations of the CD of adenine mononucleosides in which he took into account the contribution of different electronic transitions n $\rightarrow \pi^*$ and $\pi \rightarrow \pi^*$. The results indicate also that the main contribution to the optical activity of purine nucleosides can be correlated with the ϕ_{CN} torsional angle but not with the puckering of the sugar.

In conclusion, the consideration of optical activity of mononucleotides indicates that the effect of base–sugar interaction is important. It is possible that the changes in ϕ_{CN} are occurring in nucleic acids. However, these effects were not taken into account in theoretical calculations of the optical activity of polynucleotides.

4.3.3 Polymer Model

In polynucleotides and nucleic acids new bands appear not seen in mononucleotides. In these polymers the base chromophores are in a dissymmetric environment of the helical structure. To interpret the circular dichroism spectra of polynucleotides with strong electric-dipole-allowed transitions one must first consider the effect of base–base exciton interaction. The interaction of many identical (or similar) chromophores in a helix will lead to the splitting of a monomer absorption band into more than one band.

A. *Nearest-neighbour (Exciton) Interaction Theory*

The exciton theory seems to be particularly simple and suitable for explaining the optical properties of a polymer or of an aggregate composed of N identical residues with strong, electrically allowed transitions. This theory is based on the exciton idea of Davyodov[33] applied to polymers by Moffitt[34] and Tinoco *et al.*[35] In an oligomer or polymer, a light quantum is not only absorbed by a residue but migrates and leads to the excitation of any of N residues. The transfer of excitation energy occurs by resonance from residue i to the residue j and is characterized by the term V_{ij}, which is very similar to the dipole–dipole interaction energy. This resonance interaction will give rise to the splitting of N degenerate, originally singly excited states into 1, 2, 3, ..., N non-degenerate discrete states. Therefore, the excited state of a polymeric array can be considered as an exciton band of many closely spaced energy levels. A transition of energy $E_K = h v_K$ to each of these exciton levels will give rise to a rotational strength R_K.

Since the same phenomenon of resonance interaction will occur in an oligomer, the simplest case, a dimer, may be considered first. A dimer, e.g. diadenylic acid, ApA, presents the advantage of a particular simplicity in calculation and will allow correlation with experimental results.

B. *Dimer*

1. For a simple dimer composed of two identical monomers the expression for the rotational strength R will be

$$R_{\pm} = \mp \frac{\pi v_0}{2c}\left[\vec{R}_{12}\cdot\vec{\mu}_1 \times \vec{\mu}_2\right]$$

where $\vec{\mu}_1$ and $\vec{\mu}_2$ are two transition dipoles at monomer frequency v_0, and $\vec{R}_{12}$ is the distance between groups 1 and 2. This expression for a dinucleotide in a DNA B form can be simplified to

$$R_{\pm} = \mp \left(\frac{\pi v_0}{2c}\right) R_{12}\,\mu^2 \sin\alpha$$

where α is the angle between two residues. It predicts the conservative spectrum, i.e. the CD spectrum will be composed of two bands of equal magnitude and of opposite sign, that is $\sum R_K = 0$. The splitting will yield two bands with frequencies

$$v_{\pm} = v_0 \pm V_{12}/h$$

where v_0 is the frequency of the monomer band and V_{12} is the interaction energy of residues 1 and 2. V_{12} can be evaluated by theoretical calculations of transition monopoles placed at carbon and nitrogen nuclei in each purine.[36, 37]

The agreement between the calculated and observed spectrum (Fig. 3) supports the theory and the model of a stacked dimer similar to the beginning of a helix.

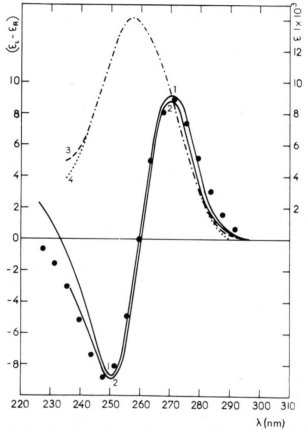

Fig. 3. The circular dichroism and absorption spectra of diadenylic acid (ApA). Curves 1 and 2: CD spectrum at pH 7·4 and 4·9, respectively. Curves 3 and 4: absorption at these two pH. The points correspond to the theoretical curve.[38]

Another way of calculating V_{12} is to apply the dipole–dipole approximation, where the dipoles involved are simply the dipole transition moments according to the expression

$$V_{12} = \frac{1}{R^3}\left[\mu_1 \cdot \mu_2 - \frac{3(\vec{R}_{12} \cdot \mu_1)(\vec{R}_{12} \cdot \mu_2)}{R^2}\right]$$

$\vec{R}_{12}$ is the vector distance between the two point dipoles, $\vec{R}_{12} = (\vec{R}_2 - \vec{R}_1)$.

A third approach for determination of the band position is semiempirical.[38, 39] If one assumes that the dimer (ApA) represents the beginning of a single-stranded helix, the interaction energy V_{12} should be approximately the same in the dimer and in the polymer. Very often this shift is small, but sufficient to be experimentally determined. On the basis of the nearest-neighbour theory,[35] the shift of the maximum in the perpendicularly polarized band ($v_\perp - v_0$) of the polymer is related to that of the oligomer ($v_K - v_0$) by

$$\frac{v_K - v_0}{v_\perp - v_0} = \frac{\cos[\pi K(N+1)]}{\cos \gamma}, \qquad (K = 1, 2, 3, \dots, N)$$

where γ is the angle of rotation of successive residues (bases) about the helix axis. One can thus calculate the absorption frequencies of any oligomer, v_K, from the observed shift in the polymer spectrum.

It is also possible to obtain the position of split bands by the decomposition of a measured CD spectrum.[40] As shown in Fig. 4, the CD of a stacked dimer is resolved into two bands, assuming their shape is Gaussian.

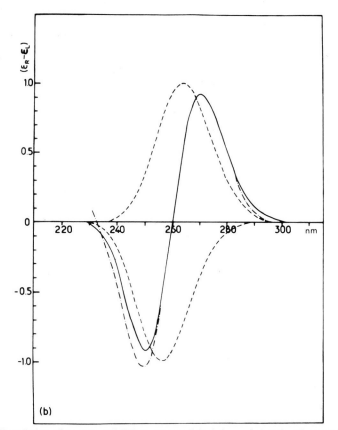

(b)

Fig. 4. Resolution of a measured CD spectrum of ApA (–·–·–) showing the contribution of two bands of equal rotational strength and opposite sign; the obtained separation of these two bands is $\Delta v \sim 1200$ cm^{-1} (ref. 40).

Figure 4 shows the resolution of a measured CD spectrum of stacked ApA (—·—·—) in arbitrary units, demonstrating the contribution of two bands of equal rotational strengths (– – –) and opposite sign, situated at different wavelengths. The obtained separation of these two bands $\Delta v \approx 1200$ cm^{-1}, is in agreement with experimental results of the derivative absorption spectrum of ApA.[40]

Since $\Delta v \ll \Gamma$, one can assume that the shape of the CD curve can be approximated by the derivative of a Gaussian (———), then the value of Γ, the half-band width, can be obtained from the intersection point and one of the extrema, v_{extr}, of the experimental curve according to the expression

$$\Gamma = (v_{extr} - v_0)\sqrt{2 \ln 2}$$

2. Non-degenerate case.—For the dimer composed of different residues, the expression for rotational strength

$$R_{OA} = \frac{\pi}{c} \frac{v_a v_b V_{1a;\, 2b}}{h(v_b^2 - v_a^2)} (\vec{R}_{12} \cdot \vec{\mu}_{10a} \times \vec{\mu}_{20b})$$

$$+ \frac{\pi}{c} \frac{v_a v_b V_{1b;\, 2a}}{h(v_b^2 - v_a^2)} (\vec{R}_{12} \cdot \vec{\mu}_{10b} \times \vec{\mu}_{20a})$$

allows the calculation of the CD spectrum when residue 1 absorbs at v_a and residue 2 at v_b while the second part gives the rotational strength for the dimer in which the residue 1 absorbs at v_b and residue 2 at v_a. Consequently, this equation predicts that the rotational strength R_{OA} will be equal in magnitude and opposite in sign to R_{OB}. Since the local sum rule is obeyed in the spectral region under consideration, this type of spectrum is called conservative by Bush and Brahms;[41] that is

$$\sum_{K}^{N} R_K = 0$$

C. Other Dinucleotides: Non-conservative Spectra

All previously examined oligoadenylate circular dichroic spectra were in good agreement with the exciton theory.[35, 42] Bush and Brahms[41] have found two types of circular dichroic spectra for a variety of $3' \rightarrow 5'$-dinucleotides at low temperatures. The first type, described previously, is called the conservative type, since the sum rule of R is conserved. In this category are the CD spectra of ApU, CpA, CpU, and the typical ApA and adenylate spectra (Fig. 4). However, a second type was found for CD spectra that essentially consist of one or two positive bands observed for GpC and GpA.

Cytidylates (Fig. 5) represent an example of a second category of non-conservative polynucleotide spectra characterized by one main positive band. The principal cause of discrepancy between calculated and observed spectra is probably due to neglecting the interaction with the 200-nm, far-UV transitions, which may be approximated using Kirkwood polarizability.[41]

By applying an approximation such as the Kirkwood polarizability for R owing to the mixing with high-energy states and the exciton theory, Johnson and Tinoco[43] derived an explicit expression for the circular dichroism of dinucleoside.

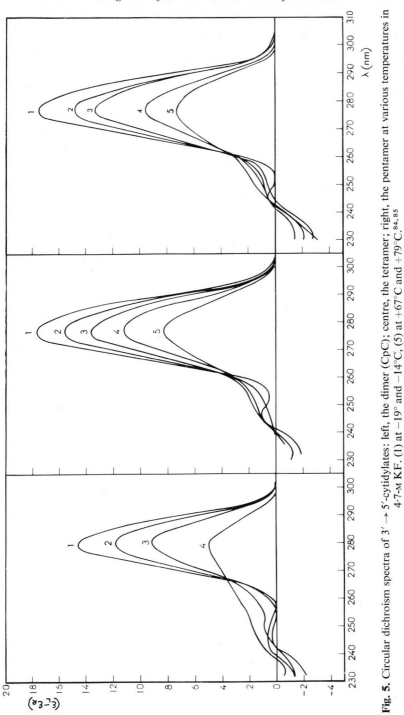

Fig. 5. Circular dichroism spectra of 3′ → 5′-cytidylates: left, the dimer (CpC); centre, the tetramer; right, the pentamer at various temperatures in 4·7-M KF. (1) at −19° and −14°C, (5) at +67°C and +79°C.[84,85]

$$(\varepsilon_L - \varepsilon_R)(v) = \frac{\pi v}{c} f(v - \bar{v}) \sum_{\substack{i,j \\ i \neq j}}' \sum_a v_{i0a} \left[\sum_{s,t} \frac{\rho_s^{i0a}}{r_{st}^3} r_{st} \right] \cdot \vec{\alpha}_t^j \times \vec{\mu}_{i0a} \cdot \vec{R}_{it}$$

$$+ \frac{\pi v}{2c} \frac{\partial f(v - \bar{v})}{\partial v} \sum_{\substack{i,j \\ i \neq j}}' \sum_a v_{i0a} \left[\sum_{s,t} \frac{\rho_s^{i0a} \rho_t^{j0b}}{r_{st}} \right] \vec{R}_{ij} \cdot \vec{\mu}_{i0a} \times \vec{\mu}_{j0b}$$

The Johnson and Tinoco equation can be used to calculate the $\pi \to \pi^*$ rotational strength of a single non-conservative band as well as that of conservative bands composed of positive and negative bands. Johnson and Tinoco's theory can be extended to high polymers. Schneider and Harris,[44] using time-dependent Hartree theory, were able to calculate correctly the CD of ApA with the simple free electron model and by taking into account the 210-nm transition.

It is concluded that the spectra of dinucleotides and also polynucleotides result from two main contributions:

(1) an exciton type contribution giving rise to the conservation of rotational strength over a limited spectral region;

(2) the non-conservative term arising from the interaction between different transitions, particularly with transitions occurring in the far UV.

D. Chain-length Effect

Qualitatively the conclusions reached from dimers can be extended to a polymer. As a function of the degree of polymerization, the rotational strength (or the intensity) of the circular dichroism band increases progressively and reaches a maximum (Fig. 6). Using an appropriate geometrical model and applying the theory, one can obtain information about the distribution of circular dichroism bands and reach some conclusion about the structure in solution, e.g. detect the presence of a single-stranded stacked chain.

CD studies of a series of homo-oligomers allow the spectra to be correlated with structure. This is particularly important for single-stranded synthetic polynucleotides which were believed to exist in an unknown, probably disordered, randomly coiled form.

The same nearest-neighbour theory can be extended to a series of longer oligomers composed of identical residues. The rotational strengths have been given by Bradley et al.[35]

The position of the maximum of the oligomer bands is related to monomer frequency v_0 by

$$v_k = v_0 + \frac{2V}{h} \cos \frac{k}{N+1}, \qquad (k = 1, 2, 3, \ldots, N)$$

Experimental results have confirmed this theory, at least for adenylates at neutral pH. The circular dichroism curves of ApA (Fig. 4) and a series of adenylates at neutral pH indicate that a pair of bands of opposite sign is present. The CD spectrum of the mononucleotide AMP is completely different and indicates the similarity in the general shape for all adenylates from the dimer to the higher polymer. The intensity of these bands increases as a function of N and there is a general shift towards lower wavelengths with increasing N (blue shift).

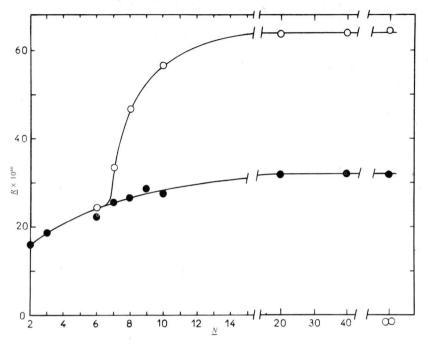

Fig. 6. Rotational strength (R) as a function of chain length N of adenylate oligomers (positive 260 nm main CD band).[39] ● pH = 7·4. ○ pH = 4·5.

The quantitative calculation of these circular dichroism properties was made using the outlined exciton theory and an appropriate model of dissymmetric ApA and adenylate structure (see Fig. 9). The geometry assumed for ApA and adenylates is that of parallel stacked purines, rotated by an angle of about 30°–45°. This can represent the start of a single-strand helix quite similar in dimension to half a double-strand DNA helix, i.e. a single strand of DNA.

Figure 6 shows the plot of rotational strength as a function of degree of polymerization. At neutral pH, the R per mole of residue increases slowly as the chain length becomes longer and reaches an asymptotic maximum for the high polymer.

E. *Double-stranded and Multiple-stranded Complexes*

The application of circular dichroism allows the double stranded and multiple stranded helices to be recognized. Poly A at acid pH is known from X-ray studies to have the structure of a double helix with parallel strand orientation.[45] The formation of the double-stranded structure is reflected in the shape of the CD spectra and in the increase of R. Oligoadenylates at acid pH exhibit a sudden increase in rotational strength at the level of heptamer indicating the formation of a double-stranded structure (Fig. 6). These spectral changes are not exhibited by small adenylates.

Another example is the formation of double- and triple-stranded helices between poly A and poly U at a neutral pH (Fig. 7). Thus the formation of these complexes

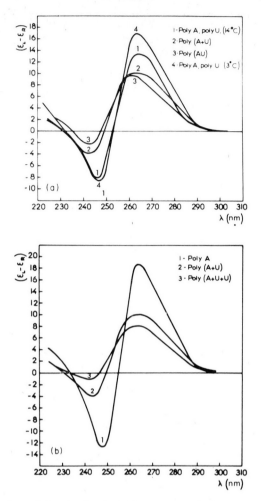

Fig. 7. Comparison of the circular dichroic spectra of single-stranded poly A (1) at pH 7·4 with poly A.poly U, the two-stranded complex, and with poly A.poly U.poly U, the three-standed complex at 2°C.[80a]

is reflected in the decrease of intensity of the CD bands and in the broadening of these bands and in the blue shift. In general the CD spectrum changes from conservative to a rather non-conservative type upon double strand formation. This may well result from the mutual cancellation of many positive and negative bands.

F. Influence of Temperature on Polynucleotide Conformation

Since rotational strength is related to the presence of dissymmetrical helical structure it is possible to use it as a very sensitive parameter to obtain thermodynamic values and correlate with structure. The experimental results for dimers and single-stranded oligomers indicate a gradual melting over a broad temperature region which suggests a nonco-operative process. A co-operative transition should give sharp melting curves.[46] There is no observable chain-length dependence. This allows the application of a very simple 'two-state' model which may suffer some conceptual limitations. An alternative explanation of some multi-state system is not supported by experimental evidence. According to the 'two-state' model, the dimer is in a stacked form at low temperature, whereas at very high temperature the unstacked form predominates.

The rotational strength at any temperature can be considered as expressing the concentration of 'stacked' dimers and one can calculate an apparent equilibrium constant and thermodynamic parameters for the unstacking process.[38, 39] For oligomers of A and of C at neutral pH it was found that the thermodynamics for unstacking are essentially not dependent upon chain length and the process is largely nonco-operative.[39, 47, 48]

The torsional oscillator model has been proposed as another alternative by Glaubiger, Lloyd and Tinoco.[49] According to this model the bases at higher temperatures are characterized by increased in-plane oscillations about the sugar phosphate backbone. This model is attractive but lacks experimental confirmation.

Neither the 'two-state' model nor the oscillating model is perfect. A re-examination of the two models, essential for the analysis of temperature dependence, was recently thoroughly carried out by Powell *et al.*[50, 51] They found that the two-state model satisfies the following criteria: (1) isosbestic points in the spectra, (2) linear van't Hoff plots, (3) comparable analysis of any optical parameters, and (4) analysis of the spectra in terms of two linear variables. This indicates the operational validity of the two-state model which is in agreement with experimental results.

It is important to conclude that the temperature of oligo- and poly-nucleotides supports the single-stranded stacked model. A completely different process characterizes the melting of the double-stranded structure which is chain-length dependent, exhibits a sharp melting curve and for which the process is co-operative.[39, 52]

4.3.4 Polydeoxynucleotides

The measurement of circular dichroism provides the basis for distinguishing polydeoxyribo- from polyribonucleotides. All the DNAs measured yielded circular dichroism spectra completely different from RNAs. It was suggested that the cause must be due to conformational differences[53].

A. Single-stranded Polydeoxyribonucleotides

The following arguments suggest that the cause must be due to conformational differences between polyribo- and deoxyribonucleotides:

1. Single-stranded deoxyoligomers all give circular dichroism spectra, which are of relatively weak intensity (Fig. 8), probably owing to weaker base–base interaction compared with corresponding ribo-oligonucleotides and to a lesser degree of dissymmetry.[54, 55]

2. The thermal 'melting' of deoxyribonucleotides gives curves with a relatively small slope indicative of weak stacking interactions in a dissymmetric array.[56]

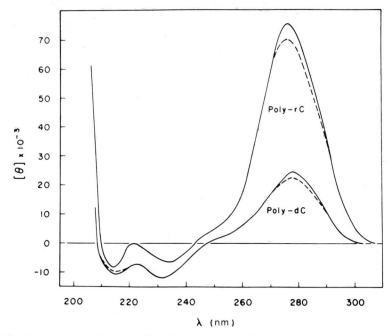

Fig. 8. Comparison of circular dichroism spectra of poly r C (upper curves) and poly d C, lower curves.[54]

3. The increase of rotational strength of oligodeoxynucleotides as a function of chain length is relatively small and reaches the plateau already at the level of the pentamer for oligo dC and oligo dT,[12] whereas for oligo dA a decrease of R^{57} is observed as a function of degree of polymerization (i.e. the rotational strength of the dimer is greater than that of the polymer).

4. The calculations of distribution of rotational strength for adenylates[12] were made using the nearest-neighbour (exciton) theory of Tinoco *et al.*[35] and assuming the geometry of a single-stranded, stacked, right-handed helix similar to one half DNA. The results obtained are shown in Fig. 9. For oligoribo there is an excellent agreement between calculated distribution of R with experimental CD spectra[39]. The predicted intersection points (shown by arrows) correspond well to the observed points (shown by circles). It should be noted that this intersection point is blue-shifted for all oligo A from the AMP. In contrast, for deoxyoligo A the intersection point (shown by X) is red-shifted relative to the monomer. Thus the circular dichroism data for a series of deoxy A oligomers does not fit the stacked model of a single-stranded, stacked helix similar to half of the DNA double helix.

The calculations of the distribution of oscillator strength[12] were made using different geometrical models and applying the same nearest-neighbour (exciton) theory. A comparison of the experimentally resolved absorption spectra using a derivative method with the calculated results indicates that neither the DNA model of 10 residues per pitch with stacked bases nor the card-stacked model of one residue per pitch (or stacked model in parallel) agrees with the experimental results.[12] Thus the stacking in a helical array cannot be considered to be satisfactorily in

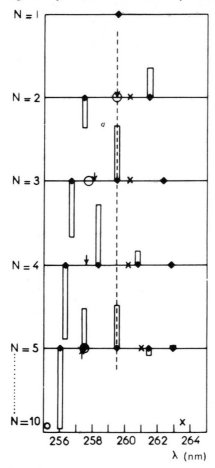

Fig. 9. Distribution of rotational strength calculated for short stacked oligoadenylates for chain length $N = 1$ to 5. Observed crossing points of the riboadenylates[39] are shown by circles and deoxyriboadenylates by crosses;[12] predicted crossing points are shown by arrows (see the text).

agreement with all reasonable geometrical models. It would thus appear that the base–base interactions are in a disordered array.

5. The semiempirical method of calculation based on the principle of additivity[58] allows the majority of ribotrinucleotides to be calculated from the known CD spectra of sixteen dinucleosides. In contrast the data for deoxytrinucleotides[59] indicate that this empirical method does not agree satisfactorily with the obtained results (example dApA and dApApA).

In conclusion, it should be emphasized that all accumulated results on the single-stranded deoxyoligomers do not support the model of a dissymmetrically ordered, stacked helix under the experimental temperature conditions. Also, all analysed models of dissymmetrical helical structure are not in agreement with experimental results. It would therefore seem that the deoxyoligomers are in a conformation more closely resembling a random coil. The dissymmetrical base–base interactions are much weaker than in ribo-oligomers and in some cases of purine deoxyoligomers are not even detectable. The experimental results suggest strongly that only a restricted rotation about the phosphodiester backbone occurs, corresponding to the conformation of minimum energy. It is conceivable that the bases may even interact without formation of a dissymmetrical, helical or partially helical structure, for example poly dA. There is no indication that the long, single-stranded DNAs adopt a conformation similar to helical polyribonucleotides.

B. Double-stranded Structure of Deoxyoligonucleotides

Recently we compared the ability to form complexes of oligodeoxyribonucleotides of various chain length with that of oligoribonucleotides.[60] The following results indicate that in dilute solution the formation of complexes is greatly facilitated in the case of deoxyoligomers and occurs for much shorter chains than in the corresponding ribo-oligomers:

1. Studies of dA_n and dT_n in solution at neutral pH, at lower temperature and deoxy C at acid pH indicate that the formation of complexes of the double-stranded type occurs with the trimer and all higher oligomers. Under identical conditions, a complex between corresponding ribo compounds ribo-A_n and ribo-U_n, rC at acid pH is detected only for oligomers longer than the hexamer. Oligoribo C yields an 'intermediate' conformation before the formation of the double-stranded structure.

2. Thermal denaturation of deoxycytidylates at acid pH, starting from the trimer, is strongly dependent on the chain length (Fig. 10) and the concentration, as one would expect for a co-operative helix coil transition. The circular dichroism spectra measured at different temperatures shows one isosbestic point and the enthalpy change is 6 kcal/mol. These properties are in agreement with the structural transition: dC_n double-stranded form → random coil for $n \geqslant 3$.

B1. Double-stranded DNA. Wells et al.[61] have studied the CD of double-stranded DNA of repeating defined sequences with complementary bases. The observed differences in the CD spectra may be explained: by the differences in the sequence-dependent nearest-neighbour interaction,[62] and by the significant geometric differences, that is differences in conformation.

The application of Gray and Tinoco's method[63] of nearest-neighbour calculation leads one to the conclusion that polymers like poly dA.dT have a different geometry from ordinary DNA in the B form. In fact Gray and Tinoco found disagreement in predicted polydeoxynucleide B-form spectra with the experimental results. The differences are taken as indicating that such polydeoxynucleotides (i.e. purine on one strand and pyrimidine on the other strand) do not have the normal B form of DNA.

Gray and Tinoco's method[63] should be appropriate to interpret the CD spectra of DNA. However, this method requires detailed knowledge of various double-stranded polydeoxynucleotides of eight different sequences which is not yet available.

It might be supposed that a similar semi-empirical approach could be used for calculating the circular dichroism of DNA for different base composition. In fact

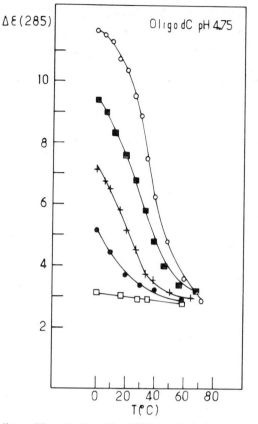

Fig. 10. Helix–coil transition of oligo dC, of different chain length (N). Changes in the positive CD band as a function of temperature for deoxyribocytidylates at acid pH (double-stranded).[60] □ $N = 2$, ● $N = 3$, + $N = 4$, ■ $N = 5$, ○ $N = 7$.

Wells *et al.*[61] obtained satisfactory agreement between the calculated and experimentally observed spectra of salmon sperm DNA. The ORD data of Samejima and Yang[64] were indicative of a linear dependence of longer wavelength Cotton effect extremum as a function of A − T base pairs.

Gratzer and collaborators[65] have shown that the data for DNA can be simply fitted on the assumption of linear dependence; extrapolation then leads to apparent circular dichroism curves for 0 % and 100 % (A + T). These extrapolated curves for 100 % A + T and 100 % G + C are not considered to have physical reality but serve as a standard for the calculation of CD curves of any given composition. It is interesting to note that the treatment of data for DNA reveals differences between absorption spectra or hypochromism and circular dichroism spectra.

It must be emphasized that all these semi-empirical calculation methods may yield very valuable information but one should be aware of the basic assumption which implies the presence of DNA in the B form but which may not be always the case.

C. *Different Conformations of DNA and RNA*

C1. Difference between RNA and DNA. The early observations of the appearance of the DNA spectrum of 'conservative' type[53] have now been extended and confirmed for all double-stranded DNAs in the B form.[65] In contrast, the RNA spectrum is of non-conservative form,[53, 66] which is also characteristic for all RNAs independently of their origin, base composition (Fig. 11a and b). X-ray data indicate that one of the major structural differences between RNA and DNA is the tilting of the bases of about 15° (see Table 1). The appearance of a non-conservative-type spectrum was recognized to be due to the interaction of the near-UV 260-nm band with far-UV transitions.[41] The exact calculations of circular dichroic spectra for different geometries and particularly for different base tilting were performed by Tinoco[67] and Johnson and Tinoco.[43] They showed that the tilting of the bases can explain the non-conservative RNA-type spectrum.

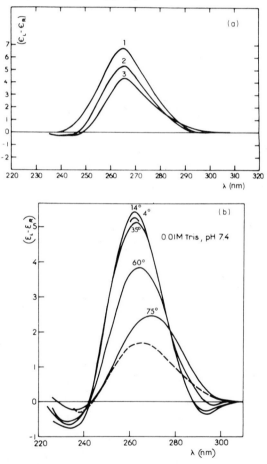

Fig. 11a. Circular dichroism spectra of RNA at different temperatures: (a) RNA from tobacco mosaic virus in 0·15-M NaCl; (b) Transfer RNA at low ionic strength after Bokès, Dirheimer and Brahms, unpublished results (1968).

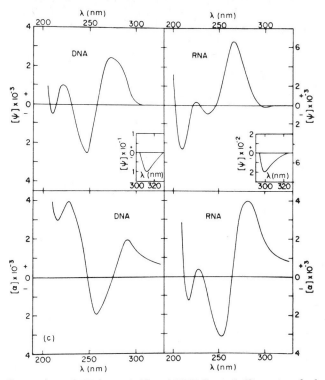

Fig. 11b. Comparison of CD (upper half) and ORD (lower half) spectra of salmon sperm DNA and ribosomal *E. coli* RNA.[65]

C2. Different form of DNA. The first experimental indication of the effect of tilting was obtained by investigations of DNA in 80% ethanol by Brahms and Mommaerts,[53] who proposed that under these conditions DNA adopts the conformation of the A form. A similar kind of spectrum, but less pronounced, with predominant positive band was observed for native DNA at premelting temperature, e.g. at about 45°C (Fig. 12, curve 2)*. It should be emphasized that these differences are not observed by conventional UV absorption spectroscopy. Further evidence of the identity with the A form of DNA came from the work of Maestre,[68, 69] who investigated DNA films under various conditions very similar to those used in X-ray diffraction studies.

Tunis-Schneider and Maestre found that the non-oriented films at high relative humidity show CD spectra identical with that of DNA in solution. At lower humidities (in the 95–81% relative humidity range) a transition occurred and the CD spectra of the DNA film became non-conservative with a larger minimum in the 280-nm region.

These conditions of salt and relative humidity correspond to those of the formation of the A form of DNA. However the form of the spectra for unknown reasons varies for different DNAs. Lithium DNA fibres at lower humidities yield CD spectra with one negative band (Fig. 13). It is also known that fibres of lithium DNA at low

* This was recently confirmed by Genis and Cantor [*J. Mol. Biol.* **65**, 381 (1972)].

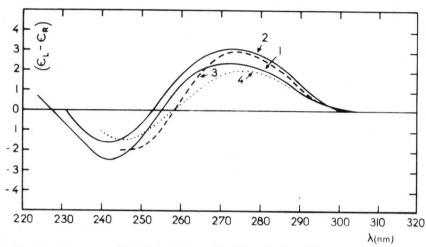

Fig. 12. CD spectra of DNA (calf thymus) in 0·1-M NaCl at different temperatures: 1, 20°C; 2, 45°C; 4, 80°C; 3, heated, followed by rapid cooling.[53]

relative humidity exhibit X-ray diffraction patterns of the C form with the bases slightly tilted (see Table 1). Similar CD spectra characterized by the reduction of the positive band are observed for DNA solutions at high NaCl or LiCl concentration of 4–6 M. Similar spectral changes were induced for DNA in concentrated CsCl solution.[70]

DNA in ethylene glycol solution also yielded CD spectra with a negative band whereas the positive band disappeared.[71, 77] From the work of Maestre on Li

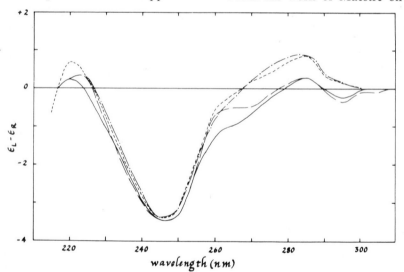

Fig. 13. Comparison of circular dichroism spectra of DNA in ethylene glycol at 20°C (———) with Li DNA film in C form from Tunis-Schneider and Maestre (– –); and DNA in 25% E.G. (v/v) (—·—) with DNA in water with 6 M-NaCl also from Tunis-Schneider and Maestre (----).[68] (After Nelson and Johnson.[71])

DNA it would appear that the geometry of DNAs in ethylene glycol is similar to that of the hypothetical C form (Fig. 13).

C3. Spectral changes in DNA-protein complexes. Similar spectral changes were observed in some DNA-protein complexes. The packing of long DNA molecules inside the virus protein coat[73] of even T phages yields a single negative Cotton effect. This may be due to distortion of DNA inside the protein coat, which may be compared to the effect of high salt concentrations on DNA.[70]

The formation of a complex between poly-L-lysine and DNA[74] and between histones and DNA[75-77] also yielded CD spectra characterized by a broad negative band. The nature of spectral changes is not yet well understood.[78, 79]

Thanks are due for permission to reproduce the following material in this chapter:

Figure 8 (ref. 54) by permission of the American Chemical Society. Figure 11b (ref. 65) by permission of Academic Press (London) Inc. Figure 13 (ref. 71) by permission of Academic Press Inc.

References

1. S. Arnott, *Prog. Biophys. Mol. Biol.* **21**, 265 (1970).
2. S. Arnott, *Science* **167**, 1694 (1970).
3. T. Sato, Y. Kyogoku, S. Higushi, Y. Mitsui, Y. Iitaka, M. Tsuboi and K. I. Miurua, *J. Mol. Biol.* **16**, 180 (1966).
4. J. Brahms, J. C. Maurizot and J. Pilet, *Biochim. Biophys. Acta* **186**, 110 (1969).
5. J. Pilet and J. Brahms, *Nature New Biol.* **236**, 99 (1972).
6. S. Arnott and D. W. L. Hukins, *Nature* **224**, 886 (1969).
7. M. Sundaralingham, *Biopolymers* **7**, 821 (1969).
8. L. B. Clark and I. Tinoco Jr., *J. Amer. Chem. Soc.* **87**, 11 (1965).
9. A. Pullman and B. Pullman, *Advan. Quantum Chemistry* **4**, 267 (1968).
10. M. Kasha, *Discuss. Faraday Soc.* **9**, 14 (1950).
11. S. F. Mason, *J. Chem. Soc.* 1240 (1959).
12. J. Brahms, H. Sellini and S. Brahms, *Third. Intern Biophys. Congr.* Abstracts, p. 171 (1969).
13. R. F. Stewart and N. Davidson, *J. Chem. Phys.* **39**, 255 (1963).
14. T. R. Emerson, R. J. Swan and T. L. V. Ulbricht, *Biochemistry* **6**, 843 (1967).
15. G. T. Rogers and T. L. V. Ulbricht, *Biochem. Biophys. Res. Commun.* **39**, 414 (1970).
16. T. Nishimura, B. Shmidza and I. Iwai, *Biochim. Biophys. Acta* **157**, 221 (1968).
17. D. W. Miles, W. H. Inskeep, W. J. Robbins, M. W. Winkley, R. K. Robbins and H. Eyring, *J. Amer. Chem. Soc.* **92**, 3872 (1970).
18(a). A. V. Lakshminarayan and V. Sasisekharan, *Biochim. Biophys. Acta* **204**, 49 (1970).
18(b). J. Donohue and K. N. Trublood, *J. Mol. Biol.* **2**, 363 (1960).
19. A. V. Haschemeyer and A. Rich, *J. Mol. Biol.* **27**, 369 (1967).
20. M. Sundaralingham and L. H. Jensen, *J. Mol. Biol.* **13**, 914 (1965).
21. H. Berthod and B. Pullman, *Biochim. Biophys. Acta* **232**, 595 (1971).
22. F. Jordan and B. Pullman, *Theor. Chim. Acta* **9**, 242 (1971).
23. I. Tinoco, R. C. Davis and S. R. Jaskunas, in B. Pullman, Ed., *Molecular Interactions.* Academic Press, 1968.
24. A. E. V. Haschemeyer and H. M. Sobel, *Acta Cryst.* **19**, 125 (1965).
25. K. Watempaugh, J. Dow, L. Jensen and S. Fuerberg, *Science* **159**, 206 (1968).
26. S. S. Tavale and H. M. Sobell, *J. Mol. Biol.* **48**, 109 (1970).
27. W. Saenger and K. H. Scheit, *J. Mol. Chem.* **240**, 2094 (1970).
28. M. P. Schweitzer, A. D. Broom, P. O. P. Ts'O and D. P. Hollis, *J. Amer. Chem. Soc.* **90**, 1042 (1968).
29. S. S. Danyluk and F. E. Hruska, *Biochemistry* **7**, 1038 (1968).
30. S. I. Chan and J. N. Nelson, *J. Amer. Chem. Soc.* **91**, 168 (1969).
31. D. W. Miles, M. J. Robbins, R. K. Robbins, M. W. Winkley and H. Eyring, **824**, 831 (1969).
32. W. H. Inskeep, D. W. Miles and H. Eyring, *J. Amer. Chem. Soc.* **92**, 3866 (1970).
33. A. S. Davyodov, *J. Exp. Theor. Phys.* **18**, 210 (1948).

34. W. Moffitt, *J. Chem. Phys.* **25**, 467 (1956).
35. I. Tinoco Jr., R. W. Woody and D. F. Bradley, *J. Chem. Phys.* **38**, 1317 (1963).
36. C. A. Bush, Ph.D. Thesis, University of California, Berkeley, 1965.
37. C. A. Bush and I. Tinoco, Jr. *J. Mol. Biol.* **23**, 601 (1967).
38. K. E. Van Holde, J. Brahms and A. M. Michelson, *J. Mol. Biol.* **12**, 726 (1965).
39. J. Brahms, A. M. Michelson and K. E. Van Holde, *J. Mol. Biol.* **15**, 467 (1966).
40. J. Brahms and S. Brahms, in G. D. Fasman and S. N. Timasheff, Eds., *Fine Structure of Proteins and Nucleic Acids.* New York, M. Dekker, 1970.
41. C. A. Bush and J. Brahms, *J. Chem. Phys.* **46**, 79 (1967).
42. I. Tinoco, Jr., *J. Amer. Chem. Soc.* **86**, 297 (1964).
43(*a*). W. C. Johnson, Jr. and I. Tinoco, Jr., *Biopolymers* **8**, 701 (1969).
43(*b*). W. C. Johnson, Jr. and I. Tinoco, Jr., *Biopolymers* **7**, 727 (1969).
44. A. S. Schneider and R. A. Harris, *J. Chem. Phys.* **50**, 1204 (1969).
45. A. Rich, D. R. Davies, F. H. C. Crick and J. D. Watson, *J. Mol. Biol.* **3**, 71 (1961).
46. B. H. Zimm and J. K. Bragg, *J. Mol. Biol.* **11**, 620 (1959).
47. M. Leng and G. H. Felsenfeld, *J. Mol. Biol.* **15**, 455 (1966).
48. D. Poland, J. N. Vournakis and H. A. Scheraga, *Biopolymers* **4**, 233 (1966).
49. D. Glaubiger, D. A. Lloyd and I. Tinoco, Jr., *Biopolymers* **6**, 409 (1968).
50. J. Powell, Ph.D. Thesis, University of London (1971).
51. J. Powell, E. W. Richards and W. Gratzer, *Biopolymers* **11**, 235 (1972).
52. J. Applequist and V. Damle, *J. Amer. Chem. Soc.* **87**, 1450 (1965).
53. J. Brahms and W. F. H. M. Mommaerts, *J. Mol. Biol.* **10**, 73 (1964).
54. A. J. Adler, K. Grossman and G. D. Fasman, *Biochemistry* **7**, 3836 (1968).
55. C. A. Bush and H. A. Scheraga, *Biopolymers* **7**, 395 (1969).
56. J. C. Maurizot, J. Brahms and F. Eckstein, *Nature* **222**, 259 (1969).
57. J. N. Vournakis, D. Poland and M. A. Scheraga, *Biopolymers* **5**, 403 (1967).
58. C. R. Cantor and I. Tinoco, Jr., *J. Mol. Biol.* **13**, 65 (1965).
59. C. R. Cantor, M. M. Warshaw and H. Schapiro, *Biopolymers* **9**, 1079 (1970).
60. J. C. Maurizot, J. Blicharski and J. Brahms, *Biopolymers* **10**, 1429 (1971).
61. R. D. Wells, J. E. Larson, R. C. Grant, B. E. Shortte and C. R. Cantor, *J. Mol. Biol.* **54**, 465 (1970).
62. G. Bernardi and S. Timasheff, *J. Mol. Biol.* **48**, 43 (1970).
63. D. M. Gray and I. Tinoco, Jr., *Biopolymers* **9**, 223 (1970).
64. T. Samejima and J. T. Yang, *J. Biol. Chem.* **240**, 2094 (1965).
65. W. B. Gratzer, L. R. Hill and R. J. Owen, *Eur. J. Biochem.* **15**, 209 (1970).
66. P. K. Sarkar, B. Wells and J. T. Yang, *J. Mol. Biol.* **25**, 563 (1967).
67. I. Tinoco, Jr., *J. Chim. Phys.* **65**, 91 (1968).
68. M. Tunis-Schneider and M. Maestre, *J. Mol. Biol.* **25**, 521 (1970).
69. M. Maestre, *J. Mol. Biol.* **25**, 543 (1970).
70. M. Tunis and J. Hearst, *Biopolymers* **6**, 1218 (1968).
71. R. G. Nelson and W. C. Johnson, *Biochem. Biophys. Res. Commun.* **41**, 211 (1970).
72. G. Green and H. R. Mahler, *Biopolymers* **6**, 1509 (1968).
73. M. Maestre and I. Tinoco, Jr., *J. Mol. Biol.* **12**, 287 (1965).
74. J. T. Shapiro, M. Leng and G. Felsenfeld, *Biochemistry* **8**, 3219 (1969).
75. V. I. Permogorov, V. G. Debabov, I. A. Shadkova and B. A. Rebentish, *Biochem. Biophys. Acta* **199**, 556 (1970).
76. A. J. Adler, B. Schaffhausen, T. A. Langan and G. D. Fasman, *Biochemistry* **10**, 909 (1971).
77. G. D. Fasman, B. Schaffhausen, L. Goldsmith and A. Adler, *Biochemistry* **9**, 2814 (1970).
78. A. J. Adler and G. D. Fasman, *J. Phys. Chem.* **75**, 1516 (1971).
79. M. Haynes, R. A. Garrett and W. B. Gratzer, *Biochemistry* **9**, 4410 (1970).
80(*a*). J. Brahms, *J. Mol. Biol.* **11**, 785 (1965).
80(*b*). W. Fuller, M. H. F. Wilkins, H. R. Wilson, L. D. Hamilton and S. Arnott, *J. Mol. Biol.* **12**, 60 (1965).
81. D. A. Marvin, M. Spencer, M. H. F. Wilkins and L. D. Hamilton, *J. Mol. Biol.* **3**, 547 (1961).
82. R. Langridge, D. A. Marvin, W. E. Seeds, H. R. Wilson, C. W. Cooper, M. H. F. Wilkins and L. D. Hamilton, *J. Mol. Biol.* **2**, 381 (1960).
83. D. R. Davies, *Ann. Rev. Biochem.* **36**, 321 (1967).
84. J. Brahms, J. C. Maurizot and A. M. Michelson, *J. Mol. Biol.* **25**, 465 (1967).
85. J. Brahms, J. C. Maurizot and A. M. Michelson, *J. Mol. Biol.* **25**, 481 (1967).

ORD and CD in Conformational Analysis of Synthetic High Polymers

P. PINO

Swiss Federal Institute of Technology
Zurich, CH

4.4.1 Introduction

The problem of the investigation of the conformational equilibria of macromolecules in solution has been approached using different experimental techniques[1] but the results obtained up to now are not satisfactory. Optical rotation, ORD and CD measurements are becoming more and more popular as experimental tools in this field.[2] These techniques can yield a set of interesting data, the difficulties encountered in the preparation of optically active polymers being largely compensated by the fact that only a small amount of polymer not fractionated according to molecular weight is, in general, needed. In fact, it has been found in the case of poly-α-amino acids[3] that when the macromolecule chain contains above five to ten monomeric units, the optical activity per monomeric unit is not appreciably influenced by molecular weight. The same trend has been observed recently[4] in the case of poly-(S)-4-methyl-1-hexene (Fig. 1).

Different types of information on the conformation of macromolecules can be obtained from optical rotation as well as from ORD and CD by comparing measurements carried out on polymers and on suitable low-molecular-weight models or by comparing measured and calculated values of optical rotation in the few cases in which such calculations are possible. In the field of synthetic high polymers semi-empirical calculations of optical activity have been successfully carried out only in the case of poly-α-olefins;[2] correspondingly, this is the only case in which information on the local conformational equilibria of single monomeric units has been obtained from simple measurements of optical activity at 589 nm and from temperature coefficients of the optical rotation. Furthermore, a reliable model has been obtained for the conformation of the macromolecules, which has shown a remarkable heuristic value.[2]

Information on the macromolecular conformation can also, in principle, be obtained from possible modifications of the chromophoric systems existing in each single monomeric unit by interaction with similar or different chromophoric systems present in the neighbouring monomeric units. This type of interaction, clearly established many years ago in the case of poly-α-amino acids,[5] has been shown

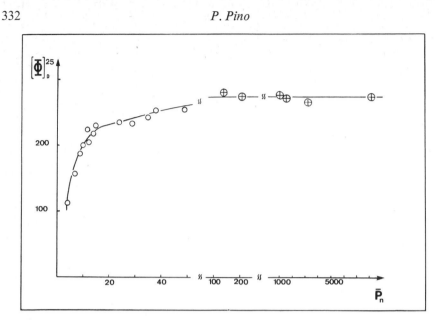

Fig. 1. Optical activity of isotactic poly-(*S*)-4-methyl-1-hexene, —⊕—, and of liquid oligomers of unknown stereoregularity, —○—.

to be very unusual in synthetic polymers. In fact, in this field some obvious cases are known in which the chromophoric systems present in the principal chain[6] are conjugated but no case has been clearly demonstrated of interactions between chromophoric systems present in lateral chains of the macromolecules. We shall consider some examples of the first type, in which—because of the possibility of conjugation—the chromophoric systems in the polymers are different from that of the monomeric unit and then some cases of the second type, in which chromophoric systems absorbing above 180 nm are present in the lateral chains.

4.4.2 Polymers having Chromophoric Systems Remarkably Different from those of the Monomeric Unit Models

Two typical examples of such polymers have recently been investigated: the linear polyacetylenes[6] and poly-isocyanates[7] having asymmetric carbon atoms in the lateral chains.

Optically active polyacetylenes, according to the method used in the synthesis[8] and to their chemical and physical properties, should have a substantially linear structure. The optical activity at 589 nm is positive and high in absolute value in poly-(*S*)-3-methyl-pentyne and negative and rather low in poly-(*S*)-4-methyl-1-hexyne (Table 1). This behaviour resembles that of (*S*)-2-(1-methyl-propyl)-butadiene[9(a)] and of (*S*)-2-(2-methyl-butyl)-butadiene[9(b)] (Table 2) which can be considered as the simplest models for the corresponding polymers. This behaviour might be taken as an indication that the conformational equilibria are of the same type in polymers and low-molecular-weight models at least with regard to the lateral chains.

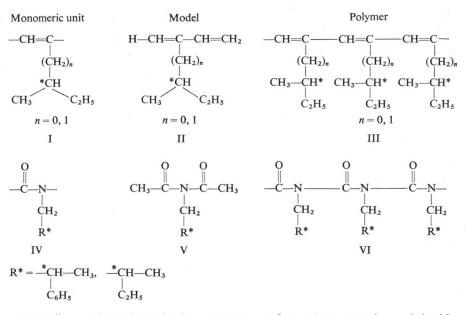

According to the polymerization catalyst used,[8] an all *trans* conjugated double bond structure should be expected for the principal chain. However, the planar structure of the principal chain, which would minimize the energy of the conjugated double-bond sequences, would involve a large steric repulsion among the lateral

Table 1

$[\Phi]_D$, UV, IR and CD data of Poly-(S)-3-methyl-pentyne and Poly-(S)-4-methyl-1-hexyne (see Reference 6)

Polymer	$[\Phi]^{a,c}$	$\frac{\Delta[\Phi]_D^{b,c}}{\Delta T}$	UV[b] λ_{max} (nm)	ε^c	IR[d] (cm^{-1})	Circular dichroism[b] Sign	λ_{max} (nm)	$[\Theta]_{max}^c$
~~—CH=C——CH=C—~~ CH$_3$—*CH CH$_3$—*CH C$_2$H$_5$ C$_2$H$_5$	+485	0·73	275	2520	1612	+	314	6300
~~—CH=C——CH=C—~~ CH$_2$ CH$_2$ CH$_3$—*CH CH$_3$—*CH C$_2$H$_5$ C$_2$H$_5$	−11·3	0·33	230 320	2905 2920	1618	+	402	300

[a] Solvent: diethyl ether. [b] Solvent: *n*-heptane. [c] Referred to one monomer unit. [d] Double-bond stretching.

Table 2

Molar Rotatory Power of Poly-(S)-3-methyl-pentyne, Poly-(S)-4-methyl-1-hexyne and of Their Model Compounds

Polymer	$[\Phi]_D^{25\ a,b}$	Ref.	Model compound	$[\Phi]_D^{25\ c}$	Ref.

⁓⁓—CH=C—⁓⁓
     |
   *CH—CH$_3$
     |
   C$_2$H$_5$
	+485	6(b)	H—CH=C—CH=CH$_2$
			       |
			     *CH—CH$_3$
			       |
			     C$_2$H$_5$
				+38·9	9(a)

⁓⁓—CH=C—⁓⁓
     |
   CH$_2$
     |
   *CH—CH$_3$
     |
   C$_2$H$_5$
	−11·3	6(a)	H—CH=C—CH=CH$_2$
			       |
			     CH$_2$
			       |
			     *CH—CH$_3$
			       |
			     C$_2$H$_5$
				−12·5	9(b)

[a] In diethylether. [b] Referred to one monomer unit. [c] Extrapolated value to 100% optical purity, neat.

groups. Therefore, a compromise should be expected corresponding to the possible slight deviation from planarity of the principal chain, which allows a sufficient release of the steric strain among the vicinal lateral chains. IR and UV data (Table 1) seem to confirm this expectation; in fact, the internal double-bond stretching frequency (1650–1660 cm^{-1}) is shifted to lower frequencies [1612 cm^{-1} for poly(S)-3-methyl-pentyne and 1618 cm^{-1} for poly-(S)-4-methyl-1-hexyne] which are rather near to the frequencies observed for conjugated double bonds (1600 cm^{-1}),[10] showing that only a partial conjugation between the double bonds exists. The UV spectra in heptane show rather flat maxima at 275 nm in the case of poly-3-methyl-pentyne and at 230 and 320 nm in the case of poly-4-methyl-1-hexyne; the absorption coefficient, ε, per monomeric unit, is about 2500 in the former case and about 3000 in the latter case. The above data show beyond any doubt that a certain degree of conjugation exists between the double bonds which, when isolated, absorb below 200 nm. However, the wavelength of the maximum, which corresponds to four or five fully conjugated double bonds, and particularly the absorption coefficient which is less than one-tenth of that of the alternated polyenes, having two to six conjugated double bonds,[11] can be clearly interpreted according to the existence of relatively long sequences of partially conjugated double bonds. CD and ORD give further information on the principal chain conformations, the Cotton effects even if occurring at longer wavelengths than the corresponding UV absorption maxima, being certainly connected with electronic transitions of the partially conjugated double bond system. In fact, to release the steric interactions both the limit conformations VII and VIII would be the most effective. It is clear that in VII and VIII the sense of skew of the dienic system would be opposite and therefore, in a long polymer chain in which VII and VIII would be randomly distributed, the optical activity arising from the dienic system should be vanishingly small. On the contrary, however, ORD and CD show that the dienic system is highly optically active, $\Delta\varepsilon_{max}$ being 10 times larger in poly-(S)-3-methyl-pentyne with respect to poly-(S)-4-methyl-1-hexyne. We must assume, therefore, that conformations with the skew

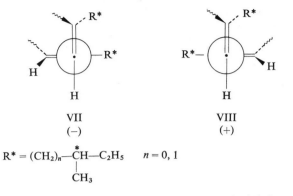

VII   (−)   VIII   (+)

$$R^* = (CH_2)_n-\overset{*}{C}H-C_2H_5 \quad n = 0, 1$$
$$\qquad\qquad \underset{CH_3}{|}$$

sense corresponding to VII or VIII largely prevail in poly-(S)-3-methyl-pentyne, and are still prevailing, even if probably to a smaller extent, in poly-(S)-4-methyl-1-hexyne. The prevalence, as in the case of optically active poly-α-olefins, might be connected with the presence of asymmetric carbon atoms, having the same absolute configuration, in the lateral chains. In fact, in this case the asymmetric induction should decrease by increasing the distance between the asymmetric carbon atom and the dienic system.

Assuming that the relationships between CD sign and skew sense of the dienic systems are the same in the case of cyclic dienes[12] and polyacetylenes we can conclude that the prevailing skew sense in the polymers investigated should be VIII. In other words, when the asymmetric carbon atom of the lateral chains has the (S) absolute configuration, right-handed helical sections should prevail in the polymer main chains. However, as the relationship between UV spectra (λ_{max} and ε_{max}) and the angle between the planes containing two consecutive double bonds is not known, it is not possible to estimate how many monomeric units are present per turn of the helical conformation.

A similar situation might exist in the poly-isocyanates investigated by Goodman and coworkers.[7] Poly-(S)-2-methyl-butyl- and poly-(+)-2-phenyl-propyl-isocyanate have been prepared by anionic polymerization of the corresponding monomers and their CD was compared with that of suitable low-molecular-weight models. Unfortunately, the polymers were soluble only in chloroform or concentrated sulphuric acid; however, the polymers which were recovered, even from the latter solvent, by dilution with methanol, showed the same properties as the starting materials.

Aliphatic poly-isocyanates are known to have a regular structure[13] as indicated in IX and X; however, probably because of steric interaction between the lateral groups, the principal chain is not expected to be planar, and, in fact, in the case of poly-*n*-butyl-isocyanate a helical structure with 8 monomer units in three turns was found in the solid state.[14] As shown in Table 3, the CD spectrum in chloroform is rather complicated, the main feature being a band with rather high ellipticity centred around 250 nm which is negative in the case of the aromatic polymer and positive in the case of the aliphatic polymer. In the aliphatic polymers the CD sign observed can be related to the configuration of the asymmetric carbon atom in the lateral chain, e.g. in the case of polyvinylketones[22] a positive CD corresponds to (S) absolute configuration of the lateral chain asymmetric carbon atom.[7] In the case of the aromatic polymers, the relationship between CD sign and absolute configura-

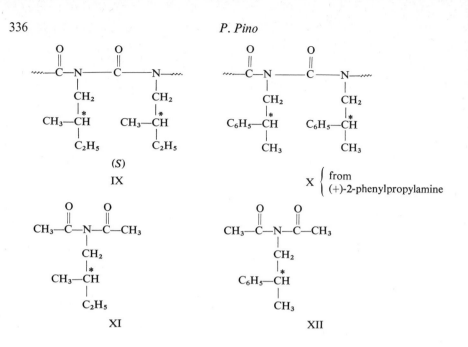

IX   (S)

X { from (+)-2-phenylpropylamine

XI

XII

tion of the asymmetric carbon atom in the monomer, and hence in the polymer lateral chain, is still unknown. The model compounds show a CD band in the same region having much lower intensity (about one-third in the case of the aromatic compounds and more than 60 times smaller in the case of the aliphatic compounds). The nature of this optically active band is not known exactly; it was tentatively attributed by Goodman[7(b)] to the $n \rightarrow \pi^*$ transition of the amide chromophore with the possible partial overlapping in the aromatic polymer of the phenyl chromophoric system.

Using H_2SO_4 as solvent, the CD maximum at about 250 nm disappears in the aliphatic polymer but is still present together with other positive CD maxima at 275, 263 and 227 nm in the aromatic polymer.

More experimental data, particularly on the UV absorption of polymers and of suitable model compounds, are needed to clarify the nature of the chromophoric

Table 3

$[\alpha]^{25}$ and CD in Chloroform of Optically Active Poly-isocyanates [see Reference 7(b)]

		CD bands	
Compound	$[\alpha]_D^{25}$ [a]	λ_{max} (nm)	Molar ellipticity
Poly-(S)-2-methyl-butyl-isocyanate (IX)	+160	253	+12,900[b]
N,N-Diacetyl-(S)-2-methyl-butyl-amine (XI)	−6	250	+192
Poly-(+)-2-phenyl-propyl-isocyanate (X)	−468·8	252	−28,000[b]
		280	+1,000
N,N-Diacetyl-(+)-2-phenyl-propyl-amine (XII)	+114·4	243	−9,100

[a] In chloroform. [b] Referred to one monomeric unit.

system absorbing at about 250 nm, taking into account that many resonance possibilities exist in the series of adjacent substituted amide groups which might influence the polymer stereochemistry.

The limit structures XIII–XV show some of the resonance possibilities in the aforementioned systems. XV might already be present in the models XI and

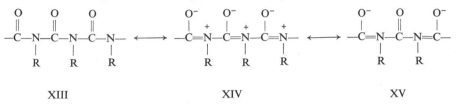

XIII   XIV   XV

XII studied by Goodman, while XIV, with the series of conjugated double bonds, closely resembles the structure of linear polyacetylenes. Only XIII might exist in a zig-zag planar form, while in both XIV and XV the main-chain double bond should not be completely planar to avoid too strong steric interaction between the lateral groups.

At the present, as a very attractive work hypothesis, particularly suggested by the order of magnitude of $\Delta\varepsilon_{max}$ and of λ_{max} of the CD, the limit structure XIV might be considered as mainly contributing to the structure of the main chain; the double bonds should be only partially conjugated, the prevailing skew sense being determined, as in the optically active polyacetylenes, by the configuration of the asymmetric carbon atom present in lateral groups.

4.4.3 Polymers in which the Chromophoric Systems are Substantially the same as in Low-molecular-weight Models

Both condensation and addition polymers of this type have been investigated but the most interesting results have been obtained in addition polymers and particularly in vinyl polymers and copolymers to which we shall restrict our discussion. The investigation of optically active vinyl polymers (poly-α-olefins, polyvinylethers, and polyvinylketones containing an asymmetric carbon atom in the lateral chain) has shown that the optical activity between 200 and 589 nm is stereoregularity dependent. Furthermore, the rotatory power is much higher than that of the most simple low-molecular-weight models when the asymmetric carbon atom of the lateral chains is in α or β position with respect to the main chain[15] (Table 4).

These effects were first discovered in poly-α-olefins,[16] and their conformational origin was postulated taking into account the following facts:

(a) The optical rotation dispersion between 589 and 200 nm follows a one-term Drude equation both in polymers and models, λ_0 being the same in both cases and corresponding to that expected for the first optically active transition in paraffins.[2, 16]

(b) The optical rotation per monomeric unit calculated according to the Brewster method,[17] which yields very reliable results in the case of paraffins,[16, 18] is in agreement with the experimental results, only admitting that the polymer main chain maintains in solution a helical conformation, similar to that assumed by the same polymers in the solid state, one of the

Table 4

Molar Optical Rotatory Power of the most Stereoregular Fractions of some Optically Active Poly-α-olefins, Polyvinylethers, Polyvinylketones and of some Low-molecular-weight Model Compounds (see Reference 15)

Polymer	n	Position of C* in lateral chain of polymer	Polymerized monomer optical purity (%)	$[\Phi]_D^{25}$ [a]	Model	n	$[\Phi]_D^{25}$ [b]
$CH_3{-}C^*H{-}(CH_2)_n{-}CH_2\text{—}$ (with C_2H_5) [d]	0	α	91	+161[f]	$CH_3{-}C^*H{-}(CH_2)_n{-}CH_3$ (with C_2H_5) [d]	0	−11.4[c]
	1	β	93	+288[f]		1	+21.3
	2	γ	95	+68.1[f]		2	+11.7
	3	δ	95	+20.4[f]		3	+14.4
$CH_3{-}C^*H{-}(CH_2)_n{-}O{-}CH{-}CH_2\text{—}$ (with C_2H_5) [d]	0	β	90	+312[f]	$CH_3{-}C^*H{-}(CH_2)_n{-}O{-}CH_2{-}CH_3$ (with C_2H_5) [d]	0	+34.5
	1	γ	>99	+6.5[f]		1	+1.1
$CH_3{-}C^*H{-}(CH_2)_n{-}C({=}O){-}CH{-}CH_2\text{—}$ (with C_2H_5) [e]	0	β	68	−118[g]	$CH_3{-}C^*H{-}(CH_2)_n{-}C({=}O){-}CH_2{-}CH_3$ (with C_2H_5) [e]	0	+34.8
	1	γ	96	−43[g]		1	+11.5
	2	δ	95	+11.7[g]		2	+15.2

[a] Referred to one monomeric unit. [b] Maximum observed value. [c] At 20°C. [d] For references see P. Pino, *Adv. Polymer Sci.* **4**, 393 (1965). [e] See O. Pieroni, F. Ciardelli, C. Botteghi, L. Lardicci, P. Salvadori and P. Pino. Paper presented at Symposium on Macromolecular Chemistry, Brussels, 1967. [f] In aromatic hydrocarbon solution. [g] *J. Polymer Sci.*, C **22**, 993 (1969). [f] In CHCl₃.

two possible helical screw senses largely prevailing. On the basis of the conformational analysis carried out on polymers, low-molecular-weight paraffins—for which only a few conformations having high rotation of the same sign are allowed—were identified and successfully synthesized.[18] These low-molecular-weight paraffins have optical rotation at 589 nm similar to that of the polymer monomeric units (Table 5).

(c) The relatively high absolute value of temperature coefficients of the optical rotation of the polymers, much higher than that of the low-molecular-weight paraffins having similar optical activity, can be reasonably explained admitting a decrease with temperature of the ratio between the number of monomeric units included in the sections of the main chain having, respectively, the thermodynamically more favoured and the less favoured helical conformation.

On the basis of these facts, a model for the poly-α-olefins in solution has been proposed[19] according to which the main chain of an ideally isotactic macromolecule assumes a helical conformation; sections spiralled in the left-handed and right-handed screw sense alternate along the main chain separated by conformational reversals which can freely flow along the chain. When asymmetric carbon atoms having the same absolute configuration are present in the lateral chains, the sections having one of the possible screw senses are longer, mainly for entropic reasons, than the sections having the opposite screw sense. The prevailing screw sense is connected with the absolute configuration of the asymmetric carbon atom of the lateral chains. The differences in length between the sections having opposite screw sense increase as the distance between the asymmetric carbon atoms and the main chain decreases, and for the same polymer the differences decrease by increasing

Table 5

Comparison of $[\Phi]_D^{25}$ and $\Delta[\Phi]_D/\Delta T$ between Optically Active Poly-α-olefins and Low-molecular-weight Model Compounds (see Reference 18)

Polymer	$[\Phi]_D^{25}$ [a]			Model	$[\Phi]_D^{25}$		
	Max. obs. value	Calc.[b]	$\dfrac{\Delta[\Phi]_D}{\Delta T}$[c]		Max. obs. value	Calc.[b]	$\dfrac{\Delta[\Phi]_D}{\Delta T}$[c]
Poly(S)-3-methyl-1-pentene	+161	+40	−0·36	(3S,5S)-2,2,3,5-Tetramethyl-heptane	−97·5	−180	+0·152
Poly(S)-4-methyl-1-hexene	+288	+60	−0·68	(3R,5S)-2,2,3,5-Tetramethyl-heptane	+137·8	+120	−0·128
Poly(S)-5-methyl-1-heptene	+68	+26	−0·34	(S)-5-Ethyl-2,2,3-trimethyl-heptane	−132	−240	+0·155
				(S)-3-Ethyl-5-methylheptane	+33·8	+60	−0·065
				(R)-5-Ethyl-2,3-dimethylheptane	+60·2	+105	−0·056

[a] Referred to one monomeric unit. [b] Average among all the allowed conformations.[17] [c] Between 25 and 110°C.

340   *P. Pino*

the temperature. For instance, in the case of poly-(S)-4-methyl-1-hexene, at 300°K, the average length of left-handed helical sections should correspond to 21–28 monomeric units, while for the right-handed helical section an average length of 1·5–2·5 is expected. The corresponding values at 500°K should be 5–6 and 1·5, respectively.

The ORD investigation of polyvinylethers[20] is much more complicated because the optically active electronic transition occurring at the highest wavelength, i.e. $n \to \sigma^*$ transition of the ethereal oxygen, is again hardly detectable with ordinary equipment. In fact, it occurs at about 190 nm and the ratio between optical rotation

Table 6

Optical Rotatory Properties of Poly-[(S)-1-methyl-propyl]-vinyl-ether, Poly-[(S)-2-methyl-butyl]-vinyl-ether and of Their Model Compounds (see Reference 21)

	Polymer[a]					Model			
	~—CH₂ ... CH₃ / ~—CH—O—(CH₂)ₙ—CH—C₂H₅ (*)					H—CH₂ ... CH₃ / H—CH—O—(CH₂)ₙ—CH—C₂H₅ (*)			
n	Optical purity[b] (%)	$[\Phi]_D^{25\ c,d}$	$\dfrac{\Delta[\Phi]_D^{c,d}}{\Delta T}$	Sign of Cotton effect[e]	n	Optical purity (%)	$[\Phi]_D^{25\ f}$	$\dfrac{\Delta[\Phi]_D^{c}}{\Delta T}$	Sign of Cotton effect[e]
0	92·5	+285	−1·20	n.d.	0	80	+29·9	−0·07	—
1	99	+7·1	+0·02	—	1	98·1	+0·84	+0·01	—

[a] Diethylether insoluble, benzene soluble fraction. [b] Of polymerised monomer. [c] In toluene. [d] Referred to one monomer unit. [e] Attributed to $n - \sigma^*$ electronic transition. [f] In isooctane.

and absorption coefficient is not very favourable. Furthermore, at least in one of the polymers, as in low-molecular-weight model compounds, the contributions to the optical rotation by the ethereal chromophoric system and the paraffinic backbone seem to have opposite sign[21] (Table 6).

This fact is not apparent in poly-|(S)-1-methylpropyl|vinyl-ether in which the contribution by the paraffinic backbone is much higher than the contribution by the ethereal chromophoric system, the asymmetric carbon atom being in the β-position with respect to the principal chain, as in the case of poly-(S)-4-methyl-1-hexene. However, it is clearly evident in the case of poly-|(S)-2-methylbutyl|vinyl-ether in which the two contributions have the same order of magnitude (Fig. 2). In this case, a maximum in ORD is observed around 260 and 220 nm while no CD band exists in this region. The position of the maximum depends on the stereoregularity of the sample, λ_{max} decreasing by increasing stereoregularity (Table 7). These data, which can be used for a relative stereoregularity determination, show that the change with stereoregularity of the positive contribution connected with the paraffinic backbone is larger than that of the corresponding negative contribution connected with the ether groups, which is overwhelming only in the region near the corresponding Cotton effect. Considering these results as well as the UV spectra of polymers and models,[21] it appears that the electronic interactions between the ethereal oxygen atoms in the polymer are very small, if any. Therefore, the optical rotation in polymers is different from that of the models mainly because of the position of the conformational equilibria. The interpretation of the results obtained in the case of poly-α-olefins and polyvinylethers has been nicely confirmed by an investigation on

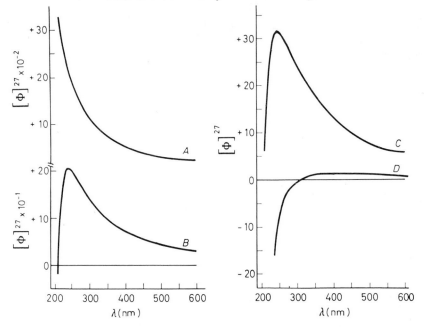

Fig. 2. (A) ORD curve of poly-[(S)-1-methyl-propyl]vinylether (monomer optical purity 90%). Acetone insoluble, ether soluble fraction. (B) ORD curve of [(S)-1-methyl-propyl]ethylether (optical purity 80%). (C) ORD curve of poly-[(S)-2-methyl-butyl]-vinyl ether (monomer optical purity 99%). Acetone insoluble, diethyl ether soluble fraction. (D) ORD curve of [(S)-2-methyl-butyl]ethylether (optical purity 99%). [From Reference 15]

Table 7

Relationship between Optical Rotation and Stereoregularity in Poly-[(S)-2-methyl-butyl]-vinyl-ether^a (see Reference 15)

Fraction^b	m.p. (°C)	IR^d crystallinity index	$[\Phi]_D^{25\ e,f}$	λ_{max}^h (nm)	$[\Phi]_{\lambda_{max}}^{27\ e,g}$
Acetone sol.	<25	0·48	+5·5	258	+21·1
Acetone ins., diethyl ether sol.	115–120^c	0·53	+5·9	244	+31·1
Diethyl ether ins., benzene sol.	135–140^c	0·87	+6·5	222	+63·8

^{a} Polymerized monomer optical purity >99%. ^{b} Obtained by boiling solvent extraction. ^{c} Determined by IR spectroscopy. ^{d} D_B 827 cm^{-1}/D_B 771 cm^{-1}. ^{e} Referred to one monomeric unit. ^{f} In toluene solution. ^{g} In n-heptane solution. ^{h} Wavelength corresponding to the maximum of the ORD curve.

polyvinylketones, which is still in progress.[15, 22] In this case the Cotton effect corresponding to the $n \rightarrow \pi^*$ transition of the carbonyl group occurs around 290 nm as in low-molecular-weight ketones and, therefore, can be thoroughly investigated.

The comparison of the UV spectra of polyvinylketones with those of the low-molecular-weight models shows (Table 8) that the maximum corresponding to the

Table 8

Ultraviolet Spectra and Features of Cotton Effect Connected with $n \to \pi^*$ Transition in Polyvinyl-ketones[a] and Low-molecular-weight Model Compounds (See Reference 22)

| | | | UV | | Cotton effect | | |
| | | | | | | Amplitude[d] $\begin{pmatrix} >\text{C}=\text{O} \\ n \to \pi^* \end{pmatrix}$ | |
		n	λ_{max} (nm)	ε_{max}	λ_0^c (nm)		Sign
Polymer		$0^{e,i}$	292	66.8^b	292	77.0	−
CH$_3$ $\qquad$ CH$_2$—⌇		$0^{f,i}$	291	56.0^b	292	221.0	−
$\mid$ $\qquad\qquad$ $\mid$		$1^{e,k}$	290	67.5^b	290	33.6	−
C$_2$H$_5$—CH—(CH$_2$)$_n$—CO—CH—⌇		$1^{f,k}$	290	60.0^b	290	66.0	−
		$2^{e,l}$	289	64.6^b	288	5.5	−
		$2^{f,l}$	288	53.5^b	288	10.8	−
Model		0^j	283	29.3	283^g	5.3	+
CH$_3$ $\qquad$ CH$_2$—H					285^h	n.d.	−
$\mid$ $\qquad\qquad$ $\mid$		1^m	282	26.5	282^g	9.5	−
C$_2$H$_5$—CH—(CH$_2$)$_n$—CO—CH—H		2^m	283	26.7	283^g	1.0	−
$\quad$ *							

[a] In CHCl$_3$ solution. [b] Referred to one monomeric unit. [c] Value taken from experimental ORD curve as $(\lambda_{trough} + \lambda_{peak})/2$. [d] Calculated from ORD curve obtained by subtracting the background rotation from the experimental ORD curve. [e] Atactic, obtained by spontaneous polymerization. [f] Stereoregular, obtained by anionic polymerization, initiator LiAlH$_4$. [g] In methanol solution. [h] In vapour phase. [i] Optical purity of the polymerized monomer 68%. [j] Optical purity 81%. [k] Optical purity of the polymerized monomer 96%. [l] Optical purity of the polymerized monomer 95%. [m] Optical purity 95%.

$n \to \pi^*$ transition occurs in polymers at wavelengths about 8 nm higher than in the models [(ε polymer/ε model) between 2·5 and 1·9]; ε, for the polymers, is slightly larger in the less stereoregular than in the more stereoregular fraction and is not temperature dependent in the small temperature range investigated (20–60°).[22] These differences are of the order of magnitude found for ketones having substituents of different bulkiness.[23] These data might be interpreted according to a stereo-regularity-dependent interaction between ketogroups in the polymer, which can obviously not exist in the monoketones used as low-molecular-weight models. However, we think that more experimental data, in a larger temperature interval, for polymers and models containing two ketogroups in 1–5 position, are needed to give a sound interpretation of the small, but perhaps significant, absorption co-efficient differences.

Despite the fact that $[\Phi]_D$ is negative for the first two members of the series ($n = 0, 1$) and positive for the third one ($n = 2$) (Table 4), the Cotton effects are negative in the three polymers in which the side chain asymmetric carbon atoms have the (S) absolute configuration. The origin of the positive rotation for the third member of the series can be easily explained taking into account that the negative Cotton effect, the amplitude of which greatly decreases going from the first member to the third, is superimposed on a positive rotation arising from other Cotton effects existing at much lower wavelengths. For this reason the optical rotation sign depends on the relative magnitude of the Cotton effect and background rotation and has no stereochemical implications.

The sign of the Cotton effect in the models corresponds to that of the polymers when $n = 1$ and $n = 2$ (Table 8). In the case of the model compound having the (S) absolute configuration, with $n = 0$, the Cotton effect is positive in methanol and in *n*-heptane but is negative in the vapour phase.[24] However, the Cotton effect at 200 nm and hence the background rotation remains positive in both cases (Fig. 3). The change of sign of the Cotton effect corresponding to the $n \to \pi^*$ transition going from heptane or methanol solution to vapour phase is probably connected with solvation phenomena of the keto group and strongly suggests that in the polymer having $n = 0$ the carbonyl group located between the main chain and the secondary butyl group is not substantially solvated.

The amplitude of the Cotton effect is much larger in the polymers than in the low-molecular-weight models, especially when the asymmetric carbon atom of the lateral chain is in the β-position with respect to the main chain. It strongly decreases with increasing distance between the asymmetric carbon atom of the lateral chain and the ketogroup; it is larger for the polymer fractions, which, on the basis of their crystallinity or of the method used for the synthesis, should be more stereoregular (Table 8). The stereoregularity degree, however, does not influence the Cotton effect wavelength. These results are in agreement with the assumptions made in the case of poly-α-olefins on the basis of the ORD following a one-term Drude equation and in the case of polyvinylethers on the basis of UV and ORD curves.

4.4.4 Vinyl Copolymers

The enhancement of the Cotton effect connected with the existence in solution of ordered conformations in which the position of the conformational equilibrium is very different from that of low-molecular-weight models suggested the investigation

Table 9

Comparison between Optical Rotation in Hydrocarbon Solution of some Samples of Copolymer[a] (S)-4-methyl-1-hexene[b]/4-Methyl-1-pentene and Mixtures of the two Homopolymers Having the Same Composition (See Reference 25)

Composition of copolymer and homopolymer mixtures.[c] Percentage of (S)-4-methyl-1-hexene	$[\alpha]_D^{25}$ of copolymer	$[\alpha]_D^{25}$ calc. for a homopolymer mixture	$[\Phi]_D^{25\ e}$	$[\Phi]_D^{25\ f,g}$
100	+292	+292	+286	—
70	+260	+204	+365	+157
40	+233	+117	+570	+162
23	+161	+67	+700	+105
13[d]	+100	+38	+755	+60

[a] Fraction extracted with cyclohexane from the product not extractable with di-isopropyl-ether if not otherwise indicated. [b] Polymerized monomer optical purity 93%. [c] Determined by IR spectroscopy. [d] Fraction extracted with di-isopropyl-ether from the product not extractable with diethyl-ether. [e] Referred to one monomeric unit of poly-(S)-4-methyl-1-hexene, calculated assuming that in the copolymer the optical rotation derives only from (S)-4-methyl-1-hexene monomeric unit. [f] Referred to one monomeric unit of poly-4-methyl-1-pentene, calculated attributing to the (S)-4-methyl-1-hexene monomeric unit in the copolymer $[\Phi]_D^{25}$ +286. [g] Value calculated by the Brewster method for the allowed conformation of 4-methyl-1-pentene monomeric unit inserted in a left-handed helical sequence $[\Phi]_D^{25}$ +240.

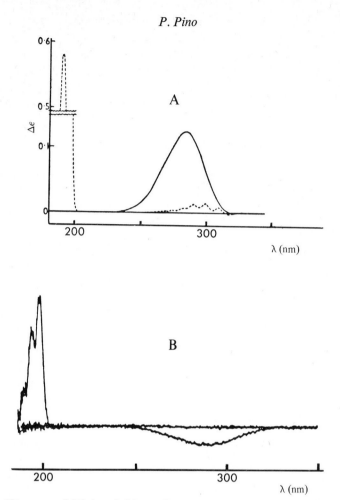

Fig. 3. CD curves of (S)-4-methyl-hexan-3-one at room temperature. (A) In solution: (———) methanol, and (–––) n-heptane. (B) In the vapour phase (path length 5 cm, sensibility 1×10^{-5} in the presence of liquid phase.) [From Reference 24.]

of stereoregular copolymers of non-asymmetric comonomers with optically active monomers to prove the existence of the aforementioned ordered conformation. In other words, it appeared possible to use the helical conformations existing in solution as an asymmetric matrix to perturb non-asymmetric chromophores. If the non-asymmetric comonomer has no chromophoric system in the accessible region of the spectrum but is included in a helical macromolecule with a predominant screw sense, the copolymer could show an optical activity different from that of the corresponding mixture of homopolymers. If a chromophore absorbing in the accessible region of the UV spectrum is present in the optically inactive comonomer, a Cotton effect should become apparent at the same wavelength as in corresponding low-molecular-weight dissymmetric compounds, if no interaction exists among the chromophoric systems present in the macromolecules.

The experiments confirmed these expectations. In fact, the optical activity of

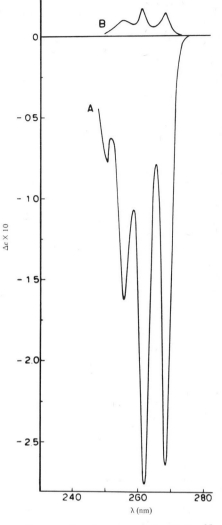

Fig. 4. CD spectra in chloroform solution at 25° of (3*S*,9*S*)-3,9-dimethyl-6-phenyl-undecane (B) and of the diethyl-ether extractable fraction of the styrene (*R*)-3,7-dimethyl-1-octene copolymer (A). Δε is based on a styrene monomer unit. [From Reference 27]

4-methyl-1-pentene/(*S*)-4-methyl-1-hexene copolymers is always much higher[25] than that of the mixture of homopolymers having the same composition (Table 9). The only possible explanation for this experimental fact is that the 4-methyl-1-pentene monomeric units, which are *per se* non-dissymmetric, being included in a polymer chain having helical conformation with a prevailing screw sense [as that postulated for (*S*)-4-methyl-1-hexene units[2]], assume optically active conformations which are thermodynamically favoured. In fact, attributing all the optical activity to the optically active comonomer present in the polymer, values of $[\Phi]_D$ per monomer unit up to 755 are obtained, which are clearly in contrast with all the experimental evidence on poly-(*S*)-4-methyl-1-hexene and low-molecular-weight models.

Styrene was chosen as an example of a monomeric unit having a chromophoric system which, if asymmetrically perturbed should give rise to a Cotton effect in an

Table 10

Circular Dichroism and Optical Rotation in Chloroform of some Highly Stereoregular Copolymers of Styrene (I) with Optically Active α-olefins[a] and of (3S,9S)-3,9-Dimethyl-6-phenylundecane[b] [see Reference 27(b)]

Compound	Units from styrene (mol. %)	$[\alpha]_D^{25}$	$\Delta\varepsilon_{262}$[c]
Copolymer of I with (R)-3,7-dimethyl-1-octene	4·4	−87	−0·24
Copolymer of I with (S)-4-methyl-1-hexene	4·0	+256	+0·18
Copolymer of I with (S)-5-methyl-1-heptene	5·3	+58	+0·06
(3S,9S)-3,9-Dimethyl-6-phenylundecane	—	+14·2	+0·02

[a] Optical purity 93–95%. [b] Optical purity ~98%. [c] Referred to one phenyl ring.

accessible region of the spectrum. If in low-molecular-weight compounds the 'styrene monomer unit' is dissymmetrically perturbed as in (3S:9S)-dimethyl-6-phenylundecane[27] a CD band between 250 and 275 nm having a $\Delta\varepsilon_{max}$ of about +0·02 is present (Fig. 4). When the same unit is included in a polymer of an optically active α-olefin, it shows a CD band in the same spectral region, but the $\Delta\varepsilon_{max}$, per styrene monomer unit, is remarkably increased.[27] This increase for copolymers containing 4–5% of styrene is more than 10 times that of the model (Table 10) if the asymmetric carbon atom of the olefin monomeric unit is in the α-position with respect to the polymer main chain, and decreases gradually if the asymmetric carbon atom is respectively in β- and γ-position (Table 10). This decrease is what we can expect according to the models we have proposed for the conformation in solution of the poly-α-olefins;[28] in fact, the prevalence of helical conformations of a single screw sense for the main chain of optically active poly-α-olefins is expected to decrease by increasing the distance between the asymmetric carbon atom of the lateral chain and the main chain. The decrease in prevalence is much smaller going from polymers having the asymmetric carbon atom in the α-position to polymers having the asymmetric carbon atom in the β-position, than going from polymers having the asymmetric carbon atom in β-position to polymers having the asymmetric carbon atom in the γ-position.[28] The fact that poly-(S)-p.sec.butyl-styrene, despite the expected helical conformation of the main chain, does not show, with respect to low-molecular-weight models, an enhancement of the $\Delta\varepsilon$ of the phenylchromophore at 260 nm ($\Delta\varepsilon \sim 0·05$)[29] is in agreement with our working hypothesis. In fact, a very rough conformational analysis shows that the sec.butyl group in the para-position is not able to induce a noticeable prevalence of a single screw sense of the helical main chain. Therefore, a practically equal number of monomeric units are included in left-handed and in right-handed main-chain helical conformations, and the only contributions to the 260 nm CD bands which do not cancel are those connected with the sec.butyl group directly bound to the phenyl ring[29] as in low-molecular-weight model compounds. The enhancement of the CD band corresponding to the phenyl group in the copolymers with respect to 2-phenyl-butane and other low-molecular-weight models[26] as well as the relationship between CD sign and absolute configuration of the asymmetric carbon atom in the aliphatic lateral chains of the copolymers (i.e. the prevailing screw sense of the helical conformation of the principal chain[28]), might be explained according to a very rough conformational analysis.

Table 11

Conformational Analysis of (S)-2-Phenyl-butane

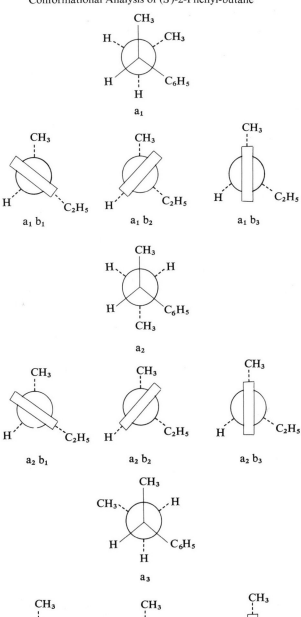

If the staggered conformations of 2-phenyl-butane are considered and, in particular the conformations originated by rotation of the phenyl ring around the bond between the phenyl group and the tertiary carbon atom, nine couples of conformations are possible (Table 11)—taking into account only the conformations in which one of the ortho carbon atoms of the phenyl ring is eclipsed, and the other is staggered, with respect to the groups bound to the tertiary carbon atom. However, because of the 1–5 interaction between the ortho carbon atoms of the phenyl ring and the methyl group in position 4 of 2-phenyl-butane, conformations a_1b_2 and a_2b_3 (Table 12) should have a larger energy than the others and can be tentatively considered as 'not allowed'. Seven couples of conformations of similar energy being

Table 12

Higher Energy Conformation of (S)-2-Phenyl Butane (Conf. $a_2 b_3$) and of a Phenyl Ring Inserted in a Laevo 3_1 Helix (Conf. c_1l) or in a Dextro 3_1 Helix (Conf. c_1d)

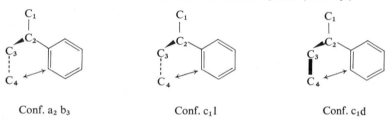

Conf. $a_2 b_3$ Conf. c_1l Conf. c_1d

allowed a small CD must be expected even if the CD of some of the allowed conformations is reasonably large.

A different situation arises in the copolymers of optically active α-olefins with styrene if we admit that the styrene units are included in left-handed or right-handed helical sections (Table 13). In fact, in this case the couple of conformations in which the plane of the phenyl ring is parallel to the helix axis (c_1l and c_1d) can be tentatively considered as 'not allowed' because of 1–5 interaction between helix and aromatic ring (Table 12), and of the two other pairs of conformations (Table 13), the ones in which an ortho carbon atom of the phenyl ring is eclipsed with the methinic hydrogen atom (c_2l and c_2d) seem to be preferred at least according to the indication given by the crystalline structure of isotactic polystyrene.[30] Obviously, each of the allowed conformations arising from the rotation of the phenyl ring in the left-handed helix (c_2l and c_3l) is enantiomorphic with respect to the corresponding conformation (c_2d and c_3d) arising from the rotation of the phenyl ring in the right-handed helix. Therefore, the position of the equilibrium between the allowed conformations arising from the rotation of the phenyl ring being obviously the same in the left-handed and in the right-handed helices, an opposite sign for the CD should be expected when the phenyl ring is inserted in a left-handed or in a right-handed helix. Furthermore, since only two pairs of allowed conformations exist in this case, and one has a prevailing statistical weight, as indicated by the crystalline structure of isotactic polystyrene,[30] a CD per phenyl ring larger than that of 2-phenyl-butane must be expected. Finally, using the same approach we hope that it will be possible to explain the large Cotton effect amplitude observed in other phenyl-containing polymers like polyisocyanates.[7]

Table 13

Conformational Analysis of a Styrene Unit Inserted in a Laevo Helix (c_1l, c_2l, c_3l) and Showing Positive CD, or in a Dextro Helix (c_1d, c_2d, c_3d) Showing a Negative CD

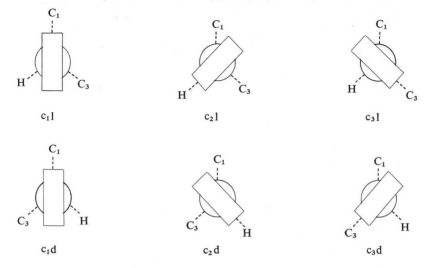

4.4.5 Final Remarks

The few examples of the application of ORD and CD to synthetic polymers reported here certainly show how fruitful this approach is in the investigation of the conformation of synthetic polymers in solution. Up to now, quantitative aspects of the conformational equilibria have been investigated only in poly-α-olefins; in all the other cases only qualitative aspects have been clarified, because of the lack of suitable theoretical or semi-empirical methods for the calculation of optical activity of single conformations, and also because of the lack of suitable approaches to conformational analysis.

The most general conclusions have been reached in the case of vinyl polymers and copolymers, in which, in order to explain the relationship between the Cotton effect sign of intrinsically non-dissymmetric chromophores and asymmetric carbon atom present in the lateral chains, the existence of ordered helical conformations of prevailingly one screw sense must be admitted. These ordered conformations are caused by the relatively small number of allowed conformations of each monomeric unit inserted in a vinyl polymer chain with respect to the closely similar low-molecular-weight models. The small number of allowed conformations causes, in the cases investigated, a remarkable increase of the amplitude of the Cotton effects connected with the paraffinic backbone of the monomeric units as well as of the Cotton effects of intrinsically non-dissymmetric chromophores present in the lateral chains. The increase of the Cotton effect amplitude is connected with the prevalence of main chain helical conformations having a single screw sense, and, therefore, they are dependent on main-chain stereoregularity.

From the aspect of progress in fundamental knowledge of CD and ORD, the enhancement of the Cotton effect amplitude in high polymers, and the use of thin films of high polymers instead of solutions, might make possible the investigation of chromophoric systems which, because of an unfavourable ratio between absorption coefficient and rotational strength, cannot be investigated in low-molecular-weight compounds.

The main aim of the research in the field of optically active polymers now is to investigate the requirements necessary to cause a sizeable electronic interaction between non-conjugated chromophoric systems; in fact, the investigation of the aforementioned interactions would improve the chances for a quantitative approach to the investigation of different factors such as type of solvent, or temperature, on the high polymer conformational equilibria.

Thanks are due for permission to reproduce the following copyright material in this chapter:

Figure 2, Tables 4 and 7 (ref. 15) by permission of I.U.P.A.C. Figure 3 (ref. 24) by permission of The Chemical Society, London. Figure 4 (ref. 27a) and Table 3 (ref. 7b) by permission of the American Chemical Society. Table 5 (ref. 18) by permission of Academic Press Inc.

References

1. See, for instance, H. Morawetz 'Macromolecules in Solution', in *High Polymers*, Vol. XXI. Interscience, 1965.
2. P. Pino, F. Ciardelli and M. Zandomeneghi, *Ann. Rev. Phys. Chem.* **21**, 561 (1970).
3. (a) M. Goodman, E. E. Schmitt and D. A. Yphantis, *J. Amer. Chem. Soc.* **84**, 1288 (1962). (b) M. Goodman, F. Boardman and I. Listowsky, *J. Amer. Chem. Soc.* **85**, 2491 (1963). (c) M. Goodman and I. G. Rosen, *Biopolymers* **2**, 537 (1964). (d) M. Goodman, M. Langsam and I. G. Rosen, *Biopolymers* **4**, 305 (1966). (e) H. Okabayashi, T. Isemura and S. Sakakibara, *Biopolymers* **6**, 323 (1968).
4. O. Bonsignori and P. Pino. In preparation.
5. (a) W. Moffit, *J. Chem. Phys.* **25**, 467 (1956). (b) W. Moffit and J. T. Yang, *Proc. Natl. Acad. Sci. U.S.A.* **42**, 596 (1956).
6. (a) F. Ciardelli, E. Benedetti and O. Pieroni, *Makromol. Chem.* **103**, 1 (1967). (b) O. Pieroni, F. Matera and F. Ciardelli, *Tetrahedron Lett.* 597 (1972).
7. (a) M. Goodman and S. Chen, *Macromolecules* **3**, 398 (1970). (b) M. Goodman and S. Chen, *Macromolecules* **4**, 625 (1971).
8. S. Kambara, N. Yamazaki and M. Hatano, *Preprints Div. Petroleum Chem.*, Amer. Chem. Soc. **9**, A-23, No. 4 (1964).
9. (a) R. Rossi and E. Benedetti, *Gazz. Chim. Ital.* **96**, 483 (1966). (b) Z. Janovic and D. Fles, *J. Polymer Sci.* A1, **9**, 1103 (1971).
10. (a) W. Oroshnik and A. D. Mebane, *J. Amer. Chem. Soc.* **76**, 5719 (1954). (b) J. L. H. Allan, G. D. Meakins and M. C. Whiting, *J. Chem. Soc.* 1874 (1955).
11. H. H. Jaffe and M. Orchin, in *Theory and Applications of Ultraviolet Spectroscopy*. John Wiley, 1962, p. 220.
12. A. Moscowitz, E. Charney, U. Weiss and H. Ziffer, *J. Amer. Chem. Soc.* **83**, 4661 (1961).
13. V. E. Shashoua, W. Sweeney and R. F. Tietz, *J. Amer. Chem. Soc.* **82**, 866 (1960).
14. U. Shmueli, W. Traub and K. Rosenheck, *J. Polymer Sci.* A2, **7**, 515 (1969).
15. P. Pino, P. Salvadori, E. Chiellini and P. L. Luisi, *Pure Appl. Chem.* **16**, 469 (1968).
16. P. Pino, F. Ciardelli, G. P. Lorenzi and G. Montagnoli, *Makromol. Chem.* **61**, 207 (1963).
17. J. H. Brewster, *J. Amer. Chem. Soc.* **81**, 5475 (1959).
18. S. Pucci, M. Aglietto, P. L. Luisi and P. Pino, in G. Chiurdoglu, Ed., *Conformational Analysis*. Academic Press, 1971, p. 203.
19. P. L. Luisi and P. Pino, *J. Phys. Chem.* **72**, 2400 (1968).
20. (a) P. Pino, G. P. Lorenzi, E. Chiellini and P. Salvadori, *Atti Accad. Naz. Lincei Rend.* [8] **39**, 196 (1965). (b) P. Pino, G. P. Lorenzi and E. Chiellini, *Ric. Sci.* Set A, **7**, 193 (1964). (c) P. Pino, G. P. Lorenzi and E. Chiellini, *J. Polymer Sci.* Part C, **16**, 3279 (1968).
21. E. Chiellini, P. Salvadori and P. Pino. In preparation.
22. O. Pieroni, F. Ciardelli, C. Botteghi, L. Lardicci, P. Salvadori and P. Pino, *J. Polymer Sci.* Part C, **22**, 993 (1969).
23. P. Maroni, *Ann. Chim.* **2**, 757 (1957).
24. L. Lardicci, P. Salvadori, C. Botteghi and P. Pino, *Chem. Commun.* 381 (1968).

25. C. Carlini, F. Ciardelli and P. Pino, *Makromol. Chem.* **119**, 244 (1968).
26. P. Salvadori, L. Lardicci and R. Menicagli, *Chim. Ind. (Milan)* **52**, 85 (1970).
27. (*a*) P. Pino, C. Carlini, E. Chiellini, F. Ciardelli and P. Salvadori, *J. Amer. Chem. Soc.* **90**, 5025 (1968). (*b*) E. Chiellini, C. Carlini, F. Ciardelli and P. Pino, *Macromolecular Preprints*, IUPAC Congress, Boston, 1971, **2**, 759.
28. P. Pino, *Advan. Polymer Sci.* **4**, 393 (1965).
29. F. Ciardelli, O. Pieroni, C. Carlini and C. Menicagli, *J. Polymer Sci.* A1. **10**, 809 (1972).
30. G. Natta, P. Corradini and I. W. Bassi, Supplements of *Nuovo Cimento* **15**, Serie X, 68 (1960).

Polypeptides and Proteins

E. R. BLOUT

Harvard Medical School
Boston, Mass., U.S.A.

4.5.1 Introduction

The main aims of recent chiroptical investigations of peptides, polypeptides, and proteins have been (a) to determine the fundamental optical properties of the various molecular groups which occur in peptides and proteins, (b) to use these optical properties to ascertain the molecular structures or 'conformations' of these compounds in solution, and (c) to investigate changes in the molecular structures of proteins under a variety of chemical and biochemical conditions. In this contribution I will in turn briefly review some of the current knowledge of the rotatory properties of peptide models for proteins, then examine the use of chiroptical information for conformational investigations of proteins, and finally present several applications of optical activity measurements of peptides and proteins.

4.5.2 Optical Properties of the Molecular Groups of Proteins

The fundamental chemical and structural unit of all proteins is, of course, the 'peptide group', and polypeptides and proteins may be considered basically as peptide polymers. Each peptide group (or peptide unit) contains at least one asymmetric centre at the α-carbon atom, except in the case of glycine. Such asymmetric centres certainly contribute to the optical properties of proteins, but it is now evident (*vide infra*) that by far the greatest influence on the optical properties of proteins is the specific arrangement of these peptide groups in three-dimensional space,[1] rather than in the inherent asymmetry due to the α-carbon atoms of the peptide units. Since the optical activity of any molecule is related to its absorptive properties, it is pertinent first to consider the absorptive properties of the peptide group and the other molecular groups found in proteins. The absorption maxima and extinction coefficients for these groupings have recently been summarized by Donovan[2] (Table 1). From this summary of many investigations, it is apparent that all the known absorptions of proteins due to peptide chains lie in the ultraviolet region, and that the strongest of these absorptions appear below 230 nm. It should be noted that, in addition to the strong absorption bands of proteins which appear in the now readily accessible ultraviolet region (185–300 nm), there are also intense protein absorption

Table 1

Chromophores of Proteins: Approximate Location, Intensity and Assignments of Singlet–Singlet Absorption Bands[a]

Residues	Chromophore	Location (nm)	$\log \varepsilon_{max}$	Assignment
Peptide bond	CONH	162	3·8	$\pi^+ \to \pi^-$
		188	3·9	$\pi^0 \to \pi^-$
		225	2·6	$n \to \pi^-$
Aspartic, glutamic	COOH	175	3·4	$n \to \pi^*$?
		205	1·6	$n \to \pi^*$
Aspartate, glutamate	COO$^-$	200	2	$n \to \pi^*$
Lysine, arginine	N—H	173	3·4	$\sigma \to \sigma^*$
		213	2·8	$n \to \sigma^*$
Phenylalanine	Phenyl	188	4·8	
		206	3·9	$\pi \to \pi^*$
		261	2·35	
Tyrosine	Phenolic	193	4·7	
		222	3·9	$\pi \to \pi^*$
		270	3·16	
Tyrosine (ionized)	Phenolic	200?	5	
		235	3·97	$\pi \to \pi^*$
		287	3·41	
Tryptophan	Indole	195	4·3	
		220	4·53	$\pi \to \pi^*$
		280	3·7	
		286	3·3	
Histidine	Imidazole	211	3·78	$\pi \to \pi^*$?
CysSH	S—H	195	3·3	$n \to \sigma^*$
CysS$^-$	S$^-$	235	3·5	$n \to \sigma^*$
Cystine	S—S	210	3	$n \to \sigma^*$
		250	2·5	$n \to \sigma^*$

[a] From reference 2.

bands which lie in the vacuum ultraviolet region; that is, below 185 nm, but these bands will not be considered here, since little is known about their properties.

Investigations of the rotatory properties of oligomeric peptides[3, 4] have shown that dramatic increases in optical activity* occur suddenly (under certain conditions) when the number of peptide units is between five and twelve. It is now clear that the observed increase in optical activity with added chain length in certain oligopeptide systems is due to the formation of periodic structures—which themselves exhibit inherent or intrinsic optical activity. Furthermore, it should be noted that recent investigations of certain model amides, due principally to the work of Dr. John Schellman and his colleagues,[5] have indicated that, when two peptide groups are held rigidly with respect to one another, similar large increases in optical activity are observed. Thus, it may be concluded that the large rotations observed with proteins

* When the terms 'optical activity', 'rotatory properties', or 'chiroptical properties' are used here, both optical rotatory dispersion (ORD) and circular dichroism (CD) are indicated. The two functions, ORD and CD, are analytically interconvertible by use of the mathematical expression known as the Kronig–Kramers transform and are, therefore, equivalent (Chapter 1.1).

are due to the fact that the peptide groups in proteins are held with a fixed geometry—either periodic or aperiodic.

The molecular groupings of proteins (other than the peptide groups), which have significant absorption in the ultraviolet and contribute to the optical activity, are the aromatic side chains of tryptophan, tyrosine and phenylalanine, and the disulphide groups of cystine residues. In addition, small contributions to the optical activity may result from the presence of carboxylate and ammonium groups, and the presence of metals in certain proteins can modify the absorptive and optical properties of the molecular groupings with which the metals are associated.[6] In general, the contributions of the above-mentioned groups to the optical spectra of proteins are small compared with the contributions of the peptide groups for two reasons; first, because the relative numbers of such groupings are small, and secondly, because the inherent optical activity of these groups is lower than that of the peptide group. A summary of the circular dichroism properties of some amino-acid residues is given in Table 2. The optical properties of the aromatic amino-acid residues may, in some cases, be used to obtain important information about the molecular conformations and interactions of peptide chains of proteins.

Table 2

Circular Dichroism Properties of Some Amino-acid Residues

Residue	Chromophore	Location[a] (nm)	Magnitude $[\theta]$ (deg cm^2 decimole^{-1})[b]	Ref.
Phenylalanine	Phenyl	255, 262, 268	-150	c, d, e
		220	$+12{,}000$	d, e, f
Tyrosine	Phenolic	276; shoulders at 270, 283	$\pm3{,}000$	g, h
		225	$+20{,}000$	f
Tyrosine (ionized)	Phenolate ion	290	$\pm2{,}000$	f
		240	$+20{,}000$	f
Tryptophan	Indole	265–300 variable	$\pm3{,}000$	g, i
		225	$+20{,}000$	f
		195	$-30{,}000$	f
Histidine	Imidazole	212–220	$+10{,}000$	e, f
Cystine	Disulphide	278	$-3{,}000$	j, k
		255	$\pm2{,}000$	j, l, m
		199	$-40{,}000$	l, m

[a] Location may not necessarily correlate with absorption maximum. [b] Intensity of $[\theta]$, as well as sign, may vary greatly.

References to Table 2

[c] J. Horwitz, E. H. Strickland and C. Billups, *J. Amer. Chem. Soc.* **91**, 184 (1969). [d] N. S. Simmons, A. O. Barel and A. N. Glazer, *Biopolymers* **7**, 275, (1969). [e] M. Goodman and C. Toniolo, *Biopolymers* **6**, 1673 (1968). [f] S. Beychok, in G. D. Fasman, Ed., *Poly α-Amino Acids*. Marcel Dekker, Inc., New York, 1967, p. 293. [g] E. H. Strickland, M. Wilchek, J. Horwitz and C. Billups, *J. Biol. Chem.* **245**, 4168 (1970). [h] J. Horwitz, E. H. Strickland and C. Billups, *J. Amer. Chem. Soc.* **92**, 2119 (1970). [i] E. H. Strickland, J. Horwitz and C. Billups, *Biochemistry* **8**, 3205 (1969). [j] S. Beychok and E. Breslow, *J. Biol. Chem.* **243**, 151 (1968). [k] E. Breslow, *Proc. Natl. Acad. Sci. U.S.A.* **67**, 493 (1970). [l] D. L. Coleman and E. R. Blout, *J. Amer. Chem. Soc.* **90**, 2405 (1968). [m] D. L. Coleman and E. R. Blout, in *Conformation of Biopolymers*. Academic Press, 1967, p. 123.

4.5.3 Polypeptide Chain Conformations

The number of theoretically possible conformations which a polypeptide chain consisting of, say, 100 amino-acid residues can assume is very large, since the principal restriction to rotation around the peptide chain bond is due to the planar

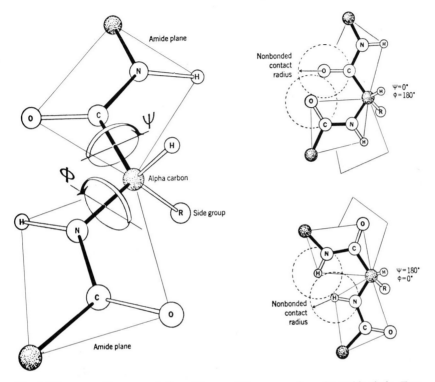

Fig. 1. Diagrammatic representation of two peptide groups of a polypeptide chain. Two amide planes are joined by the tetrahedral bonds of the α carbon. The only easy movement is rotation about the C_α—C and C_α—N single bonds. The rotation parameters are $\phi(C_\alpha$—N bond) and $\psi(C_\alpha$—C). Positive rotation for ϕ and ψ is clockwise when viewed from the α carbon. The zero position in both ϕ and ψ occurs with the two peptide planes themselves coplanar as shown in the large-drawing (above left). Some positions of ϕ and ψ are not permitted because of too close approach of unbonded atoms. The drawing at the top right shows the maximum forbidden overlap of carbonyl oxygens at $\phi = 180°$, $\psi = 0°$. Below it is shown the maximum forbidden overlap of hydrogens at $\phi = 0°$, $\psi = 180°$. [From R. E. Dickerson and I. Geis, *The Structure and Action of Proteins.* Harper and Row, Publishers, New York, 1969.]

nature of the C—N bond of the peptide group. The restriction of rotational movement about the C_α—C and C_α—N bonds is relatively minor (Fig. 1). If the peptide bond is planar, then the polypeptide chain has two degrees of freedom per residue, the twist about the C_α—N bond axis, ϕ, and that about the C_α—C axis, ψ. Thus, if one knew all the ϕ, ψ values for all residues of a peptide chain, it would completely define the geometry of the chain.

In synthetic polypeptides and in certain proteins, there are several periodic arrangements of peptide groups which contribute markedly to the optical properties of these substances. The periodic structures found most widely distributed in proteins are (a) the helix, (b) the polyproline-II helix, (c) extended sheet structures, (d) double-helical structures, such as those found in the muscle protein, myosin, and (e) triple-helical conformations present in the structural protein, collagen. Diagrammatic representations of some of these structures are shown in Fig. 2. In addition to the periodic structures existing in proteins, there are significant regions of the peptide chains in which the peptide groups are not in periodic array but yet have definite fixed arrangements with respect to one another. Both the periodic and aperiodic regions of peptide chains make significant contributions to the observed rotatory properties.

A. The α-Helix

One of the important milestones in the investigations of the absorptive and optical properties of polypeptide chains was the elegant work of the late William Moffitt who introduced the idea of exciton splitting of helical polypeptide absorption bands (Fig. 2).[7] The basic idea behind Moffitt's work was that the rotatory properties of polypeptides and proteins in the visible spectrum result from optically active absorption bands which lie in the ultraviolet region, and that these absorption bands will differ in position and magnitude depending on the molecular structure of the polypeptide or the protein. This concept of exciton splitting led to the formulation of a semi-empirical equation useful in characterizing the optical rotatory dispersion of helical peptide molecules *outside* their absorption bands.[8] One of the constants of this equation, b_0, proved useful as a semi-quantitative measure of the α-helical content of such molecules. At the present time, however, with the general availability of instruments to measure the ultraviolet Cotton effects directly, the use of an inferential treatment, like the Moffitt equation (and other such equations), has in the view of most workers in the field become obsolete,[9] except for those situations in which the far ultraviolet is obscured by solvent or other extraneous absorptions.

Impetus was given to investigations of the chiroptical properties of proteins by the development of polarimeters capable of measurement below 230 nm and by the experimental discovery in the late 1950s that certain polypeptides and proteins exhibit a relatively large Cotton effect in the spectral region around 225 nm.[10] This Cotton effect has been shown both to be related to the n $\rightarrow$ π* transition of the peptide group and to be conformation-dependent. Destruction of the α-helical conformation of synthetic polypeptides by means of pH changes, solvent changes, or thermal changes results in the loss of this Cotton effect. Following the discovery of this 225 nm Cotton effect, other absorption bands of peptides lying at still shorter wavelengths were investigated, and other Cotton effects related to periodic peptide structures were discovered and investigated—initially by optical rotation measurements[11] and more recently by circular dichroism measurements. Optical rotatory dispersion data in the ultraviolet region for α-helical polypeptides are shown in Fig. 3.

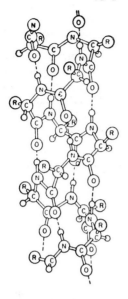

Helical
[α]

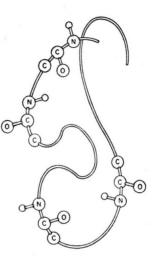

Random

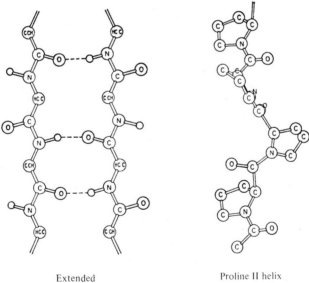

Extended
[β]

Proline II helix

Fig. 2. Diagrammatic representation of some periodic (and 'random') conformations which have been shown to exist in protein chains. [From E. R. Blout, 'Conformations of Proteins', in *The Neurosciences*. Rockefeller University Press, New York, 1967.]

B. β-Conformations

Following the characterization of the rotatory properties of the α-helix, several investigations were performed to establish the rotatory properties of other periodic conformations found in polypeptides and proteins. A common structural motif in proteins is the presence of short segments of β or extended chain conformations. The optical properties of synthetic polypeptides known to exist in such conformations have now been examined, and some typical data are shown in Fig. 3.

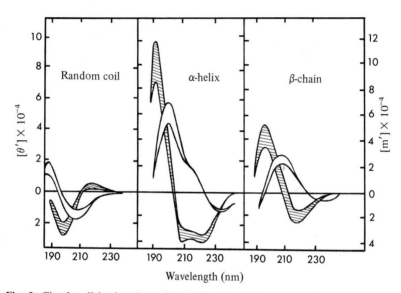

Fig. 3. Circular dichroism (cross-hatched) and optical rotatory dispersion of homopolypeptides in the random coil, α-helical and β-conformations. The enclosed areas indicate the range of values reported in the recent literature. [From Gratzer and Cowburn.[9]]

C. 'Random' Polypeptide Chains

With the characterization of the two ordered polypeptide structures cited above, the next step was to determine the optical properties of an unordered polypeptide chain, and the assumption was made that a charged chain, such as poly-L-glutamic acid or poly-L-lysine, would serve as a model for this conformation. It has been recently pointed out, both on the basis of experimental results and theoretical arguments, that such chains may have 'local' structure.[12] It has been shown, however, that it is possible to obtain charged polypeptides in an essentially unordered state by treatment of such substances with various concentrated salt solutions. However, the CD spectra obtained, while of a characteristic qualitative form, are not quantitatively identical for all synthetic polypeptides. The experimental fact is that different circular dichroism spectra are found for charged random chain synthetic polypeptides and for denatured proteins.

D. Proline Helices

Two different helical forms of polyproline are known, designated polyproline I and polyproline II. Due to the steric constraints imposed by the proline residue, these helical proline structures differ markedly from the α-helix. Polyproline I is a right-handed helix containing *cis*-peptide bonds; polyproline II is a left-handed helix with *trans*-peptide bonds. The rotatory properties of the two different polyproline conformations are shown in Fig. 4. Polyproline I may be reversibly converted to

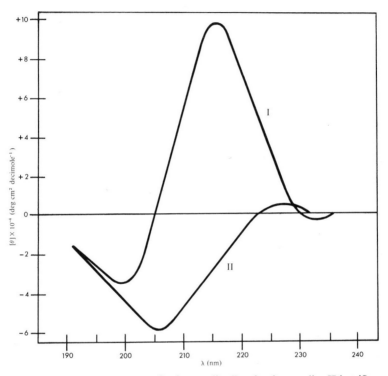

Fig. 4. Circular dichroism spectra of poly-L-proline I and poly-L-proline II in trifluoro-ethanol solution. [The data are redrawn from F. A. Bovey and F. P. Hood, *Biopolymers*, **5**, 325 (1967).]

polyproline II via an acid-catalysed reaction,[13] and this transformation has been monitored by rotatory measurements. The polyproline-II helix is a major structural motif of the collagen class of proteins (see below).

E. Quantitative Determination of Periodic Conformations of Proteins

After the determination of the optical parameters of the α-helical and β-structures with synthetic polypeptides, a logical further step was to attempt to use these data in order to make quantitative (or semi-quantitative) estimates of the percentages of such ordered structures in proteins. The most extensive work in this area has been performed by Dr. G. D. Fasman and his colleagues.[14] The basic assumption (made with reservations) is that unique circular dichroism curves can be used for the α-helical, β-conformation, and random coil segments of proteins from the corresponding data of homopolypeptides. Figure 3 shows CD and ORD curves of homopolypeptides in these three different conformations.[9] The enclosed areas indicate the range of values from recent literature data based on modern instruments. It is possible, perhaps likely, that the spread of values is due not only to real variability of different polymers in different solvents, but also to experimental errors; for example, possible contamination of one conformation by another, as well as instrumental errors. Some average values of optical rotatory dispersion and circular dichroism of several polypeptide chain conformations are shown in Table 3.

Table 3

Optical Properties of Various Polypeptide Chain Conformations (in the Region of Peptide Bond Absorption)

Conformation	Optical Rotatory Dispersion $[R]$ = deg cm² decimole⁻¹ in parentheses			Circular Dichroism λ_{max} $[\theta]$ = deg cm² decimole⁻¹ in parentheses
	Trough	Peak	Crossover	
α-Helix	233 (−15,000)		224	222 (−36,000)
		218 (shoulder, +20,000)		208 (−33,000)
		199 (+77,000)	189	191 (+77,000)
β-Structure (antiparallel?)	230 (−6,000)		~220	217 (−18,000)
		205 (+22,000)		195 (+32,000)
Poly-L-proline I	208 (−18,000)	223 (+28,000)	217	215 (+99,000)
				199 (−34,600)
Poly-L-proline II	217 (−32,000)			226 (+3,000)
		195 (+19,000)	205	206 (−59,000)
Collagen				221 (+8,000)
	207 (−36,000)	190 (+37,000)	197	198 (−56,000)
	238 (−1,500)			238 (−150)
Random (?) chain				217 (+4,600)
	205 (−18,000)	190 (+18,000)	198	197 (−42,000)

Wavelengths in nm (±1 nm); magnitudes ±10%.

With the reservations mentioned above, the experimental circular dichroism curves of several proteins, whose three-dimensional structures are known from X-ray diffraction studies, have been fitted by a linear combination of α-helical, β and random structures in the 208–240 nm region. The results obtained show that if the protein possesses a high percentage of periodic structure (e.g. myoglobin), the agreement between the calculated and the X-ray diffraction determined structure is good. If the protein contains large percentages of aperiodic structures, the results are less satisfactory.

More recently, D. B. Wetlaufer[15] has combined experimental CD spectra of three proteins with estimates of the content of peptide chain structural modes from X-ray diffraction studies of the same protein. Solution of the simultaneous equations at a series of wavelengths permitted the construction of a CD spectrum for the three structural modes: α-helix, β-structure, and 'random' chain. The CD spectra obtained in this way are compared with those obtained from polypeptide models (Fig. 5). The

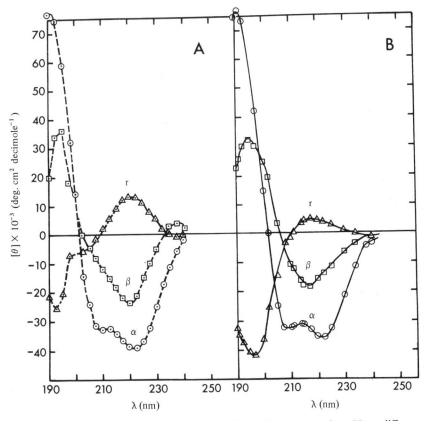

Fig. 5. A. Circular dichroism spectra of three polypeptide structures from X-ray diffraction structural data and experimental circular dichroism spectra of lysozyme, myoglobin and ribonuclease. B. Experimental circular dichroism spectra of three polypeptide structures obtained for the three forms of poly-L-lysine by Greenfield and Fasman.[14(b)] [From Saxena and Wetlaufer.[15]]

results indicate that the α-helical spectra from the two approaches are nearly congruent, the β-structure spectra are in fair agreement, and the 'random' forms are quantitatively substantially different, although qualitatively similar. Very recently it has been shown that the use of poly-L-serine in high salt solution gives a CD spectrum which corresponds better to that of a random protein chain.[16]

The reasons for the failure of such analyses to determine periodic structures in proteins quantitatively (except for α-helix contents) may be due, in large part, to the fact that the aperiodic portions of proteins contribute strongly, in an as yet unknown manner, to the overall optical properties of the protein. In addition, there are undoubtedly contributions, in the region of the spectrum analysed, from aromatic amino-acid residues and from disulphide bonds of the proteins. Furthermore, there is the additional problem that the varying environments of any particular peptide group in the protein may have somewhat different contributions to the overall optical spectrum. It is possible that such problems could be overcome, provided sufficient time and effort were expended, but interest in this approach has lessened, since protein chemists now generally desire more detailed structural information than can be provided by total periodic conformation estimates. There are many other questions, which appear more relevant with respect to protein chemistry, that can be answered by CD and ORD determinations, some of which will be discussed below.

4.5.4   Some Applications of Chiroptical Measurements

One of the earliest uses of the optical properties of proteins was to determine whether a protein changed in structure upon changing the chemical or physical environment surrounding the protein. 'Denaturation' is the term commonly employed which encompasses the structural and functional changes observed when proteins are subjected to such treatments. It is now evident that an important use of optical activity measurements of proteins is to follow both major and minor changes in the conformation of peptide chains with chemical or physical treatment—even though the observed changes cannot always be interpreted in terms of absolute molecular structure.

A. Major Conformational Changes in Proteins

An example of a major conformational change in a protein which can be effectively monitored by optical measurements is the thermal denaturation of collagen. The characteristic circular dichroism of native collagen and that of heat-treated collagen is shown in Fig. 6. The characteristic strong negative circular dichroism band at 198 nm (and the weaker positive band at 221 nm) is lost upon 'denaturation' via heating at 40°C for short periods of time. The temperature dependence of the native (ordered) collagen structure may be determined by measuring the magnitudes of these two circular dichroism bands as a function of temperature. Examples of such data are shown in Fig. 7.[17] It will be readily seen that a sharp temperature transition (at approximately 37°C) can be measured in this manner. One of the present uses for rotatory measurements is the determination and monitoring of major structural changes in proteins.

Another type of major structural change in proteins that has been detected via chiroptical measurements is that occurring when some proteins are exposed to detergents.[18] Treatment of protein mixtures with detergents such as sodium dodecylsulphate (SDS) is a common practice; for example, in the isolation of proteins from cell walls and cell membranes. We have recently reported the effects of sodium dodecylsulphate treatment on the rotatory properties and conformations of several proteins.[19] An example of the effects of such treatment is shown in Fig. 8. Treatment of elastase with small amounts of SDS changes the circular dichroism spectrum of native elastase markedly, and this new spectrum can be interpreted as indicating a conformation having considerably higher α-helical content than is present in the native molecule. Removal of most, or all, of the sodium dodecylsulphate by dialysis again changes the observed circular dichroism spectrum—this time to a spectrum which indicates a considerable amount of β-structure. Evidently, major conformational changes have occurred upon treatment with this detergent, and these changes can be followed via circular dichroism measurements.

B. *Minor Conformational Changes in Proteins*

As noted above, the aromatic amino-acid residues and the disulphide bonds of proteins often give rise to characteristic rotatory spectra in the region 240–300 nm.

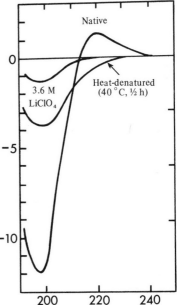

Fig. 6. Circular dichroism spectra of native rat tail collagen in 3·6 M-lithium perchlorate. [From Tiffany and Krimm.[12]]

On the one hand, the presence of such groups is a complication for quantitative measurements of periodic structures in the shorter wavelength ultraviolet region, but on the other hand, the presence of such groups may provide a valuable probe for minor conformational changes involving, particularly, tyrosine or tryptophan residues. An example of this type of investigation is the recent work of Dr. John Griffin in our laboratory,[20] who has been studying the binding of substrates and inhibitors to the enzyme, aspartate transcarbamylase (from *E. coli*). This enzyme is a multi-subunit protein; that is, the native enzyme consists of six polypeptide chains (subunits) which are held into one active enzyme molecule by non-covalent bonds. There are three catalytic subunits and three regulatory subunits. Dr. Griffin has found that the binding of substrates and inhibitors to native aspartate transcarbamylase and to the catalytic and regulatory subunits isolated from the native enzyme gives rise to characteristic circular dichroism difference spectra between 250 and 310 nm. CD difference spectra, which reflect changes in the asymmetric structure or environment of tyrosyl and tryptophanyl residues, have been used to characterize optical activity changes which arise during binding of carbamylphosphate (a substrate of the enzyme) and succinate (a substrate analogue). The carbamylphosphate CD difference spectra of the native enzyme show a CD peak at 278 nm with shoulders at 272 and

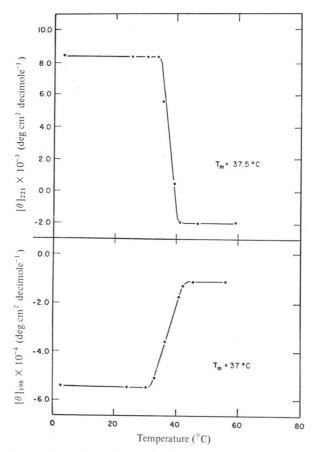

Fig. 7. Temperature dependence of ordered collagen structure. Guinea pig skin collagen in water, concentration = 0·5 mg/ml. [From Brown *et al.*[17]]

285 nm. These difference spectra do not occur in the isolated catalytic subunit. Since the 285 shoulder and the 278 peak are tyrosine transitions, it can be concluded that the binding of the substrate, carbamylphosphate, perturbs tyrosine residues in the native enzyme, but not in the isolated catalytic subunit. In contrast, succinate CD difference spectra of *both* the native enzyme and the catalytic subunit show perturbation of the tryptophan transition at 282 nm. This finding implies that these tryptophanyl perturbations are inherent features of the binding of succinate, both to the native enzyme and its catalytic subunit.

It is only recently, with the improved circular dichroism instruments now available, that such small changes can be measured in protein CD spectra. The possibility of

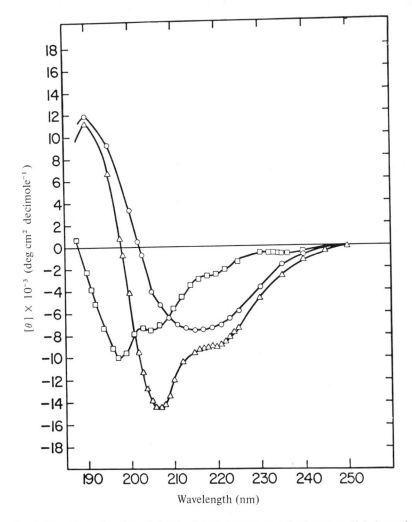

Fig. 8. The effect of sodium dodecyl sulphate treatment and subsequent dialysis on the circular dichroism spectrum of elastase. Solid sodium dodecyl sulphate was added to 0·025% elastase and then circular dichroism spectra were obtained after 1 hour. Similar results were obtained with 0·2% and 2% sodium dodecyl sulphate: elastase (□–□) plus sodium dodecyl sulphate (△–△) and subsequent dialysis (○–○). [From Visser and Blout.[19]]

making such measurements opens new areas for the biochemist interested in examining the details of peptide chain–peptide chain interactions and peptide chain–small molecule interactions involving aromatic amino-acid residues.

C. Collagen and Synthetic Tripeptide Analogues

Collagen is the most prevalent protein in all mammalian systems and, in addition, possesses a unique and characteristic triple-helical structure. The collagen molecule consists of three peptide chains, each of which has the polyproline II conformation, twisted together into a right-handed super-helix.[21] Extensive chemical work with collagen indicates that it is unique in another aspect; namely, the amino-acid sequence is such that glycine appears at every third residue in each of the three component peptide chains, and that the imino acids, proline and hydroxyproline, account for 20–30% of the total amino-acid content.

These findings have suggested that synthetic polytripeptides having the repeating sequence, X-Y-Gly, where X and/or Y are proline, might form the triple-helical structure found in native collagen. Circular dichroism measurements have been obtained on synthetic polytripeptides in order to examine this possibility and to compare the rotatory properties of these substances with native collagen. As noted above, native collagen exists as a triple-helical molecule, and it can be seen from Fig. 9 that its circular dichroism spectrum differs from that of polyproline II, the single-chain model compound for the triple-helical collagen structure.[22] On the other hand, the polytripeptides, $(Pro-Ser-Gly)_n$ and $(Pro-Ala-Gly)_n$, show almost identical circular dichroism spectra to that of native collagen (Fig. 10),[23] strongly suggesting that these synthetic polytripeptides assume the same conformation in solution as if found in collagen.

D. Induced Optical Activity

Until this point we have been discussing the optical activity intrinsic to polypeptide chains and amino-acid residues of proteins. A related, but different, phenomenon has been observed when certain chromophoric substances are bound to polypeptide chains. Several years ago Dr. Lubert Stryer observed that certain dyes (which were inherently symmetric and, therefore, not optically active) when bound to some polypeptides or proteins, showed optical activity in the absorption band of the dyes.[24] This phenomenon was explained in terms of 'induced' optical activity* of a symmetric molecule brought about by its close spatial relationship to the dissymmetric polypeptide chain.

Similar phenomena are also observed in protein systems; e.g. in haemoglobin,[25] myoglobin[26] and rhodopsin.[27] These proteins consist of polypeptide chains and non-peptide moieties—prosthetic groups, such as the haeme group of haemoglobin and myoglobin. The haeme group of myoglobin by itself possesses a characteristic absorption spectrum in the visible region but shows no rotatory properties. Conversely, the protein moiety alone, apomyoglobin, of the myoglobin molecule shows no absorption in the visible but does show optical rotation. Adding haeme to apomyoglobin results in the recovery of the original rotatory properties of myoglobin.[26] It appears that the fit of the haeme group into the apomyoglobin molecule

---

* 'Induced' optical activity is a term which describes the optical activity observed in chromophores which are not asymmetric and not part of the peptide chains of proteins. Such chromophores are often termed 'extrinsic', and the rotatory phenomena observed with them are often termed 'extrinsic Cotton effects'.

is such that 'induced' optical activity occurs when the combination of the haeme and the protein is exactly correct. Several other recent investigations that are related to this phenomenon of 'induced' optical activity in proteins have been described.[28]

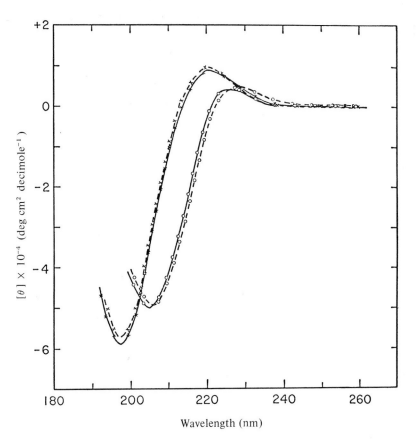

Fig. 9. Circular dichroism spectra of collagen (–×–×–) and poly-L-proline II (–○–○–) in ethylene glycol/water, 2:1 (v/v), at +24° (-----) and −112° (———). [From Brown *et al.*[22]]

E. *Magnetic Circular Dichroism*

The application of magnetic circular dichroism to investigations of amino acids and proteins has recently been reported by Dr. Carl Djerassi and his colleagues.[29] They have found that, of the naturally occurring amino acids, only tyrosine and tryptophan give intense magnetic circular dichroism bands. Tryptophan shows strong magnetic circular dichroism bands that are about 30 to 50 times more intense than its circular dichroism bands. Tryptophan shows an absorption band with a maximum at 279 nm and its characteristic strong magnetic circular dichroism band at 290 nm (Fig. 11). This is a spectral region in which there is negligible overlap from bands belonging to other amino acids. The intensity of this tryptophan band seems to be independent of the position of tryptophan in proteins, as well as the con-

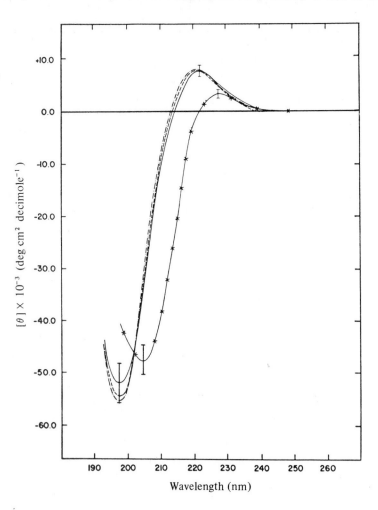

Fig. 10. Circular dichroism spectra of (Pro-Ser-Gly)$_n$ (-----), (Pro-Ala-Gly)$_n$ (-··-··-··-), and (Pro-Gly-Pro)$_n$ (-×-×-) compared with guinea pig skin collagen (———). In all cases the solvent = 1,3-propanediol, concentration = 1·25 mg/ml, and temperature = +24°C. [From Brown et al.[23]]

formation of the protein. Therefore, it is suggested that this magnetic circular dichroism of tryptophan can be used for its quantitative determination, and this suggestion has been verified by examining many well-characterized proteins.[29]

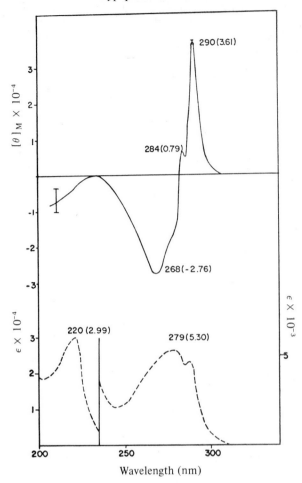

Fig. 11. Magnetic circular dichroism (———) and ultraviolet (-----) spectra of L-leucyl-L-tryptophan amide acetate in 0·01 M phosphate buffer (pH 6·9). [From Barth *et al.*[29(b)]]

F. Cyclic Peptides

The synthesis and examination of the rotatory properties of small cyclic peptides have been reported recently.[30-34] Such compounds are of interest because, among other reasons, they provide peptide structures in which the peptide groups may be held in relatively restricted conformations. Examples of such compounds are cyclo(tri-L-prolyl) and cyclo(L-Pro-L-Pro-L-Hypro) whose CD spectra are shown in Fig. 12. Cyclic peptides may prove to be useful models for the structured, but non-periodic, regions of proteins. At the moment it is not possible to interpret the circular dichroism spectra of such compounds unequivocally, but hopefully, further investigations of this type of compound will provide a link between rotatory theory and experiment.

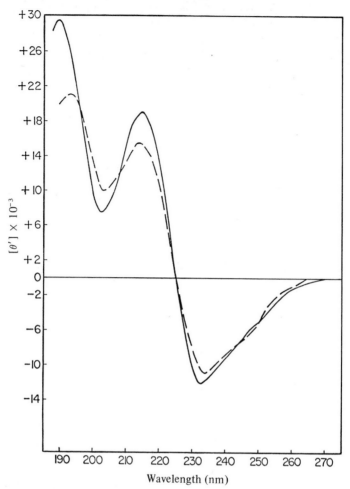

Fig. 12. Circular dichroism spectra of cyclo(tri-L-prolyl) and cyclo(L-Pro-L-Pro-L-Hypro) in methanol. [From C. M. Deber, F. A. Bovey, J. P. Carver and E. R. Blout, in E. Scoffone, Ed., *Peptides 1969*. North Holland Publishing Company, 1971, p. 189.]

4.5.5 Summary

1. The circular dichroism and optical rotatory dispersion spectra of α-helical, prolyl helix and triple-helical (collagen-like) polypeptides are well characterized and show distinctive rotatory properties. Those of another periodic conformation—the β (extended) form—are less well characterized but also appear to be distinctive. There is still greater uncertainty about the uniqueness of the circular dichroism and optical rotatory spectra of 'random' chain polypeptides and the non-periodic portions of polypeptide chains in proteins. Different types of polyproline helices can easily be distinguished via chiroptical measurements.

2. The quantitative determinations of periodic conformations in proteins appear to be possible for helical conformations, at least.

3. Chiroptical measurements have been shown to be valuable for monitoring major changes in protein conformations upon treatment with chemical or physical agents.

4. The present indications are that, using rotatory data, in some cases it will be possible to ascertain and perhaps explain minor conformational changes in proteins, especially those involving aromatic amino-acid residues.

5. Recent work on the magnetic circular dichroism of proteins indicates that it will be possible to determine tryptophan contents of proteins quantitatively via this method.

6. In order to reconcile theory and experiment, model peptide compounds—especially cyclic peptides with relatively restricted conformations—should prove useful.

In any field as large and vital as the one reviewed above, it is impossible to include all significant work. I trust my scientific colleagues in this area will recognize that the many omissions on my part were due to space and time limitations.

I am pleased to acknowledge the many years of fruitful collaboration with students and postdoctoral fellows who performed some of the work reported here; without their determined and imaginative efforts little would have been accomplished.

I also wish to acknowledge the continued support of our work by the National Institutes of Health, particularly via U.S. Public Health Grant AM-07300.

Thanks are due for permission to reproduce the following material in this chapter:

Table 1 (ref. 2) by permission of Academic Press Inc. Figure 1 by permission of Harper & Row Inc. Figure 3 (ref. 9) by permission of Macmillan Journals Ltd. Figure 4 and Figure 6 (ref. 12) © John Wiley and Sons Inc. Reprinted by permission of the copyright owner. Figure 5 (ref. 15) by permission of the U.S. National Academy of Sciences. Figure 11 (ref. 29*b*) by permission of the American Chemical Society.

References

1. C. Cohen, *Nature* **175**, 129 (1955).
2. J. Donovan, in S. Leach, Ed., *Physical Principles and Techniques of Protein Chemistry*. Academic Press, 1969, p. 109.
3. See for example: H. Okabayashi, T. Isemure and S. Sakakibara, *Biopolymers* **6**, 323 (1968).
4. C. M. Deber, F. A. Bovey, J. P. Carver and E. R. Blout, *J. Amer. Chem. Soc.* **92**, 6191 (1970).
5. V. Madison and J. Schellman, *Biopolymers* **9**, 65 (1970).
6. For references see: B. L. Vallee and W. E. C. Wacker, in *The Proteins*, Second ed., Vol. 5. Academic Press, New York, 1970, pp. 104–120.
7. W. Moffitt, *Proc. Natl. Acad. Sci. U.S.A.* **42**, 736 (1956).
8. W. Moffitt and J. T. Yang, *Proc. Natl. Acad. Sci. U.S.A.* **42**, 596 (1956).
9. W. B. Gratzer and D. A. Cowburn, *Nature* **222**, 426 (1969).
10. (*a*) N. S. Simmons and E. R. Blout, *Biophys. J.* **1**, 55 (1960). (*b*) N. S. Simmons, C. Cohen, A. G. Szent-Gyorgyi, D. B. Wetlaufer and E. R. Blout, *J. Amer. Chem. Soc.* **83**, 4766 (1961).
11. E. R. Blout, I. Schmier and N. S. Simmons, *J. Amer. Chem. Soc.* **84**, 3193 (1962).
12. M. L. Tiffany and S. Krimm, *Biopolymers* **8**, 347 (1969).
13. I. Z. Steinberg, W. F. Harrington, A. Berger, M. Sela and E. Katchalski, *J. Amer. Chem. Soc.* **82**, 5263 (1960).
14. (*a*) N. Greenfield, B. Davidson and G. D. Fasman, *Biochemistry* **6**, 1630 (1967). (*b*) N. Greenfield and G. D. Fasman, *Biochemistry* **8**, 4108 (1969).
15. V. P. Saxena and D. B. Wetlaufer, *Proc. Natl. Acad. Sci. U.S.A.* **68**, 969 (1971).
16. H. Rosenkranz and W. Scholtan, *Hoppe-Seyler's Z. Physiol. Chem.* **352**, 896 (1971).
17. F. R. Brown, III, A. J. Hopfinger and E. R. Blout, *J. Mol. Biol.* In press.
18. B. Jirgensons and S. Capetillo, *Biochim. Biophys. Acta* **214**, 1 (1970), and references therein.

19. L. Visser and E. R. Blout, *Biochemistry* **10**, 743 (1971).
20. J. H. Griffin. To be published.
21. (*a*) G. N. Ramachandran and G. Kartha, *Nature* **174**, 269 (1954). (*b*) G. N. Ramachandran and G. Kartha, *Nature* **176**, 593 (1955).
22. F. R. Brown, III, J. P. Carver and E. R. Blout, *J. Mol. Biol.* **39**, 307 (1969).
23. F. R. Brown, III, A. di Corato, G. P. Lorenzi and E. R. Blout, *J. Mol. Biol.* In press.
24. (*a*) E. R. Blout and L. Stryer, *Proc. Natl. Acad. Sci. U.S.A.* **45**, 1591 (1959). (*b*) L. Stryer and E. R. Blout, *J. Amer. Chem. Soc.* **83**, 1411 (1961).
25. S. Beychok, C. de Loze and E. R. Blout, *J. Mol. Biol.* **4**, 421 (1962).
26. S. C. Harrison and E. R. Blout, *J. Biol. Chem.* **240**, 299 (1965).
27. (*a*) F. Crescitelli, W. F. H. M. Mommaerts and I. T. Shaw, *Proc. Natl. Acad. Sci. U.S.A.* **56**, 1729 (1966). (*b*) T. P. Williams, *Vision Res.* **6**, 293 (1966). (*c*) A. S. Waggoner and L. Stryer, *Biochemistry* **10**, 3250 (1971).
28. Some recent references are: (*a*) G. Scheibe, O. Wörz, F. Haimerl, W. Seiffert and J. Winkler, *J. Chim. Phys.* **65**, 146 (1968). (*b*) M. Martinez-Carrion, D. C. Tiemeier and D. L. Peterson, *Biochemistry* **9**, 2574 (1970). (*c*) A. Conway-Jacobs, B. Schechter and M. Sela, *Biochemistry* **9**, 4870 (1970). (*d*) J. H. Perrin and M. Wilsey, *Chem. Commun.* **14**, 769 (1971).
29. (*a*) G. Barth, R. Records, E. Bunnenberg, C. Djerassi and W. Voelter, *J. Amer. Chem. Soc.* **93**, 2545 (1971). (*b*) G. Barth, W. Voelter, E. Bunnenberg and C. Djerassi, *J. Amer. Chem. Soc.* In press.
30. M. Rothe, R. Theysohn, K.-D. Steffen, M. Kostrezewa and M. Zamani, in E. Scoffone, Ed., *Peptides 1969*. North-Holland Publishing Company, 1971, p. 179.
31. V. T. Ivanov, V. V. Shilin, G. A. Kogan, E. N. Meshcheryakova, L. B. Senyavina, E. S. Efremov and Yu. A. Ovchinnikov, *Tetrahedron Lett.* No. 30, 2841 (1971).
32. F. Naider, E. Benedetti and M. Goodman, *Proc. Natl. Acad. Sci. U.S.A.* **68**, 1195 (1971).
33. A. E. Tonelli, D. J. Patel, M. Goodman, F. Naider, H. Faulstich and Th. Wieland, *Biochemistry* **10**, 3211 (1971).
34. U. Ludescher and R. Schwyzer, *Helv. Chim. Acta* **54**, 1637 (1971).

Special Topics

Faraday-effect Spectroscopy

B. BRIAT*

E.P.C.I.
10 rue Vauquelin
Paris 5^e, France

5.1.1 General Theory with Applications to Organic Molecules

A. General Theory

A1. Introduction. The general name 'Faraday-effect spectroscopy' is intended for magnetically induced optical activity and covers both magnetic circular dichroism (MCD) and magneto-optical rotatory dispersion (MORD). These phenomena can be measured by means of a dichrometer (MCD) or a spectropolarimeter (MORD), provided a magnetic field is induced in the sample compartment, parallel to the direction of the light beam. The origin of the Faraday effect lies basically in the 'helical symmetry' of the magnetic field. The material under investigation thus responds differently to optical stimulation with right or left circularly polarized light. The induced activity is frequency dependent and (generally) proportional to the magnetic field strength. Finally, the method is applicable—at least in principle—to any optically inactive or active molecule.

The reader may refer to recent review articles[1-3] for a historical background. Suffice it to say here that the interest in Faraday-effect spectroscopy has been renewed in the recent years. This is dramatically illustrated in Fig. 1 by the rapid increase since 1963 in the number of publications concerned with the applications in this field. To a great extent, this interest has been motivated by instrumental progress (Chapter 5.2) as well as by the development of a general theory[1] which explained previous experimental studies and stimulated further extensive work. As a result, the theory can be presented in a much more tractable form and the potential validity of Faraday effect spectroscopy can be exemplified in the fields of organic or biological chemistry (Section 5.2.1) and inorganic chemistry (Section 5.2.2). Reference 4 may be consulted for a number of interesting discussions on magneto-optical effects.

Finally, a few comments will be made regarding the potential interest of magnetic linear dichroism (Voigt–Cotton–Mouton effect).

A2. Definitions. (*a*) *Practical units.* Natural and/or magnetic optical activity can be defined in two different ways according to the method of measurement employed. If

* E.R. Nº 5 du C.N.R.S.

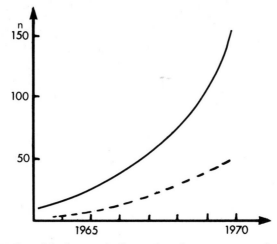

Fig. 1. Illustration of the increase in the number of papers concerned with the Faraday effect: ——— theory and inorganic; ———— organic.

circularly polarized light is used (left and right components), one can define circular dichroism as $\Delta\varepsilon = \varepsilon_L - \varepsilon_R$ or $\Delta k = k_L - k_R$ and circular birefringence as $\Delta n = n_L - n_R$ where ε, k and n stand for the molar extinction coefficient, the extinction index and the refractive index of the medium, respectively; n and k are the real and imaginary parts of the complex index of refraction $\tilde{n} = n - jk$. If plane polarized light is employed, it becomes elliptically polarized after travelling through the sample. It can be shown that the ellipticity θ, and the angle α between the long axis of the ellipse and the initial direction of planar polarization, constitute a means of measuring CD and ORD, respectively.

In practice, commercial instruments provide $\Delta\varepsilon$ (or better ΔD which is a difference in optical density units) or θ on the one hand and α on the other hand. When a magnetic field H is added, and since the phenomena are proportional to H, measured values should be standardized to 1 G if not otherwise stated. We suggest as units the use of the following quantities.

$$\Delta D_M = \Delta D/\beta H \quad \text{molar magnetic dichroic optical density} \qquad [1]$$

$$\Delta\varepsilon_M = \Delta D/\beta Hcl \quad \text{molar magnetic circular dichroism} \qquad [2]$$

where c and l stand for the concentration (in mole 1^{-1}) of the solution and the length of the cell (in cm) respectively, and β is the Bohr magneton.

$$[\phi]_M = 100 \, \frac{\alpha}{\beta Hcl} \quad \text{molar magnetic rotation (α in degrees)} \qquad [3]$$

$$[\theta]_M = 100 \, \frac{\theta}{\beta Hcl} \quad \text{molar magnetic ellipticity (θ in degrees).} \qquad [4]$$

It should be stated that $\Delta\varepsilon_M$, $[\phi]_M$ and $[\theta]_M$ are molar quantities and thus suitable for comparisons on a mole-for-mole basis. Furthermore, it is interesting to be able to switch easily from one system of units to the other. As for natural optical activity, one has $[\theta]_M = 3300 \, \Delta\varepsilon_M$.

(*b*) *Sign convention.* Provided the light propagates in the direction of the magnetic field, it follows from the definition of α and $\Delta\varepsilon$ that the magnetic rotation for water is negative in the visible region and the MCD through, say, the 500 nm band of co-baltous salts, is also negative.

(*c*) *Calibration of instruments.* ORD and CD instruments may be calibrated with standard solutions such as cholestandione in methanol[5] and epiandrosterone in dioxane ($\Delta\varepsilon = +3310 \pm 0.007$ at 304 nm). Commercial instruments are available for the determination of the magnetic field. For MORD, however, it is preferable to measure the rotation of water ($\alpha = V \int H \, \mathrm{d}l$) and to take the value of the Verdet constant V from the literature.[6]

For CD as well as MCD the experimentalist would find it useful to have at his disposal a stable, solid secondary calibrant which could be used to check the apparatus with greater regularity. In our laboratory we use a piece of europium-doped glass sealed between the pole pieces of a small, permanent, horseshoe magnet, a system which is easily aligned in the light beam. A piece of glass of thickness 2 mm containing about 20 % Eu_2O_3 will, if the permanent magnet gives a field of about 1 kG, give two peaks at 4641 Å and 4669 Å which are sufficiently strong and sharp to enable evaluation of the wavelength and intensity scales and the resolution of the instrument to be checked.

(*d*) *Technical details.* MCD machines operate with a superconducting magnet, or a permanent magnet, or else an electromagnet. As will be realized in the next section, low-temperature work is frequently needed, especially when inorganic materials are under investigation. Details of magnetic or cryogenic devices used in our laboratory have been given elsewhere (reference 4, p. 27).

Low-temperature MCD work is generally conducted on oriented crystals. We have also made a number of experiments on rigid glasses, e.g. various cytochromes in sucrose-saturated water (down to 15°K) or else porphyrins in ethanol. Finally, we have recently[7] commented upon the use of polymer films. Table 1 is a list of a limited number of mixtures which we have successfully employed. A solution of the polymer and the material is evaporated on a silica window (e.g. with polyvinyl alcohol) or at the bottom of a Petri dish (all other polymers).

Table 1
Examples of Usable Polymer Films

Polymer	Solvent
Polyvinyl alcohol	H_2O
Polyvinyl acetate	Dioxane
	Methylene chloride
Polyvinyl chloride	Tetrahydrofuran
Cellulose diacetate	Acetone
	Acetonitrile
	Methylene chloride
Polystyrene	Acetonitrile
	Methylene chloride
Polymethylmethacrylate	Acetone
Nitrocellulose	Alcohol + ether

*A*3. *Dispersion of the Faraday effect.* MCD has a non-zero value through absorption bands only. Considering an isolated band, the MCD dependence versus the energy v

(in cm^{-1}) or the wavelength can be approximately described[8] by means of the following equation

$$R = \frac{\Delta\varepsilon_M}{\varepsilon_m} = \frac{\Delta k_M}{k_m} = \frac{\Delta D_M}{D_m} = a\frac{dF}{dv} + \left(b + \frac{c}{kT}\right)F \qquad [5]$$

where F is some mathematical function which describes the shape of the absorption curve (e.g., lorentzian or gaussian) and $\varepsilon_m(D_m, k_m)$ is the maximum molar extinction coefficient (optical density, extinction index) at the centre of the band. According to this equation, an MCD curve can be described as a linear combination of the absorption curve in zero magnetic field and its first derivative. It is also worth noting that the R parameter which is characteristic of magneto-optical activity is in many respects similar to Kuhn's factor for natural optical activity.

In general, the extraction of MCD parameters from MCD data requires a knowledge of the temperature dependence of R. It should also be noted that for any reasonable shape function, the first term in equation [5] is inversely proportional to the width of the band. Thus b and c terms are favoured for wide bands while the magnitude of (adF/dv) is enhanced for sharp lines (e.g., rare earths).

MORD and MCD (and vice versa) are related through the Kramers–Kronig relationship and one has

$$[\phi]_M/\varepsilon_m = 3300aKK\left(\frac{df}{dv}\right) + \left(b + \frac{c}{RT}\right)KK(f) \qquad [6]$$

where the simplified notation KK means 'take the Kramers–Kronig transform of'. The wavelength dependence of $\Delta\varepsilon_M$ and $[\phi]_M$ for positive a and b values is illustrated in Fig. 2. If a and b were negative, one would obtain curves symmetrical to the above ones versus the wavelength axis.

A4. Comparison between MCD and MORD. It follows from equations [5] and [6] that MCD and MORD should, at least in principle, provide the same information, i.e. the sign and value of a, b and c. However, it is usually highly advantageous to work with MCD data for a number of reasons. These are illustrated in Fig. 3 where we considered hypothetical MCD and MORD curves corresponding to three individual absorption bands. It appears that the contribution of each band is reasonably well isolated in MCD whereas the MORD terms strongly overlap. This is so because MORD curves are more complicated than MCD ones and they possess tails outside the region of absorption. In view of the previous argument, one has also to add a background rotation (the so-called Drude term) arising from the contribution of bands located outside the range of available data.

Figure 3 also serves to illustrate the interest of MORD measurements in the transparency region. Although this has not always been recognized in the past, the rotation (e.g. at λ_1) is generally the sum of many contributions of different origins. This severely restricts the possibility of a detailed interpretation of the spectra. Thus such measurements are of interest when absorption bands are not within reach of the spectral range of the instrument or when the compound is too highly absorbing (e.g. magnetic materials).

In the subsequent sections, the main emphasis will be MCD, since a basic understanding of the significance of Faraday-effect parameters is easy in this case.

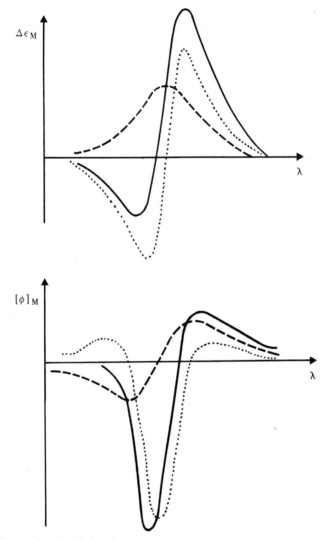

Fig. 2. Shape of MCD [$\Delta\varepsilon$] and MORD [ϕ]$_M$ curves through an isolated absorption band: ——— experiment; ...... a term; – – – – b term.

A5. Significance of MCD parameters. (a) Phenomenological approach. The dispersion curves can be accounted for by considering the perturbation of the various states and electronic transitions by a magnetic field. In the absence of H, an electronic transition at a frequency ν_0 corresponds to an absorption band. When the magnetic field is applied, three perturbations may occur:

(i) The ground and/or excited state (s) may be split and transitions with different circular polarizations observed at different frequencies. This is the Zeeman effect and leads to the observance of an S-shaped MCD curve (a term). It should be stated, however, that, unlike Zeeman experiments

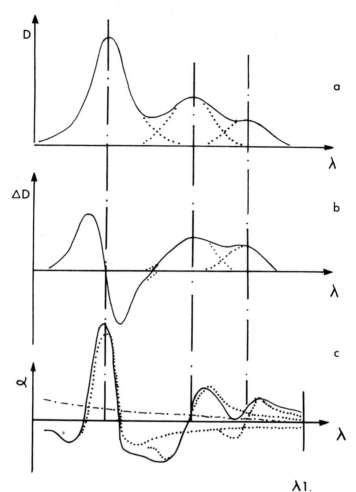

Fig. 3. Wavelength dependence of the optical density D, the magnetic dichroic optical density ΔD and the magnetic rotation α in a spectral range where three optical transitions are present.

which require sharp lines (gas or low temperature), MCD measurements can be performed on bands, the width of which may be 1000 times larger than the Zeeman splitting (e.g. solids or solutions at room temperature). This is because the difference in wavelengths between the two peaks of an S-shaped MCD curve is of the order of magnitude of the width of the absorption band.

(ii) The eventual sublevels in the ground state (paramagnetic molecule or ion) are differently populated, according to the Boltzman law (c terms).

(iii) Right and left transitions may have different intensities even when the ground state is non-degenerate (b terms).

(*b*) *Basic principles for the calculation of MCD parameters.* We first assume an isotropic centre or an anisotropic centre with H parallel to the optic axis. For an isolated transition from the ground state a (degeneracy d_a) to an excited state j, the optical density D may be expressed as follows

$$\frac{D}{v} = \frac{K}{2}\left\{\sum_{+} N_+ I_+ f(v.v_+) + \sum_{-} N_- I_- f(v.v_-)\right\} \qquad [7]$$

Now, from the definition of MCD, one has

$$\frac{\Delta D_M}{v} = K\left\{\sum_{+} N_+ I_+ f(v.v_+) - \sum_{-} N_- I_- f(v.v_-)\right\} \qquad [8]$$

where K is a constant $(108 \cdot 9cl \times 3/d_a)$, $f(v.v_0)$ is the shape function of the absorption curve satisfying:

$$\int f\,dv = 1, \qquad \int fv\,dv = \bar{v}, \qquad \int f'v\,dv = -1 \qquad [9]$$

$\bar{v}$ is the mean frequency (cm^{-1}) of the band, $f' = \partial f/\partial v$ and β is the Bohr magneton. $I_\pm = |\langle j_\pm| m_\pm |a_\pm\rangle|^2$ stands for the probability of transition* with circular $(\sigma_\pm)$ polarization, and $m_\pm$ are the appropriate electric dipole moment operators; $N_\pm$ are the relative populations of the sublevels of the ground state from which $\sigma_\pm$ transitions originate.

One has finally

$$\frac{\Delta D_M}{D} = \frac{\displaystyle\sum_{+} N_+ I_+ f(v.v_+) - \sum_{-} N_- I_- f(v.v_-)}{\displaystyle\frac{1}{2}\left\{\sum_{+} N_+ I_+ f(v.v_0) + \sum_{-} N_- I_- f(v.v_-)\right\}} \qquad [10a]$$

This equation provides the key to understanding of Sub-section (*a*) of Section *A*5, since a, b and c parameters are obtained by making successively $v_+ \neq v_-$, $I_+ \neq I_-$ and $N_+ \neq N_-$. A good example is that of a doublet → doublet transition. With the notations shown above, one easily obtains

$$a = -(s_e + s_g) \qquad \text{and} \qquad c = s_g \qquad\qquad [10b]$$

when the following sign conventions are used: s_g is positive if σ_+ originates from the lowest sublevel in the ground state; s_e is positive when σ_+ attains the highest sublevel in the excited state. In more complicated situations, $\sigma_\pm$ transitions occur in pairs with intensity I_α and the parameters for the whole band are obtained by weighting the individual parameters with the appropriate intensities (see Section 5.1.2) as follows

---

* It follows from our reasoning that the z component of the magnetic dipole moment operator is diagonal in $|a \pm\rangle$ and $|j \pm\rangle$.

$$a = \sum_\alpha a_\alpha I_\alpha / \sum_\alpha I_\alpha \qquad \text{and} \qquad c = \sum_\alpha c_\alpha I_\alpha / \sum_\alpha I_\alpha \qquad [10c]$$

In equation [10], we implicitly assumed that H was applied along the z axis of the molecule. The comparison with experiment (laboratory axes) suffers no difficulty as long as we are considering randomly oriented isotropic molecules (solutions) or a properly oriented uniaxial centre with H along its optic axis. When we are dealing with randomly oriented anisotropic molecules and σ polarized transitions the experimental value for $\Delta D_M/D$ proves to be too low by a factor of 2 with respect to the calculated quantity in a molecule-fixed axes system.

A6. *Data analysis.* (a) *Formalism in use in the literature.* For practical purposes, D and ΔD_M may be expressed as

$$\frac{D}{\nu} = K' \mathscr{D} f \qquad [11]$$

$$\frac{\Delta D_M}{\nu} = -2K' \left\{ \mathscr{A} f' + \left(\mathscr{B} + \frac{\mathscr{C}}{kT} \right) f \right\} \qquad [12]$$

where $K' = 108 \cdot 9cl$ and $\mathscr{D}$ is the dipole strength of the transition. It follows that:[3]

$$\frac{\Delta D_M}{D} = a \frac{f'}{f} + (b + c/kT) \qquad [13]$$

where $a = -2\mathscr{A}/\mathscr{D}$, $b = -2\mathscr{B}/\mathscr{D}$, and $c = -2\mathscr{C}/\mathscr{D}$.

The $\mathscr{A}$, $\mathscr{B}$, $\mathscr{C}$ and $\mathscr{D}$ parameters are just those encountered in many papers on MCD.[1,2] We note here that $\mathscr{A}/\mathscr{D}$, for example, is given in Bohr magnetons.

$\mathscr{D}$ is easily extracted from experimental data, since

$$\mathscr{D} = 9 \cdot 18 \times 10^{-3} \int \frac{\varepsilon}{\nu} \, d\nu \qquad [14]$$

(b) *Extraction of MCD parameters from experiment.* (i) Equation [5] can be used for a crude estimate, F being an approximate expression for f; F can be taken* as $\exp(-X^2)$ for a gaussian shape or as $1/(1 + x^2)$ for a lorentzian shape. The $(b + c/kT)$ term is obtained as the value of R at $v = \bar{v}$, while a is derived from the peak-to-peak magnitude of R.[9] (ii) Equations [11] and [12] have been used extensively and reference should be made to the original literature[1,2] for further comments. (iii) Billardon *et al.*[10] have proposed an elegant method based on the assumption that equation [13] is valid. (iv) Finally the method of moments will be considered further, as it has been recommended[11] for data analysis and should be extensively used in future work (see Section 5.1.2).

Let us define

$$\langle D \rangle_0 = \int \frac{D}{\nu} \, d\nu \qquad \text{and} \qquad \langle D \rangle_1 = \int \frac{D}{\nu} \, \nu \, d\nu$$

---

* $X = (v - \bar{v})/\delta$ and $x = (v - \bar{v})/\gamma$, where δ and γ stand for the half-widths at $1/e$ and one-half of the peak maximum.

as the zeroth and first moment of the absorption band. The ratio $\langle D \rangle_1 / \langle D \rangle_0 = \bar{v}$ is the mean frequency of the band.

Now,

$$\langle \Delta D_M \rangle_0 = \int \frac{\Delta D_M}{v} \, dv \qquad \text{and} \qquad \langle \Delta D_M \rangle_1 = \int \frac{\Delta D_M}{v} (v - \bar{v}) \, dv$$

are the zeroth and first moment of the MCD curve.

From equations [11–13] and the properties of f and f' functions, the following identities are easily established

$$\mathscr{D} = \frac{1}{K'} \langle D \rangle_0$$

$$\Delta M_0 = \langle \Delta D_M \rangle_0 / \langle D \rangle_0 = b + c/kT \qquad [15]$$

$$\Delta M_1 = \langle \Delta D_M \rangle_1 / \langle D \rangle_0 = -a \qquad [16]$$

When only b ($\mathscr{B}$) terms are observed, it might be useful to consider the rotational strength $\mathscr{R}$ of the transition. As for natural optical activity, one has

$$\mathscr{R} = \frac{1}{K'} \langle \Delta D_M \rangle_0 = \frac{1}{K'} \int_0^\infty \frac{\Delta D_M}{v} \, dv = \frac{1}{K'} \int_0^\infty \frac{\Delta D_M}{\lambda} \, d\lambda$$

Then $\mathscr{R} = -2 \mathscr{B}$, i.e. a positive rotational strength (b and ΔD positive) corresponds to a negative $\mathscr{B}$ term.

(c) *Limits to the validity of the analysis.* The derivation of equation [13] from equation [10] is only possible under two conditions:

(i) The magnetic field causes a rigid shift of the shape function $f(v, v_\pm)$ in circular polarizations (f' function).

(ii) The expression of $N_\pm$ is linear as a function of the magnetic field. This means that the exponential in the Boltzman distribution law may be expanded and requires that H/T be not too high. In practice this condition is often satisfied.

It should be stated that condition (i) is no longer necessary when the method of moments is used for data analysis. Also, when condition (ii) is not satisfied, $\langle \Delta D_M \rangle_0$ is not linear in H/T and the MCD parameters lose their significance; equation [10] must be reconsidered with the appropriate expression for $N_\pm$. For example, if we have a doublet ground state with total separation Δ between the extreme components, the temperature-dependent MCD term will be given as

$$\frac{N_+ - N_-}{\frac{1}{2}(N_+ + N_-)} = \frac{e^{+x} - e^{-x}}{\frac{1}{2}(e^{+x} + e^{-x})} = 2 \tanh x$$

when $x = \Delta/2 \, kT$, and equations [10a] and [15] are employed. This situation is encountered, for example, for certain magnetic materials or when studying ions with a zero-field splitting in the ground state. Of course, Δ is just what we called the c term when x is small.

*A*7. *Conclusion.* For comparison of the experimental parameters with a theoretical model, the procedure may be as follows:

(i) Determine the Zeeman pattern. This requires the evaluation of the eigenfunctions and eigenvalues of the Zeeman hamiltonian. The selection rules in circular polarization are then used in order to complete the scheme. Finally, the intensity of $\sigma_\pm$ transitions are evaluated.

(ii) Use equation [10], since the various $v_\pm$, $N_\pm$ and $I_\pm$ are now fully known. See Section 5.1.2 for a complete evaluation of the three MCD parameters in particular cases.

B. *Applications to Organic Molecules*[12,13]

*B*1. *Introduction.* It is worth noting that degenerate excited states (thus a terms) are predicted only when the molecule under study possesses at least a three-fold axis of symmetry. This, of course, severely restricts the number of eventual candidates.

On the other hand, *all* compounds exhibit b terms with presently available magnetic fields. This term originates in the 'scrambling'—via the magnetic field (helical symmetry)—of the orbitals and thus the electronic states arising from a given repetition of electrons in the orbitals. This means that the shape of an orbital distorted by the field can be described by adding the proper amounts of the shapes of certain unperturbed orbitals of the set. In fact, it is found that the mixing orbitals must possess certain symmetry properties in order to overlap and their energies should not be too different; this appears as an energy denominator in the expression of the Faraday effect.

MCD c terms are expected for molecules having an orbitally degenerate ground state or a spin degenerate ground state with substantial spin-orbit coupling (see Section 5.1.2). Thus, most organic free radicals do not show a paramagnetic MCD behaviour, since the latter condition is eventually not satisfied.

*B*2. *Comparison between natural and magnetic optical activity.* It is already clear that an MCD a term has no counterpart in natural optical activity; this means that MCD provides new information. The resemblance, if any, of the two phenomena arises from the apparent similarity between an MCD b term and a natural Cotton effect. Both occur since there is a difference among the probabilities of transition for the two circular polarizations, due to a mixing of states. The cause of this mixing, however, is different for the two phenomena. In particular the perturbation is inherent in the molecule in the case of CD and external to it in the case of MCD.

Finally, CD and MCD have completely distinct physical origins and this is why their quantum mechanical expressions differ. This also means that the two quantities are additive. When both kinds of measurements are made on an optically active molecule, there is no *a priori* reason to believe that one of them should be much larger than the other. Actually, it may even be found that the two techniques are sometimes complementary.[14]

*B*3. *Study of porphyrin-like molecules.* (*a*) *Theoretical arguments.* Metalloporphyrins [Fig. 4(a)] have an approximate symmetry D_{4h} and their visible spectrum shows the intense B (Soret) band near 400 nm and the much weaker Q band near 580 nm. The two excited states are orbitally doubly degenerate and each can be described by two functions transforming as $|x\rangle$ and $|y\rangle$. In the presence of a magnetic field perpendicular to the molecular (x,y) plane, new eigenfunctions are found transforming as $x \pm iy$ (or $m \pm$) under the symmetry of the group. The separation between the two states is $2\beta HMz$ where Mz is the magnetic moment in the excited state. The Zeeman pattern is thus easily established and comparison of equations [10] and [13] leads to $a = -Mz$, since we are dealing with randomly oriented anisotropic molecules.

In base-free porphyrins [Fig. 4(b)] the approximate symmetry is D_{2h}. $|x\rangle$ and $|y\rangle$ states are now nondegenerate in the absence of H; although the two states for the

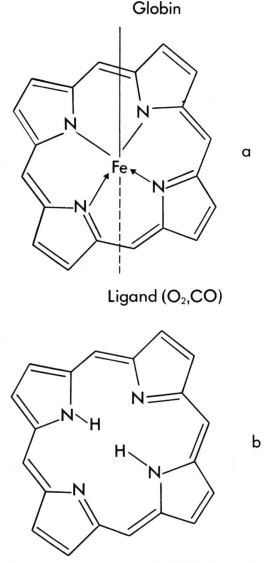

Fig. 4. Formulae for a particular metalloporphyrin (a) and a base-free porphyrin (b).

B band remain almost degenerate. The orbital magnetic dipole moment operator is able to mix $|y\rangle$ into $|x\rangle$ to a small extent, the perturbed wave function being

$$|x'\rangle = |x\rangle + \frac{\langle y|\,Lz\beta H\,|x\rangle}{Ex - Ey}\,|y\rangle = |x\rangle + \varepsilon i|y\rangle \quad |y'\rangle = |y\rangle - i\varepsilon|x\rangle$$

where ε is a real quantity. This means that the transitions to $|x'\rangle$ and $|y'\rangle$ become partly circularly polarized and b terms occur. The expressions for b and ΔD are:

$$|b_{0x}| = 2\,\frac{\langle y|\,Lz\,|x\rangle}{Ex - Ey}\left(\frac{\mathscr{D}_{0y}}{\mathscr{D}_{0x}}\right)^{1/2} \qquad [17]$$

$$\Delta D_{0x} = 2\,\frac{\vec{\mu}_{xy}(\vec{m}_{0x} \wedge \vec{m}_{y0})}{Ey - Ex} \qquad [18]$$

The numerator in ΔD involves the triple cross product of three vectors which are electric $(\vec{m})$ or magnetic $(\vec{\mu})$ moments for the various transitions. Equation [18] shows that $\Delta D_{0x} = -\Delta D_{0y}$; thus MCD for the two transitions is the same, regardless of their dipole strengths.[3]

(b) *Practical use of MCD.* All the arguments just set forth have been checked on a number of planar porphyrin-like molecules[4, 15] possessing D_{4h} or D_{2h} symmetry. (i) Substantial a terms are observed for metalloporphyrins (e.g. phthalocyanines) with a being about nine times larger for the Q band than for the B band, in good agreement with the free electron network model. It follows that deviations from the 9:1 ratio occur from metal to metal, and MCD provides the theoretician with a stringent test for his calculations. (ii) Large b terms are observed in the free-base porphyrins. It follows from equation [18] that MCD predicts the relative polarization (not the absolute one) of the various transitions (B_x, B_y, Q_x, Q_y). Actually, a large number of overtones are observed for the Q bands, due to a coupling of vibrational modes to the electronic part of the wave functions. Again, MCD tells us something about the symmetry of the modes. (iii) Low-temperature MCD experiments have shown the paramagnetism (c terms) of the ground state of ferrihaems.

Even from a qualitative point of view, MCD can play an important role. (i) Substantial quenching of the a parameters from the above predicted values means a possible pseudo-degeneracy, i.e. a lowering of symmetry due to substituents on the haems or on the metal. (ii) A weak absorption band may show a large MCD and vice versa. This is the case for example in chlorins[16] for the peak around 540 nm. It has further been shown that the large magnitude of the observed b term is very much dependent upon the nature of the substituents on the ring. (iii) MCD is very sensitive to the degree of oxidation of the metal in iron-containing porphyrins. This is so since the ferrous compound is diamagnetic and gives rise to a large a term through the Q band while the ferric compound is paramagnetic and shows much smaller ($b + c/kT$) terms at room temperature. Faraday effect spectroscopy is thus a very powerful tool for studying the kinetics of reactions involving porphyrin-like molecules. (iv) Finally, since b terms are positive or negative, MCD is of great help in resolving overlapping bands.[3]

B4. Study of carbonyl compounds. Many MCD studies have been motivated in part by the possibility that the technique may provide information about the stereochemistry of organic compounds, and particularly of molecules containing the carbonyl chromophore. Djerassi and his group[4] have run the spectra of a large number of such molecules and have found that b terms are often small but their strength and sign for the individual components are highly dependent on the structure of the compounds. The reason for this lies basically in the fact that we are dealing with electric dipole forbidden transitions and many coupling mechanisms (vibrations, solvent) may play a very important role regarding the sign of b terms. The experimental facts have recently been rationalized by Professor Moscowitz and his student Seamans, who derived a theoretical framework.

B5. Miscellaneous. (*a*) *Use of* a *terms.* There have been a number of practical applications pertaining to the assignment of excited states and to the experimental determination of their magnetic moments. These data allow in turn a quantitative verification of various molecular orbital calculations and give significant support for the theoretician. Investigated systems range from triphenylene or coronene[17] to annulenes[9] or ferrocene[18] derivatives.

(*b*) *Use of* b *terms.* b terms have already been used extensively. Although they are difficult to estimate theoretically, their existence (and sign) or non-existence is very significant by itself. For example, absorption bands which are hidden in the UV spectrum can sometimes be revealed by means of MCD measurements. Examples include various[14] annulene systems,[19] vitamin B_{12} derivatives,[20] or purine and pyrimidine nucleosides or cyclonucleosides.[21] In the former case, some of the transitions are electric-dipole forbidden and the action of the solvent upon the sign of the b terms has been demonstrated. A large number of hydrocarbons has also been investigated.[22] It should be noted however that although their MCD has been correlated with the Hammett parameter, these data are unlikely to be of fundamental interest.

5.1.2 Some Applications to Inorganic Compounds

A. Some Useful Group Theoretical Arguments

Before dealing with practical situations where MCD has its main application, we will consider a few examples where the ideas presented in Section 5.1.1, A7, may be worked out fully. The free-ion model is very instructive in that, it is a good introduction to the practice of MCD spectroscopy.

A1. Wigner-Eckart theorem. Once the transformation properties of eigenfunctions and operators are known in a particular group, the W.E. theorem allows the evaluation of (i) all matrix elements such as

$$\int \phi_i^* \, h_j^i \, \theta_k \, d\tau = \langle \phi_i | \, h_j | \theta_k \rangle$$

in terms of constant factors (thus chosen as units); (ii) the selection rules of, for example, electric dipole transitions. Actually, *these are just the conditions required to establish the Zeeman pattern and calculate MCD terms* by means of equation [10] in Section 5.1.1.

(*a*) *Free ion model and weak (intermediate) field scheme.* (*see* Ref. 17 *for the full derivation*). Considering the free ion model first, ϕ_i^* and θ_k are replaced by $\langle K' M_K'|$ and $|KM_K\rangle$, respectively, where K' and K are any pair of angular momentum vectors of the same kind (e.g., J' and J). In order that the W.E. theorem may be applied, the operators h_j must transform in an identical fashion to some set of states $|kq\rangle$, where $q = k, k-1, ..., -k$. This is guaranteed if the operators which we now write as $T_q^{(k)}$, transform like the spherical harmonics. Thus for k = 1 we require

$$T_{\pm}^{(1)} = \frac{\pm 1}{(2)^{1/2}} (Tx \pm iTy) \qquad \text{and} \qquad T_0^{(1)} = Tz$$

In this particular case (the only one subsequently required), the W.E. theorem states that

$$\langle K' M_K' | T_q^{(1)} | KM_K \rangle = (-1)^{K'-M_K'} \begin{pmatrix} K' & 1 & K \\ -M_K' & q & M_K \end{pmatrix} \langle K' \| T^1 \| K \rangle \qquad [19]$$

This means that any matrix element of $T_q^{(1)}$ can be written as the product of a factor which is independent of M_K and M_K' (reduced matrix element written with double bars) and a numerical factor (called the 3j symbol) which can be taken from tables.[23]

Before dealing with any calculation, it is therefore first necessary to consider which required matrix elements are non-vanishing. This is done by looking at the properties of the 3j symbols. It follows from theory that they are zero unless (i) a triangle can be formed with K, k and K', this being equivalent to the condition that the representation $\mathscr{D}_K$ occurs in the decomposition of $\mathscr{D}_k \times \mathscr{D}_{K'}$; (ii) that $M_K' + q = M_K$.

Let us apply these ideas further in the case of a free ion when J, M_J are good quantum numbers (in the presence of spin orbit coupling) and stand for K, M_K in equation [19]. The Zeeman operator is already under the form of an irreducible tensor and its z component may be written $T_q^{(K)} \equiv Z_0^1$. Thus, one must have $M_J' = M_J$ (since $q = 0$) and the Zeeman effect is purely diagonal. Now the dipole moment operators $m_{\pm}$ for circular polarizations may be written $M_{\pm 1}^1$ (since a vector transforms as $\mathscr{D}_1$) so that the 3j symbol becomes

$$\begin{pmatrix} J' & 1 & J \\ -M_J' & \pm 1 & M_J \end{pmatrix}$$

where J and J' are associated with the ground and excited states respectively. It follows that $J' - J = 0, \pm 1$ (triangular condition) and $M_J' - M_J = \pm 1$ for $\sigma_{\pm}$ polarization. These are well-known selection rules of course, but it was important to recall their origin.

Finally, the W.E. theorem may be expressed in a slightly different way when one considers the Zeeman effect. As $\mathscr{D}_K$ occurs only once in the decomposition of $\mathscr{D}_k \times \mathscr{D}_{K'}$, the matrix elements of the components of $L + 2S$ are proportional to those of corresponding components of any other vector. Since the states are labelled by J it is very convenient to choose J for this role. One thus has, for example,

$$\langle JM_J | L_z + 2S_z | JM_J \rangle = g \langle JM_J | J_z | JM_J \rangle = gM_J \qquad [20]$$

where g is the Lande factor given by

$$g = 1 + \frac{J(J+1) + S(S+1) - L(L+1)}{2J(J+1)}$$

in terms of the quantum numbers J, L, S.

We note finally that, in the weak (or intermediate) field scheme (e.g., rare earths ions), wave functions will generally be expressed in the form:

$$|\phi_i\rangle = \sum C_{\alpha i} |L, M_L, S, M_S\rangle$$

or

$$|\phi_j\rangle = \sum C_{\beta j} |J, M_J\rangle$$

C_i and C_j standing for coefficients.

The arguments given above to provide selection rules and relative intensities for the Zeeman components will still be valid, each intensity being weighted with the appropriate $C_{\beta j} C_{\beta i}$ or $C_{\beta j(i)}^2$ factor.

(*b*) *Cubic groups and strong field scheme.* The W.E. theorem applies to cubic (and other) groups as well, but it should be reformulated in a slightly different way. If we consider the strong field approximation (see, for example, reference 24) the good 'quantum numbers' are now the irreducible representations of the group. Using Mulliken's notations, these are A_1, A_2, E, T_1 and T_2, if the total spin multiplicity is odd. Following Griffith,[25] for example, (hereafter referred to as GI), the W.E. theorem may now be written

$$\langle a\alpha| g_c |b\beta\rangle = [-1]^{a+\alpha} V \begin{pmatrix} a & b & c \\ -\alpha & \beta & \gamma \end{pmatrix} \langle a\| g^c \|b\rangle \qquad [21]$$

when α, β and γ are complex components of a, b, c (e.g. $|a\alpha\rangle = |T_1 1\rangle$) and

$$[-1]^\zeta = 1 \quad \text{if } \zeta \text{ is } A_1, A_2 \text{ or } E \text{ (or their components)}$$

$$= -1 \quad \text{if } \zeta \text{ is } T_1 \text{ or } T_2$$

$$= (-1)^\zeta \quad \text{if } \zeta \text{ is one component of } T_1 \text{ or } T_2$$

The correspondence with equation [19] can be checked on an example. In the tetrahedral group, the electric dipole moment operator transforms as T_2. Thus from say, a A_1 ground state, only transitions to T_2 excited states are allowed due to the triangular condition (b $\otimes$ c contains a). If we choose a $= T_2$ and b $= A_1$, the selection rules for circular polarizations $\sigma_\pm$ will be found from the V coefficient, namely from the condition $\alpha = \beta + \gamma$. Thus from $\gamma = 0$, the transitions to the ± 1 components of T_2 will be polarized $\sigma_\pm$. The relative intensities of transitions are just proportional to the square of V and these are tabulated in GI. The above results also apply to a $A_1 \rightarrow T_1$ transitions in the octahedral group.

For a transition involving one U' state (double group) more care must be taken and equation [21] must be modified. Two parameters (instead of one reduced matrix element) might then be required to describe fully the relative intensities of the various Zeeman components and the Zeeman splittings. If we consider, for example, the electronic transition $^4A_2(U') \rightarrow {}^4T_1(U'\,5/2)$ for the tetrahedral $CoBr_4^{2-}$ ion[26] the spacing between the λ and μ components of $U'_{5/2}$ will be different from that between the λ and ν (or μ and K) components. Moreover, the spectroscopic splitting factor will depend upon the orientation of H with regard to the axes of the tetrahedron.

A2. MCD parameters for a free ion with an orbital singlet ground state. (a) $^1S_0 \rightarrow {}^1P_1$ *transition.* This transition is allowed since the condition of the triangle is satisfied in the 3j symbol. Under the action of H, the orbital triplet splits into three sublevels with eigenfunctions $|1, 0$ or $\pm 1\rangle$ and eigenvalues 0 or $\pm g$ (see equation [20]). We already know that the transitions to $M_J = \pm 1$ are polarized $\sigma_\pm$ but it is also found in the tables that their intensities (3j symbol squared) are equal. Application of equation [10], Section 5.1.1 then leads to

$$a = -2g = -2\langle {}^1P_1\,1|\,Lz\,|{}^1P_1\,1\rangle \qquad\qquad [22]$$

since S is zero here.

From what we recall about the V coefficients above, a similar result is obtained for transitions $A_1 \rightarrow T_{1(2)}$ in cubic groups

$$a = -2\mu$$

where

$$\mu = \langle T_{1(2)}|\,Lz|T_{1(2)}\rangle$$

is the *magnetic moment* in the excited states.

(b) $J \rightarrow J, J \pm 1$ *transitions (spin singlet ground state).* (i) The energies of the various sublevels of the ground and excited states are easily calculated using equation [20]. (ii) The Zeeman pattern may be drawn (apart for I_+) using the selection rules $\Delta M = \pm 1$ for $\sigma_\pm$ components (M stands for M_J hereafter). (iii) For each Zeeman component, $I_\pm$ could be taken from tables for particular values of J and M. However, they have already been expressed as a function of these quantum numbers,[27] and this saves time (Table 2).

Table 2

Transition	$I\pm$
$J \rightarrow J+1$	$\{(J+1)(J+2) + M^2 \pm M(2J+3)\}\,A$
$J \rightarrow J-1$	$\{J(J-1) + M^2 \mp M(2J-1)\}\,A'$
$J \rightarrow J$	$\{J(J+1) - M^2 \mp M\}\,B$

A, A' and B are different; they contain a function of J and a reduced matrix element squared.

$$A = \mathcal{M}_A^2\{(2J+1)(2J+2)(2J+3)\}^{-1}$$
$$A' = \mathcal{M}_A^2\{(2J-1)\,2J(2J+1)\}^{-1}$$
$$B = \mathcal{M}_B^2\{2J(J+1)(2J+1)\}^{-1}$$

One interesting feature of Table 2 is that transitions are always associated in pairs, the intensity being the same for the two members of a given pair. This argument is of major importance in the application of equation [10c].

As an illustration we will consider the alkali metal atom model (Fig. 5) where the 2P excited state splits under the action of spin orbit coupling into levels with $J = \frac{1}{2}$ and $J = \frac{3}{2}$. From the Zeeman pattern we find

(i) Transition $^2S_{1/2} \rightarrow {}^2P_{1/2}$: $a = -(g_1 + g_2)$, $c = +g_1$.

(ii) Transition $^2S_{1/2} \rightarrow {}^2P_{3/2}$.

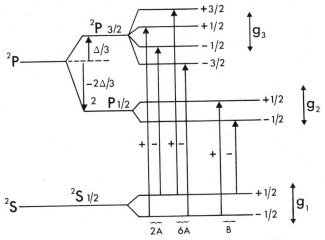

Fig. 5. Zeeman scheme for the alkali atom model.

First $\sigma_{\pm}$ pair (to $M = \pm\frac{1}{2}$) $= a_1 = -(g_1 + g_3)$

$$c_1 = +g_1$$

Second pair (to $M = \pm\frac{3}{2}$) $= a_2 = -(3g_3 - g_1)$

$$c_2 = -g_1$$

Altogether $a = (g_1 - 5g_3)/2$

$$c = -g_1/2$$

The b terms arising from the mixing of the two spin orbit states can also be calculated easily. We note however that not only the absolute value of 3j symbols but also *their signs are required here*.

For any transition $J \rightarrow J, J \pm 1$ (except $0 \rightarrow 0$), the a and c parameters can be derived by means of Table 2 and the sum rule

$$\sum M^2 = \tfrac{1}{6}J(J + 1)(2J + 1) \qquad [23]$$

where the summation extends from $M = \frac{1}{2}$ to $M = J$ (J half integer) or from $M = 1$ to $M = J$ (J integer). The results are given in Table 3 and the reader may find it good practice to carry out some of them for himself.

Table 3

Transition	a	c	$\mathscr{D}$	$\mathscr{D}^*/M^2$
$J \rightarrow J+1$	$-(J+2)g_e - Jg_g$	$-Jg_g$	$|\langle J+1\|m\|J\rangle|^2$	$2J+3$
$J \rightarrow J$	$-(g_e + g_g)$	$+g_g$	$|\langle J\|m\|J\rangle|^2$	$2J+1$
$J \rightarrow J-1$	$-(J+1)g_g - (J-1)g_e$	$+(J+1)g_g$	$|\langle J-1\|m\|J\rangle|^2$	$2J-1$

B. MCD Studies of Charge Transfer Bands

So far, the most spectacular and fruitful applications of MCD are probably in the study of allowed charge transfer bands of transition metals. I have chosen to discuss the tetrahedral compounds of the 3d series at some length, since they present all types of theoretical difficulties.[26]

Table 4 shows the ground state and the allowed excited terms in the absence of

Table 4

Compound	Ground configuration	Ground state	Allowed excited terms
$TiX_4\text{-}VS_4^{3-}$	d^0	$^1A_1$	$^1T_2$
FeX_4^-	d^0	$^6A_1$	$^6T_2$
CoX_4^{2-}	d^0	$^4A_2$	$^4T_1$
NiX_4^{2-}	d^0	$^3T_1$	$^3A_2, {}^3E\ ^3T_1\ ^3T_2$
CuX_4^{2-}	d^0	$^2T_2$	$^2A_1, {}^2E_1\ ^2T_1\ ^2T_2$

spin-orbit coupling for various compounds (X stands for Cl, Br, I), in the strong field approximation.

$\mathcal{D}$ stands for the dipole strength of the various transitions. The derivation of the reduced matrix elements (such as $\mathcal{M}_A$, $\mathcal{M}_B$ and $\mathcal{M}_{A'}$) is beyond the scope of this paper. Suffice it to say here that vector coupling techniques (W.E. theorem) allow them to be expressed in terms of the same reduced matrix element M by means of a 6j (group of rotations)[17] or a W symbol (cubic groups) (see GI).

An important particular case is when the ground state is an orbital singlet ($L = 0$). The 6j symbol is then expressed very simply in terms of the quantum number J only. The last column of Table 3 gives the dipole strengths $\mathcal{D}^*$ in this case. Now if we sum the individual c and a terms over the three spin-orbit components with the appropriate weight for $\mathcal{D}^*$ we obtain:

$$\frac{\sum c_i \mathcal{D}_i^*}{\sum \mathcal{D}_i^*} = 0 \qquad [24]$$

and

$$\frac{\sum a_i \mathcal{D}_i^*}{\sum \mathcal{D}_i^*} = -2g_e \qquad [25]$$

Thus, two conclusions are reached:

(i) The sum of c terms is zero over the spin-orbit components when the ground state is spin (but not orbital) degenerate. This means that c is zero in the absence of spin-orbit coupling.

(ii) The sum of a terms gives the magnetic moment in the excited state. Thus it is predicted that g_e will be contained in the first moment of the MCD curve (see following section).

B1. Study of $TiCl_4$ *and* VS_4^{3-}. (*a*) $TiCl_4$. This is the simplest case encountered. Only a and b terms are expected, since the ground state is non-degenerate. Experimentally, the first absorption band in the UV indeed shows an almost symmetrical a term with a positive. It follows on the ground of *symmetry arguments only* (see preceding section) that

$$\mu = \langle {}^1T_2\, 1|\, Lz\, |{}^1T_2\, 1 \rangle$$

is negative.

In order to check this against theory it is now necessary to consider the molecular orbital scheme more carefully (Fig. 6). All transitions are charge transfer in origin since they imply the promotion of an electron from a molecular orbital of ligand

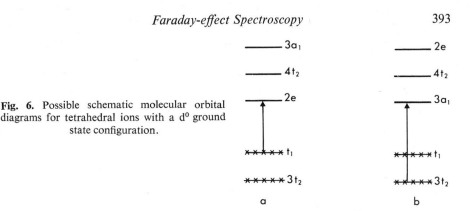

Fig. 6. Possible schematic molecular orbital diagrams for tetrahedral ions with a d^0 ground state configuration.

character (t_1 or $^3t_2$) to an orbital mainly localized on the metal. We call a^6 the ground-configuration and $a^5 b$ one excited configuration.

The full calculation of μ is beyond the scope of this paper. I wish, however, to show how this can be made rather simply.

(i) Using Griffith's book again,[25] i.e. group theoretical arguments only, one derives

$$\mu = \langle a^5 b, {}^1T_2 \, 1| \, Lz |a^5 b, {}^1T_1 \, 1\rangle$$

$$= k_1 \langle a| \, Lz|a\rangle + k_2 \langle b| \, Lz|b\rangle \qquad [26]$$

where k_1 and k_2 can be taken from tables.[25]

(ii) We now have to deal with monoelectronic matrix elements such as $\langle a| Lz|a\rangle$. The a and b wave functions are first expressed as linear combinations of atomic metal and ligand orbitals (characterized with the quantum numbers l, m_1) while the Lz operator is expressed in atoms fixed axes systems. Then calculations are made using the operators lz and $l_\pm = lx_\pm ily$, as well as their properties:

$$lz|l, m_1\rangle = m_1 \, |l, m_1\rangle$$

$$l_\pm |l, m_1\rangle = \{l(l + 1) - m_1(m_1 \pm 1)\} \, |l, m_1 \pm 1\rangle$$

Finally, it is found that μ is generally expressed as a linear combination of *molecular orbital coefficients*. Note that there is an exception for the $t_2^5 e$ configuration since an e orbital has no magnetic moment and t_1 is a purely ligand (thus *non-bonding*) orbital; μ is here always -0.25, whatever the compound is.

It is now clear that MCD will provide an answer to such a question as: Which is the nature of the first excited configuration? In other words: Which is the first empty orbital? The question has long been debated and e.g. $t_1^5 2e$ or alternatively $3t_2^5 3a_1$ have been suggested as possible candidates. MCD rules out the latter since the calculated μ value is found positive contrary to experiment.[4] However, *MCD strongly supports the former*, since the theoretically estimated sign and value for μ agree with experiment.

(b) VS_4^{3-}. This compound shows many optical transitions in its visible and near UV spectrum. The configurational origin of the excited states, however, has been a matter for controversy. Again, it has been possible[30] to locate the bands more accurately and assign the excited states to given configurations from the *signs* of the various MCD a terms only.

Finally, I wish to point out the following fact: since a is a combination of molecular orbital coefficients, its experimental value tells us something about these, i.e., about the *nature of the chemical bond*.

B2. Study of FeX_4^-. It follows from the arguments given in Section 5.1.2, *A2(b)* that only a terms would be expected in the absence of spin–orbit coupling; in that case the theoretical treatment would be identical to that of VS_4^{3-}. Actually, low-temperature experiments on polymer films[7] have shown that all MCD terms have mainly a c character, even at room temperature. This definitely *demonstrates* that *spin-orbit coupling* is effective on the $^6T_2$ cubic terms.

The ground state may then be characterized by its 'effective' *J* quantum number and, according to Table 3, three transitions must be observed for a given excited configuration. However, the table also provides the signs and values of individual c terms and dipole strengths ($\mathscr{D}^*$) if one uses $J = \frac{5}{2}$ and $g_g = 2$ (spin-only value). It is clear in particular that, since c is negative for the $\frac{7}{2}$ component, *MCD is able* not only *to predict the approximate position* of the spin-orbit components, but also *their nature* (in terms of *J*), i.e. the sign* of the spin orbit coupling parameter Δ (total spread of S.O. components).

This is indeed the case, since the theoretically estimated sign for Δ is in fair agreement with that found from MCD, at least for the two first configurations. It should be noted, however, that the experimentally obtained c terms for individual components are always too low (specially in the case of $FeCl_4^-$). This can be understood since we are dealing with overlapping c terms of opposite signs. This overlapping is very effective in $FeCl_4^-$ since the spin-orbit coupling constant is about 10 times smaller for Cl^- than for Br^-.

It appears from the above arguments as if we had lost all information about the orbital moment in the $^6T_2$ excited states. This was because we were trying to fit individual S.O. components to the theory. This is not the case however if we consider the three components arising from a given $^6T_2$ state as a single entity. The method of moments is very profitable here. We call $\bar{v}_0$ the mean frequency of the whole band ($\bar{v}_0 = \langle D \rangle_1 / \langle D \rangle_0$) and $\bar{v}_i$ those of the three individual components i. Using equations [15] and [16] it can be demonstrated that

$$\Delta M_0 = \frac{\sum (b_i + c_i/kT)\mathscr{D}_i}{\sum \mathscr{D}_i} \qquad [27]$$

$$\Delta M_1 = \frac{-\sum a_i \mathscr{D}_i + \sum (\bar{v}_i - \bar{v}_0)(b_i + c_i/kT)\mathscr{D}_i}{\sum \mathscr{D}_i} \qquad [28]$$

Once the various parameters have been expressed in terms of their theoretical values (a_i and c_i can be taken i.e., from Table 2), one obtains

$$\Delta M_1 = 2\mu - \frac{35}{36}\frac{g_g}{kT}\Delta \qquad [29]$$

* Δ is positive if the $(J + 1)$ component has higher energy.

Thus a plot of ΔM_1 *against the temperature* provides both the *total spread* (Δ) of the spin-orbit components, and *the magnetic moments* μ, for the excited $^6T_2$ state. The comparison of the latter with theory then proceeds as for $TiCl_4$. Finally, it is interesting to note that the derivation of equation [29] is independent of the coupling mechanism and thus of the wave functions in the excited state, as long as these satisfy certain conditions (unitary transform). This is known as the principle of spectroscopic stability.

B3. Study of other tetrahedral ions.[26] $CoBr_4^{2-}$ for example, can be treated as $FeBr_4^-$ in a first approach since it has an orbital singlet ground state. However, the experiment shows four MCD c terms under the first absorption band instead of the three expected (Table 3). This can be rationalized in terms of second-order spin-orbit coupling. The situation is even more complicated for CoI_4^{2-} where interaction between excited configurations must be considered. In these examples the fact that experimental MCD b and c terms have *definite signs* is used to find the best approximate theoretical model. This also applies, for example, to $CuBr_4^{2-}$, which is a distorted tetrahedron.

The low-temperature MCD spectrum of $NiBr_4^{2-}$ for example is much more complicated than the above ones. This is due to the fact that several transitions are allowed from the $^3T_1$ ground state to the various spectroscopic terms arising from one given excited configuration. Addition of spin-orbit coupling to the above model results in a considerable number of MCD paramagnetic terms within a rather short spectral range. We did observe overlapping c terms but were nevertheless able to demonstrate that the spin-orbit coupling in the ground state is small, in contradiction with certain previous assumptions for the interpretation of paramagnetic susceptibility measurements. Detailed MCD measurements on the sharp d–d bands of tetrahedral nickel complexes are now indicated. These would clarify the situation in the ground state and lead to a better understanding of the MCD through charge transfer bands.

C. MCD Studies on Magnetic Materials

C1. Interest of MCD. We recall first that magnetic materials under thin films are of great technological importance. We note then that a substantial amount of the compound is needed to perform EPR or magnetic susceptibility experiments; thus such measurements are not feasible on thin films. I wish to emphasize that MCD is not only capable of providing the same information as EPR on such films, but also leads to additional data regarding excited states.

We shall confine our attention to ferro- and antiferro-magnetic materials and provide very rough examples (Fig. 7) in order to illustrate the above arguments. The case of ions with an orbital singlet ground state is chosen for convenience ($^{2S+1}A_1$ in an Oh field where S is the spin degeneracy).

C2. Ferromagnetic materials. $CrBr_3$ single crystals possess a hexagonal axis, and the light should be propagated along it for magneto-optic measurements. The ground state is $^4A_{2g}$ for the Cr^{3+} ion and as was shown for CoX_4^{2-} compounds, transitions are allowed to the spin-orbit components of excited states which would be $^4T_{2u}$ in an Oh field. We do not need to bother about the detailed coupling mechanism in these excited states; suffice it to say that MCD is expected via the process of spin-orbit coupling.

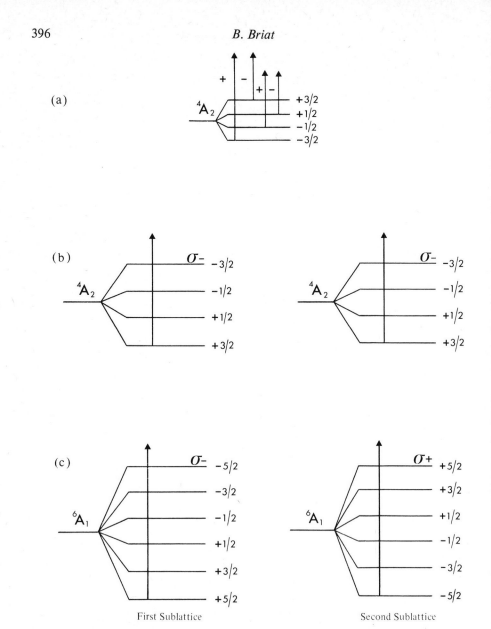

Fig. 7. Circularly polarized transitions arising from the ground state of Cr^{3+} in the paramagnetic (a) or ferromagnetic (b) phase, and Mn^{2+} below the Néel temperature (c).

Under the Curie temperature ($T_C = 33°K$ here), the material becomes ferromagnetic. This means that a low external magnetic field along the six-fold axis (a few thousand gauss) is sufficient to align the spins along the field (and axis). Put in other words, the state with $M_s = +\frac{3}{2}$ is considerably stabilized and therefore has the lowest energy [Fig. 7(b)]. The total separation Δ of the spin levels may be expressed as $\Delta = 6\beta H_e$, where β is the Bohr magneton and H_e (exchange field) is here of the order of 200,000 Øersteds. This means that Δ is about 30 cm^{-1}. According to the Boltzman law it is thus clear that only the $M_S = +\frac{3}{2}$ states will be appreciably populated below T_C. Now it can be checked from Table 2 that for a transition $J \to J$, for example, only the σ_- component is allowed from the $M_S = +\frac{3}{2}$ component. Thus, *MCD becomes enormous below T_C and comparable to the absorption* in zero magnetic field. We note also that Δ is independent of the external field as long as it is sufficient to orient the spins.

The above example was of the perfect type. In many other situations (e.g. for EuO) the orientation of the spins depends upon the external field,[31] and the MCD which is temperature and field dependent is not as large as for CrBr$_3$. It follows that such experiments on, for example, thin films of EuO or EuS allow the precise determination of the *Curie temperature* since the behaviour of the material is so much different in the paramagnetic and ferromagnetic phases. Also, subtle variations of the MCD often reveal the *exchange interactions* in the excited states.

C3. Antiferromagnetic materials. A perfect type is MnO ($^6A_1$ ground state) where two types of magnetic domains occur below the transition Néel temperature (T_N): those with the spins oriented along the external field and those with the spins oriented against the field. A simple diagram [Fig. 7(c)] illustrates where the $M_S = +\frac{5}{2}$ state is the lowest in one domain and the highest in the other. These lowest sublevels are the only ones appreciably populated below T_N but the situation is now very different from that in the previous section since one σ_+ and σ_- component originates from the two states. It is thus clear that MCD should be zero on averaging over all domains.

In practice it is not so since, for a number of reasons, the two transitions may have different intensities. Nevertheless, the observed MCD is much smaller than in the ferromagnetic case and advantage is here taken from the sensitivity of our instruments to determine T_N and learn much about excited states. This has, for example, been done in EuTe[32] in our laboratory. We have also gained much spectroscopic information from measurements on single crystals such as KNiF$_3$ or RbCoF$_3$.

D. Miscellaneous Applications

D1. Study of strongly forbidden lines. Under certain circumstances, a dichrometer is equivalent to a very sensitive spectrophotometer. Consider an absorption line having a maximum optical density of 10^{-3}; its precise location and study (e.g. shape) is practically impossible with an ordinary spectrophotometer. Suppose now that the ground state is degenerate, i.e. with a g factor of 2. If MCD measurements are conducted with a high magnetic field (typically 50 kG) at liquid helium temperature, the relative population among the lowest and highest sublevels in the ground state is practically infinity, i.e. only one transition is allowed with pure σ_+ or σ_- polarization. The recorded magnetic dichroic optical density is thus 10^{-3}, that is at least hundred times larger than the smallest signal detectable. It follows that the error on the absorption curve, as measured with a dichrometer, is only 1 % in this case. The argument has been used to study forbidden lines in tetrahedral compounds,[33] rare-earth ions[34] or else chromic ion pairs in Al$_2$O$_3$.[4]

In general, MCD is of considerable help in the study of vibrationally assisted (otherwise parity forbidden) electric dipole transitions. If we consider, for example, an A$_{1g} \to$ T$_{1g}$ transition for an ion belonging to the 0h group, the magnitude of the observed a term will be unaffected but its sign will be different according to the symmetry (t_{1u} or t_{2u}) of the active vibrational mode. Studies along these lines are being pursued in many laboratories.[35,36] Finally, MCD investigations are of great potential interest in the study of magnon side bands in antiferromagnetic materials such as MnF_2.[37]

D2. Study of low-energy levels. Consider some low-energy levels in an interval of a few hundred wave numbers, and assume that transitions are allowed from these levels to particular excited states. Actually, in order to see absorption bands, the levels should be populated, i.e. the temperature should not be too low. Let us consider a few examples in order to show the merit of MCD experiments in this case.

(*a*) Sm^{2+} *in cubic* CaF_2 (*or the isoelectronic* Eu^{3+} *ion.*)[8b,38] The two lowest levels in the ground state are the $J = 0$ and $J = 1$ spin-orbit components of the ^7F multiplet. The $^7F_1$ state is not appreciably populated, even at room temperature. It turns out however that MCD tells us something about it, since the observed b terms arise from the mixing of $^7F_0$ and $^7F_1$ under the action of the magnetic field.

(*b*) Pr^{3+} *in* $AlLaO_3$.[39] In this crystal there are a number of doublet and singlet states of low energy and MCD complements Zeeman experiments for their study. The latter require sharp lines, i.e. low temperatures. Under such circumstances, however, the upper levels suffer depopulation, and the sensitivity of spectrophotometers is again too low to determine the Zeeman pattern with a good accuracy. This is not so with MCD, due to a greater sensitivity. Thus it has been possible to extract the g factors of upper levels from such experiments.

D3. Some analytical applications. MCD studies have shown the occurrence of ions with unusual valencies (Cu^-, Ag^-) in electrolytically reduced, Cu^+ or Ag^+ containing alkali halide matrices, by comparison with the behaviour of isoelectronic ions such as Pb^{2+}.

Thin films of rare earths chalcogenides (i.e. EuTe) are also currently being checked by means of the MCD technique.[32] Sm^{2+} or Yb^{2+} have also been identified by our group in thin films containing samarium or ytterbium, and tellurium or selenium.

MCD provides a good method of analysing tripositive rare earth ion mixtures[3] from a quantitative as well as qualitative point of view. This is due to the facts: (i) that RE^{3+} ions show very large MCD terms since they are paramagnetic and have sharp lines; and (ii) these lines are numerous and at least one of them for each ion is reasonably well isolated from those of other rare-earth ions. Actually, we have succeeded[3] in detecting one part of Pr^{3+} among 200 million parts of water, using a 50-kG field and a 5-cm-long cell at room temperature.

E. Notes on Magnetic Linear Dichroism (MLD)

We think it appropriate to make a few comments on MLD in a paper mainly devoted to MCD spectroscopy. The reason is that the two techniques are in many respects complementary.

Assuming the light propagation is along the Z axis and the magnetic field H is applied along X, MLD (the so-called Voigt–Cotton–Mouton effect) may be defined as:

$$\Delta K = K_X - K_Y$$

or

$$\Delta D = D_X - D_Y$$

We have offered a basic phenomenological theory[4, 40-42] for the interpretation of the MLD spectra of certain paramagnetic materials. Without entering into the details of the derivation, we can summarize our conclusions as follows: (i) ΔD is proportional to H^2 if the Zeeman splitting is small compared to KT; (ii) ΔD is, in general, a linear combination of the absorption curve and its first and second derivatives, the former and latter terms being the largest for wide and sharp lines respectively; and (iii) MLD is equivalent to the longitudinal Zeeman effect when direct measurements are not feasible (broad bands). We have so far accumulated a number of experimental data on rare-earth ions and extracted the perpendicular spectroscopic splitting factors of many excited states.[43]

Figures 7b and 7c are appropriated to describe the MLD of magnetic materials below their transition temperature. It can be shown that the phenomenon is proportional to the square of the magnetization of the medium and therefore insensitive to an opposite polarization of the magnetization. MLD is thus expected to be of the same order of magnitude for ferro- and antiferro-magnets and this was actually observed in $RbNiF_3$ (ferro) and $KNiF_3$ (antiferro)[44] through the absorption band corresponding to the $^3A_2 \rightarrow {}^1E$ transition (15,000–16,000 cm^{-1}). Unlike MCD, MLD spectroscopy proves most useful for antiferromagnets since the phenomena are large. It allows the precise determination of the Néel temperature T_N; moreover, something can be learnt of the exchange field in the excited states from subtle variations of ΔD around T_N. Finally, MLD provides detailed information on the magnetic anisotropy of materials. Numerous investigations along these lines have recently been conducted in our laboratory on $KNiF_3$ by R. Pisarev and J. Ferre.

MLD is not expected to lead to accurate quantitative experimental data (for individual transitions) when wide bands overlap significantly in a spectrum (e.g. charge transfer bands). However, the qualitative information thus available may still be very useful in checking a theoretical model.[45] As an illustration, Fig. 8 shows the low temperature absorption, MCD and MLD spectra of the $FeBr_4^-$ ion (polymer film) in the 350–450 nm region. From the arguments given earlier in this contribution, we know that the MCD should be positive and negative for the $\frac{3}{2}$ and $\frac{7}{2}$ spin-orbit components of the $^6T_2$ excited state respectively. From the signs of the experimental c terms we were thus able to determine the sign of the spin-orbit coupling parameter corresponding to the second excited configuration. However, the absorption and MCD contributions being positive for both the $\frac{3}{2}$ and $\frac{5}{2}$ states, these cannot be clearly resolved in the spectra since they are too close in energy. Actually, we have calculated the MLD corresponding to our model. Terms proportional to the absorption band shape are largely predominant, since the bands are wide and the temperature is low. Our main conclusion is that ΔD corresponding to the $\frac{5}{2}$ state is opposite in sign to that corresponding to the two extreme states. This is indeed observed experimentally (Fig. 8) and strongly supports our assignment.

5.1.3 Conclusion

I have not intended in this contribution to cover all the applications of Faraday-effect spectroscopy, nor have I claimed that the technique may, by itself, replace any other. I hope however that I have made clear that it is one of the most fruitful tools in the hands of the inorganic chemist and spectroscopist, as well as certain solid-state

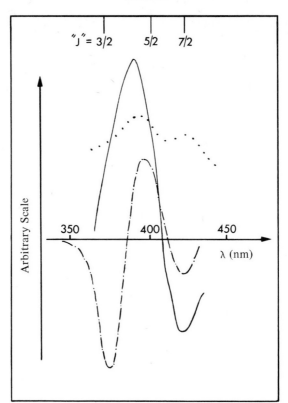

Fig. 8. Absorption ...., magnetic circular dichroism ——— and magnetic linear dichroism —·— of FeBr$_4^-$ in the 350–450 nm spectral range at low temperature.

physicists. I am also convinced that magnetic linear dichroism experiments should prove very useful for qualitative checking of certain spectroscopic assignments.

Numerous investigations on organic materials remain to be done, since the possible role of MCD for structural or conformational studies is not yet definitely established. However, recent experimental and theoretical work by Djerassi's group on the one hand, and Moscowitz on the other, tends to indicate that one should be now reasonably optimistic.

Main emphasis has been placed here on studies conducted in our laboratory. My contribution, of course, owes much to all of my colleagues in Paris and could not have been written without their most qualified and friendly assistance. I am specially indebted to Professor Badoz and Dr. Billardon for their constant and very stimulating interest in my work. Finally, I express my deep gratitude to Professor Mathieu who first pointed out to me the potential value of Faraday-effect spectroscopy.

References

1. A. D. Buckingham and P. J. Stephens, *Ann. Rev. Phys. Chem.* **17**, 399 (1966).
2. P. N. Schatz and A. J. McCaffery, *Quart. Rev. Chem. Soc.* **4**, 552 (1969).

3. B. Briat, *Method. Phys. Anal.*, (*GAMS*) **6**, 19 (1970).
4. *Symposia of the Faraday Society*; *Magneto Optical Effects*, No. 3, 1970.
5. P. J. Stephens, W. Suetaka and P. N. Schatz, *J. Chem. Phys.* **44**, 4592 (1966).
6. R. de Mallemann, P. Gabiano and F. Guillaume, *J. Phys. Red.* **5**, 41 (1944).
7. B. Briat and J. C. Rivoal, *C.R.H. Acad. Sci.* **271**, 1166 (1970).
8. See, for example, (*a*) J. Margerie, *Ann. Phys.* (*Paris*) **5**, 18 (1970). (*b*) J. Margerie, Ph.D. Thesis, Paris, 1966. *Publications scientifiques et techniques du Ministère de l'Air*, No. N.T. 155.
9. B. Briat, D. A. Schooley, R. Records, E. Bunnenberger and C. Djerassi, *J. Amer. Chem. Soc.* **89**, 7062 (1967).
10. M. Billardon, F. Sicart, J. Badoz, J. Chapelle and L. Taurel, *J. Phys.* (*Paris*) **31**, 219 (1970).
11. (*a*) C. H. Henry, S. E. Schnatterly and C. P. Slichter, *Phys. Rev.* A, **137**, 583 (1965). (*b*) P. J. Stephens, *J. Chem. Phys.* **52**, 3489 (1970). (*c*) P. J. Stephens, *Chem. Phys. Lett.* **2**, 241 (1968).
12. B. Briat, in *Houben Weyl*, *Methodicum Chimicum*, Vol. 1, Chapter 5.9. Georg Thieme, Verlag, Stuttgart, 1973.
13. C. Djerassi, E. Bunnenberg and D. L. Elder, *Pure Appl. Chem.*, **25**, 57 (1971).
14. B. Briat and C. Djerassi, *Nature* **217**, 918 (1968).
15. E. A. Dratz, Ph.D. Thesis, University of California, Berkeley, 1966.
16. B. Briat, D. A. Schooley, R. Records, E. Bunnenberg and C. Djerassi, *J. Amer. Chem. Soc.* **89**, 6170 (1967).
17. B. R. Judd, *Operator Techniques in Atomic Spectroscopy*. McGraw-Hill, p. 154, 1963.
18. H. Falk, *Monatsh. Chem.* **100**, 411 (1969).
19. B. Briat, D. A. Schooley, R. Records, E. Bunnenberg, C. Djerassi and E. Vogel, *J. Amer. Chem. Soc.* **90**, 4691 (1968).
20. B. Briat and C. Djerassi, *Bull. Soc. Chim. Fr.* 135 (1969).
21. (*a*) W. Voelter, R. Records, E. Bunnenberger and C. Djerassi, *J. Amer. Chem. Soc.* **90**, 6163 (1968). (*b*) W. Voelter, G. Barth, R. Records, E. Bunnenberg and C. Djerassi, *J. Amer. Chem. Soc.* **91**, 6165 (1969).
22. J. G. Foss and M. E. McCarville, *J. Chem. Phys.* **89**, 30 (1967).
23. M. Rotenberg, R. Binns, N. Metropolis and J. K. Wooten, *The 3-j and 6-j Symbols*. M.I.T. Press, 1959.
24. J. S. Griffith, *The Theory of Transition Metal Ions*. Cambridge University Press, 1964.
25. (G. I.) J. S. Griffith, *The Irreducible Tensor Method for Molecular Symmetry Groups*. Prentice Hall, Englewood Cliffs, N.J., 1962.
26. J. C. Rivoal, Ph.D. Thesis, Paris, Dec. 1971.
27. B. G. Wybourne, *Spectroscopic Properties of Rare-earths*. Interscience Publishers, 1965.
28. B. D. Bird, B. Briat, P. Day and J. C. Rivoal, *Symposium of the Faraday Society* 3, 70 (1969).
29. B. Briat, J. C. Rivoal and R. H. Petit, *J. Chim. Phys. Physicochim. Biol.* **67**, 463 (1970).
30. R. H. Petit, *Thèse 3ème cycle*. Paris, 1970.
31. J. Ferre, J. Badoz, C. Paparoditis and R. Suryanarayanan, *Proc. Intl. Conf. on Magnetism*, Denver, 1971.
32. B. Briat, M. Billardon, R. Suryanarayanan and D. Paparoditis, *Phys. Status Solidi*, **35**, 963 (1969).
33. J. A. Lomenzo, B. D. Bird, G. A. Osborne and P. J. Stephens, *Chem. Phys. Lett.* **9**, 332 (1971).
34. B. Briat, M. Billardon, J. Badoz and J. Loriers, *Anal. Chim. Acta* **34**, 465 (1966).
35. S. B. Piepho, J. R. Dickinson and P. N. Schatz, *Phys. Status Solidi* **47**, 225 (1971).
36. M. J. Harding, S. F. Mason, D. J. Robbins and A. J. Thomson, *J. Chem. Soc. A* 3047 (1971).
37. F. L. Scarpace, M. Y. Chen and W. M. Yen, *J. Appl. Phys.* **42**, 1655 (1971).
38. A. C. Boccara, *C.R.H. Acad. Sci.* **270**, 804 (1970).
39. J. Ferre, A. C. Boccara and B. Briat, *J. Phys.* (*Paris*) **31**, 631 (1970).
40. A. C. Boccara, J. Ferre, B. Briat, M. Billardon and J. Badoz, *J. Chem. Phys.* **50**, 2716 (1969).
41. J. Badoz, *Ann. Phys.* (*Paris*) **5**, 22 (1970).
42. B. Briat, A. C. Boccara, N. Moreau, M. Billardon and J. Badoz, *Proceedings of the XVIth Congress A.M.P.E.R.E.*, Bucharest, Sept. 1–5, 1970.
43. (*a*) N. Moreau and A. C. Boccara, *Phys. Status Solidi* **45**, K 69 (1971). (*b*) A. C. Boccara and N. Moreau, *Phys. Status Solidi* **45**, 573 (1971).
44. P. V. Pisarev, I. G. Siny and G. A. Smolensky, *Solid State Commun.* **5**, 959 (1967).
45. J. C. Rivoal and B. Briat. To be published.

Current Problems and Future Developments in ORD and CD Instrumentation

J. BADOZ*

E.P.C.I.
10, rue Vauquelin
Paris 5e, France

5.2.1 Current Problems in ORD and CD Measurements

The use of half-shadow devices was a major development in visual polarimetry[1] although their various advantages and basic underlying principles had been pointed out for a long time.[2] Modern apparatus for measuring ORD or CD can be more or less related to these long-known basic principles, but greater sensitivity and extended spectral range have been achieved since the pioneering work of Laurent, Bruhat and others.

Progress is due mainly to technological advances in three domains:

   (i) radiation detectors, with the discovery of the photomultiplier tube;

  (ii) electronics, with the use of synchronous detection which allows the enhancement of a noise-drowned signal;

 (iii) sources technology, with increase in brightness (e.g. xenon arc lamps).

A. Basic Principles[3]

Suppose we wish to measure the rotation α of the plane of polarization of a light beam. To be easily detected it must be transformed into a light flux ϕ or, better, a photoelectric current I proportional to ϕ. The simplest way to perform this is to place the sample exhibiting optical rotatory power between two crossed polarizers P_1 and P_2 and to measure the light flux emerging (Fig. 1). It is easily seen that the corresponding photoelectric current is

$$I \approx I_0 \alpha^2 + I_0 \varepsilon^2 \qquad [1]$$

where I_0 is the photocurrent without the sample when the two polarizers are set parallel. $I_0 \varepsilon^2$ is a parasitic current due to the imperfections of the optical device.

Unfortunately, every physical system of measurement is troubled by noise. Here, this is the erratic fluctuations of the signal I (shot noise) due to the photocell. We shall measure it by its r.m.s. value $n = I_N$. For a photocell

---

* Equipe de recherche du C.N.R.S. (N° 5).

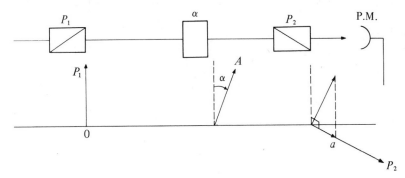

Fig. 1

$$I_N = k_B I^{1/2}$$

where k_B is a constant.

Thus we have:

$$\frac{s}{n} \approx \frac{I_0^{1/2}}{k_B} \frac{\alpha^2}{\varepsilon} \tag{2}$$

This equation shows that the sensitivity $d(s/n)/d\alpha$ is very poor, because it goes to zero with α and is dependent on ε (thus on the quality of the optical device).

In the half-shadow polarimeter, however, the two crossed polarizers are retained but a rotation α_m (the 'shadow' angle) is superimposed on the rotation α to be measured (Fig. 2). The photoelectric current is then

$$I \approx I_0(\alpha + \alpha_m)^2 + I_0 \varepsilon^2 \approx I_0(2\alpha\alpha_m + \alpha_m^2) \tag{3}$$

(we suppose $\alpha_m \gg \varepsilon, \alpha$).

The resulting signal to noise ratio is

$$\frac{s}{n} = \frac{2\alpha}{k_B} I_0^{1/2} \tag{4}$$

i.e. independent of α and ε and much greater than in the first case [2]. Actually, a few 10^{-4} of a degree is a standard limit for a spectropolarimeter instead of about

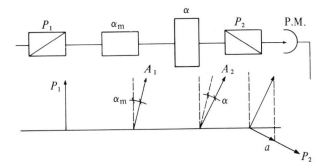

Fig. 2

10^{-2} degree for the first device. Considering expression [3], the reasons for the improvements can be understood:

    (i) the signal $2I_0\alpha\alpha_m$ is linearly dependent upon α (and not upon α^2 as in [2]). This gives a constant sensitivity when $\alpha \to 0$;

    (ii) the mean current $I_0\alpha_m^2$ is quite independent of the parasitic current $I_0\varepsilon^2$.

Finally, any device which obeys such a law for the photoelectric current is going to exhibit the same qualities. A good example is the Legrand–Grosjean dichrograph. The photoelectric current is here expressed by

$$I = \frac{I_0}{2}[2 - 2 \cdot 3\,\Delta D \sin \varphi_m] + I_0\,\varepsilon^2 \tag{5}$$

where we can neglect the parasitic current $I_0\varepsilon^2$ against the mean current I_0. The signal to noise ratio is:

$$\frac{s}{n} = \frac{2 \cdot 3}{2}\,\frac{I_0^{1/2}\sin\varphi_m\,\Delta D}{k_B}$$

This discussion is based upon two hypotheses. Firstly, that the system is noise limited and this noise is of a photoelectric origin; the noise of the electronics must be negligible. We shall see that this is realized only with photomultiplier tubes. Secondly, that we are able to measure the signal, i.e., the phenomenon-dependent part in the photoelectric current. This can be accomplished by a modulation of the 'shadow angle'. Synchronous detection allows the best use of this modulation.

B. *The Importance of Technological Improvements.*

B1. The fundamental importance of the discovery of the photomultiplier cell must be emphasized. To measure the photocurrent, we use an electronic amplifier. The photocurrent flows through a resistor R and we amplify the voltage $V = RI$.

    However, even for $I = 0$, there is a noise voltage (r.m.s, ΔV_N) due to the resistor R (or the first stage of the amplifier). Our first hypothesis assumes that the photoelectric noise is bigger than this electronic noise, thus:

$$k_B\,I^{1/2}\,R \gg \Delta V_N$$

$$k_B\,I^{1/2} \gg \Delta V_N/R$$

Photomultipliers should be distinguished from photocells. A photocell is chiefly a layer of metal K (cathode) emitting electrons when light falls on to it and an anode A collecting the photoelectrons (Fig. 3). The corresponding photocurrent is

$$i = s\phi$$

where s is the photoelectric sensitivity of the metal.

    The noise $i_N = (2e\Delta f.i)^{1/2}$ where e is the electronic charge, and $\tau = 1/\Delta f$ is the time constant of the apparatus used to measure the current (Δf is its band-width).

    A photomultiplier possesses a cathode but the photoelectrons impinge secondary

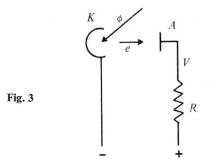

Fig. 3

electrodes (dynode D) and are multiplied by secondary emission before reaching the anode A (Fig. 4). The final current is then

$$I = sG\phi$$

G is the gain of the photomultiplier, and is typically 10^5 to 10^7.

Yet, the main difference between photomultipliers and single photocells is in the expression of the noise which for a photomultiplier is:

$$I_N = (2eG\,\Delta f.I)^{1/2}$$

This is due to the fact that the amplification of the photocurrent flowing from the cathode K is practically performed without superimposed noise. *The photomultiplier is an amplifier working practically without any noise.*

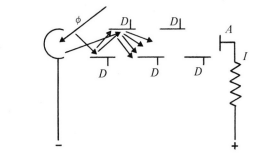

Fig. 4

The condition 'photoelectric noise $\gg$ electronic noise' cannot practically be satisfied for a photocell, since

$$(2e\,\Delta f.s)^{1/2}\,\phi^{1/2} < \frac{V_N}{R} \qquad [6]$$

Alternatively, it may be written

$$(2e\,\Delta f.s)^{1/2}\,\phi^{1/2}\,G \gg \frac{V_N}{R} \qquad [7]$$

for a photomultiplier and is easily fulfilled, due to the presence of the G factor (the value of G is 10^5 to 10^7). *This is the key for the success of modern ORD and CD apparatus.*

B2. The use of electronic synchronous detection, first used in radar techniques, and now widely used in spectrometers, allowed a drastic decrease of Δf, the electronic band-width of the electronic measuring device. A lowering of Δf results in a decrease of the noise and an increase of s/n or the sensitivity, since

$$\sigma = \frac{A}{k_B} = \frac{A}{(2eG\,\Delta f)^{1/2}}$$

B3. The last factor for improving the sensitivity is $I_0 = \phi_0 s$. I_0 is proportional to the sensitivity s of the photocathode and to the mean light flux ϕ_0. ϕ_0 is proportional to optical factors which we will not consider here, and to the brightness of the light source.

An increase in this brightness is thus important and has been obtained by the use of xenon arc lamps.

C. Practical Devices

As we have seen, the best conditions in ORD and CD measurements are obtained:

  (i) when a term proportional to the phenomenon P (rotatory power or dichroism) appears in the light flux;
  (ii) when this term is modulated and synchronously detected.

C1. Polarimeters[3-5] (*Fig. 5*). The monochromatic linearly polarized vibration $0A$ issued from a polarizer P_1 is rotated through an angle α_m by a 'shadow angle' modulator, then through an angle α (to be measured) and finally through α_c by a compensator. A polarizer P_2 crossed with P_1 gives a vibration $0a$ and the light flux impinging the photomultiplier is

$$\Phi = 0a^2 = 0a^2 \sin^2(\alpha_m + \alpha + \alpha_c)$$

$$\phi \approx 0A^2\alpha_m^2 + \underline{2\,0A^2\,\alpha_m(\alpha + \alpha_c)} + 0A^2(\alpha + \alpha_c)^2$$

if $\alpha_m = \alpha_M \sin \omega t$, the underlined term $2\,0A^2(\alpha + \alpha_c)\alpha_M . \sin \omega t$ is properly modulated [frequency $\omega/2\pi = f$] and a selective amplifier eliminates constant or second harmonic terms.

The modulation is achieved, for example, by oscillating the polarizer P_1 (Perkin

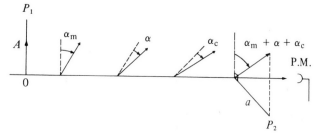

Fig. 5

Elmer, Jasco J20), or using magneto-optical rotation (Faraday cell fed with a.c. current: Bendix, Cary, Fica, Jasco, Jouan, Zeiss).

The measured signal $2\,0A^2(\alpha + \alpha_c)\alpha_M \sin \omega t$ cancels when $\alpha_c = -\alpha$ and this provides a null measurement (good condition for stability).

The compensation angle α_c can be introduced by means of mechanical rotation of the second polarizer P_2 (Cary, Jasco, Perkin Elmer, Zeiss), or magneto-optical rotation (Faraday cell fed with direct and adjustable current: Bendix, Fica, Jouan).

Standard sensitivity is such that, between 190 and 600 nm rotation, as low as a few 10^{-4} of a degree can be detected.

C2. Dichrometers: direct measurement[6-8] (*Fig. 6*). A monochromatic linearly polarized light beam $0A$ is periodically transformed (frequency $\omega/2\pi$) by means of a birefringent plate M_0 into a right and a left circularly polarized vibration. The dichroic sample

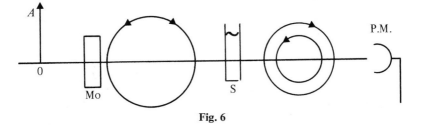

Fig. 6

absorbs right and left vibrations differently (Fig. 6). Then, if dichroism is present, the amplitude of the light is modulated at the same frequency $\omega/2\pi$. This rippling of the light flux is proportional to the dichroism ΔD to be measured and can be detected.

The main problem is the production of periodically left, right, left, ..., vibrations. This can be achieved with a birefringent plate, the birefringence angle φ_m being periodically varied by means of either the well-known electrooptic plate or Pockel's cell (Jouan, Cary, Jasco), or, alternatively, a photoelastic modulator[9] which possesses several main advantages over the Pockel's cell. An isotropic medium periodically stressed ($F\sin \omega t$) exhibits a birefringence $\varphi_M \sin \omega t$ proportional to the stress.

The standard sensitivity corresponds to a dichroism of $\Delta D \approx 10^{-5}$ in the spectral range 185–600 nm.

C2. Dichrometers: indirect measurement.[2,7] It has long been known that a dichroic medium transforms a linearly polarized vibration into an elliptic one, the ellipticity being proportional to the dichroism of the sample. A quarter wave plate transforms this ellipticity into a rotation which can be measured with a photoelectric polarimeter. The measured signals are then independent of the rotatory power and proportional to the dichroism.

Attention must be paid to two points:

(1) The quarter wave plate must be achromatic (its angle of birefringence must be independent of wavelength); this is best achieved with a Fresnel rhomb.
(2) Stray birefringence in optical parts of the apparatus must be avoided.

These conditions are now properly fulfilled in commerical instruments.

5.2.2 Future Developments in ORD and CD

Present apparatus has reached a high point of technical achievement. However, some improvements can still be hoped for in the near future.
   Three points will be reviewed:

   A. Extension of the spectral range of apparatus.
   B. Improvement of the sensitivity.
   C. New facilities provided by differential CD accessories and kinetic studies capabilities.

A. Extension of the Spectral Range

   This improvement is mainly dependent on the transparency of optical materials (in the UV) and the spectral sensitivity of detectors (in the infrared).

(*i*) *Towards the far UV*.[10, 11] Operating in a vacuum, using an MgF_2 Rochon polarizer and a photoelastic modulator, fairly good results are claimed (spectral range extended down to 135 nm, noise level less than 10^{-5} optical density units for a 1·6 nm spectral slitwidth and 10-s time constant).

(*ii*) *Towards the red edge of the visible spectrum*. New trialkaline photocathodes now allow measurements with the same phototube from 185 nm up to at least 800 nm. The older ones are limited to 600 nm.

(*iii*) *Farther into the infrared*. Photomultipliers with a Cs–O–Ag cathode allow measurements from 0·5 to 2 μm. The sensitivity, however, is low, due to the poor quantum efficiency of this type of photocathode.
   To go farther in the infrared it is necessary to use quite different detectors. Thus we built a dichrometer[12] with a Ge photodiode for the 1–2 μm range and an In/Sb cell between 2 and 5·7 μm. The modulator is a photoelastic one. Preliminary results show a sensitivity of $10^{-4}/10^{-5}$ optical density units between 1 and 2 μm and about 10^{-3} optical density units between 2 and 5 μm.
   Similar apparatus has also been built by S. F. Mason at King's College (London, U.K.), by G. Holzwarth and I. Chabay at Chicago[13] and by P. J. Stephens at Los Angeles. (See Notes added in proof, p. 411.)
   The application of Fourier transform spectroscopy to the measurement of CD has also been proposed[14] but no result has yet been given although the method seems particularly promising.

B. Improvement of Sensitivity

   If we recall the expression of the signal-to-noise ratio for a dichrometer

$$\frac{s}{n} = \frac{2 \cdot 3}{2} \frac{I_0^{1/2} \sin \varphi_m . \Delta D}{k_B}$$

the factor which can be changed significantly in the future may be I_0, which is proportional to the brightness of the source. Thus the introduction of tunable lasers (parametric or chemical lasers) can drastically transform the situation, by improving the brightness of the source by several orders of magnitude.

However, there are at present severe limitations: the spectral range is very limited for a CW mode (525–700 nm), and the price is too high.

C. New Facilities

C1. Differential CD. If we reverse the sense of polarization of the light between two samples, the dichrometer gives us the difference between the CD of these two samples. Other means may be used to reverse the sense of circular polarization of the light beam; for example

(i) a half-wave birefringent plate, which transforms a right light into a left one, and vice versa;

(ii) the properties of reflection on a suitably designed mirror (Cary).

C2. Kinetic studies. In order to improve the sensitivity of ORD or CD measurements it is necessary to decrease the electronic band-width $\Delta f = 1/\tau$, i.e. to increase the time constant τ. Typically, τ is chosen between 1 and 10 s, but this prevents measurement as the phenomenon changes significantly during this time.

If we want to measure such a phenomenon (e.g. to follow a chemical reaction taking place in 10^{-2} s) it is necessary that τ be as low as 10^{-3} s. Then, the sensitivity $\sigma = A/\Delta f^{1/2}$ decreases by a factor of 10^2. Also, if $\tau \approx 10^{-3}$ s, the frequency $f = \omega/2\pi$ of the modulator must be sufficiently high so that several periods $T = 1/f$ take place during τ.

C3. Low-temperature measurements. Since the previous report,[15] commercial accessories, which operate easily at variable temperature down to liquid nitrogen, have become available. Experiments at low temperatures down to liquid helium present no particular difficulty—theoretically, at least.

The substance to be studied can be dispersed in a polymer film[16] or in a solvent giving a glass at low temperature (e.g. EPA).

5.2.3 Other Measurements

Polarimeters or dichrometers can be used to study many physical phenomena besides ORD and CD.

A. Magnetic Circular Dichroism (MCD)

This can be readily measured if a magnetic field parallel to the light path is superimposed on a sample. Induced optical activity is exhibited proportional to the field (Faraday effect). Thus a field generator must be located in the sample compartment. Permanent magnets (7 kG with a 4-mm air gap) or superconducting solenoids (50 kG or more) are now currently being used for this purpose.

Shielding problems are easily solved and such solenoids can operate safely.

B. Linear Dichroism

Optical anisotropy gives rise to optical birefringence and linear dichroism. For example, the absorption of a linear dichroic sample is different for two orthogonal linearly polarized vibrations π and σ (Fig. 7).

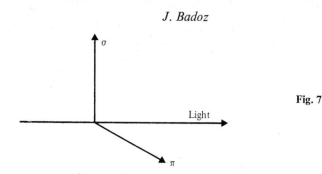

Fig. 7

Linear dichroism is naturally exhibited by a number of anisotropic crystals such as quartz. It may also be induced by, for example,

    (i) a uniaxial stress on an isotropic solid;
    (ii) a magnetic field perpendicular to the direction of propagation of the light (Voigt Cotton–Mouton effect);
    (iii) the flow of liquids containing large molecules;[17, 18]
    (iv) orienting anisotropic molecules in polymer films.

The measurement of such linear dichroism may be easily performed with a slightly modified dichrometer or a polarimeter.[19]

(a) A birefringent quarter-wave plate transforms circular left C_L and right C_R vibrations into two linear mutually orthogonal vibrations L_R and L_L (Fig. 8).

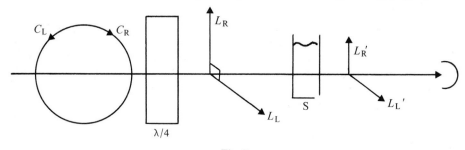

Fig. 8

We thus have periodically two orthogonal linear vibrations which are unequally absorbed by the dichroic sample. The ripple of the light flux emerging from the sample is proportional to the linear dichroism and recorded electronically by the dichrometer. In practice, one just uses achromatic quarter wave plates (Fresnel rhombs) located behind the modulator of the dichrometer.

(b) In another method[17] the optical device of a circular dichrometer is retained, but the electronics are modified. In the Fig. 6 device, the modulator is operated on a $\pm\lambda/2$ mode (instead of $\pm\lambda/4$ as in a circular dichrometer). The amplitude of the second harmonic $2f$ of the modulation frequency f, is then proportional to the linear dichroism of the sample if the principal directions of modulator and sample are parallel.

(c) A spectropolarimeter allows linear dichroism measurements. When the principal directions of the sample exhibit a $\pi/4$ angle with the polarization directions of the two crossed polarizers, the rotation angle given by the polarimeter is proportional to the dichroism to be measured.[19]

C. Studies by Reflection

(i) A spectropolarimeter or a spectrodichrometer allows certain other spectroscopic problems to be dealt with. The azimuth α_i of a linearly polarized vibration is changed into α_r by the reflection at the surface of a dielectric material (Fig. 9). The rotation of the vibration $\alpha = \alpha_r - \alpha_i$ is a function of the refractive index of the medium.

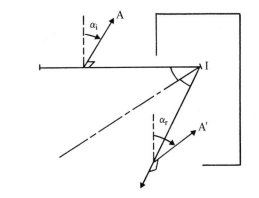

Fig. 9

The variation of α with λ is a determination of the dispersion of the refractive index of the reflecting sample.[20, 21]

(ii) A dichrometer (circular or linear) is also suitable for measuring linear or circular dichroism by reflection on highly absorbing materials. This has been achieved on magnetic samples in our laboratory.

Notes added in Proof

I. Since the Tirrenia A.S.I., Badoz *et al.* have made substantial progress in the detection of CD by means of Fourier transform spectroscopy [*Appl. Opt.* **11**, 2375 (1972)].

A Michelson interferometer is followed by a photoelastic modulator (frequency f) and by the dichroic sample (ΔD).

In the photocurrent of the detector, retaining only the first harmonic (I_f) and the term independent of $f(I_0)$, we have shown that

$$\Delta D = \frac{1}{2 \cdot 3\, J_1} \cdot \frac{TF^{-1} I_f}{TF^{-1} I_0}$$

where TF^{-1} stands for inverse Fourier transform and J_1 for the Bessel function $J_1(\phi_M)$; ϕ_M is the maximum birefringent angle of the modulator.

For practical reasons, our preliminary results have been limited to the visible part of the spectrum. They were successful (e.g. MCD spectrum of praseodymium chloride) and may now be extended towards the infrared.

II. Several papers have recently been devoted to infrared dichrometers: R. J. Dudley, S. F. Mason and R. D. Peacock, *Chem. Commun.*, 1084 (1972); I. Chabay,

E. C. Hsu and G. Holzwarth, *Chem. Phys. Lett.* **15**, 211 (1972); G. A. Osborne, J. C. Cheng and P. J. Stephens, *Rev. Sci. Instrum.* **44**, 10 (1973).

We acknowledge the support given for the infrared part of this research by the Direction des Recherches et Moyens d'Essais, under DRME Contract No. 666/68.

References

1. H. Laurent, *J. Phys. Theor. Appl.* **3**, 183 (1874).
2. G. Bruhat, *Traité de Polarimétrie*, Paris, 1930.
3. J. Badoz, *J. Phys. A* **17**, 143 (1956).
4. Rudolph, Spectropolarimeter Model 200.
5. E. J. Gilham, *Nature* **178**, 1412 (1956).
6. M. Grosjean and M. Legrand, *C.R.H. Acad. Sci.* **251**, 2150 (1960).
7. L. Velluz, M. Legrand and M. Grosjean, *Optical Circular Dichroism*. Verlag Chemie and Academic Press, 1961.
8. M. Billardon, J. C. Rivoal and J. Badoz, *Rev. Phys. Appl.* **4**, 353 (1969).
9. M. Billardon and J. Badoz, *C.R.H. Acad. Sci.* **262 B**, 1972 (1966).
10. O. Schnepp *et al. Rev. Sci. Instrum.* **41**, 1136 (1970).
11. W. C. Johnson, Jr. *Rev. Sci. Instrum.* **42**, 1283 (1971).
12. M. F. Russel, N. Moreau, M. Billardon and J. Badoz, *26th Symposium on Molecular Structure and Spectroscopy*, Columbus, Ohio, 14-18 June, 1971.
13. Discussion on instrumentation held during the Advanced Study Institute on ORD and CD in Tirrenia (Pisa) Sept. 1971.
14. J. E. Stewart, *Appl. Opt.* **10**, 1464 (1971).
15. *ORD and CD in Organic Chemistry*, G. Snatzke, Ed., Heyden, London, 1967, p. 235.
16. B. Briat and J. C. Rivoal, *C.R.H. Acad. Sci.* **271**, 1166 (1970). See also Chapter 5.1 of the present work.
17. S. Wooley and G. Holzwarth, Advanced Study Institute on ORD and CD, Pisa, Sept. 1971.
18. J Hofrichter and J. A. Schellman, Advanced Study Institute on ORD and CD, Pisa, Sept. 1971.
19. A. C. Boccara, J. Ferre, B. Briat, M. Billardon and J. Badoz, *J. Chem. Phys.* **50**, 2716 (1969).
20. J. C. Canit, D. Berger, M. Billardon, *Opt. Acta* **13**, 255 (1966).
21. J. C. Canit, *Opt. Acta* **16**, 237 (1969).

INDEX

413